Building a Successful
Ambulatory Care Practice

A COMPLETE GUIDE FOR PHARMACISTS

MARY ANN KLIETHERMES, BS, PharmD

Vice-Chair of Ambulatory Care, Associate Professor
Chicago College of Pharmacy
Midwestern University
Downers Grove, Illinois

TIM R. BROWN, PharmD

Director, Clinical Pharmacotherapy
Center for Family Medicine and Department of Pharmacy
Akron General Medical Center
Professor, Northeast Ohio Medical University
Akron, Ohio

American Society of Health-System Pharmacists®

Bethesda, Maryland

Any correspondence regarding this publication should be sent to the publisher, American Society of Health-System Pharmacists, 7272 Wisconsin Avenue, Bethesda, MD 20814, attention: Special Publishing.

The information presented herein reflects the opinions of the contributors and advisors. It should not be interpreted as an official policy of ASHP or as an endorsement of any product.

Because of ongoing research and improvements in technology, the information and its applications contained in this text are constantly evolving and are subject to the professional judgment and interpretation of the practitioner due to the uniqueness of a clinical situation. The editors, contributors, and ASHP have made reasonable efforts to ensure the accuracy and appropriateness of the information presented in this document. However, any user of this information is advised that the editors, contributors, advisors, and ASHP are not responsible for the continued currency of the information, for any errors or omissions, and/or for any consequences arising from the use of the information in the document in any and all practice settings. Any reader of this document is cautioned that ASHP makes no representation, guarantee, or warranty, express or implied, as to the accuracy and appropriateness of the information contained in this document and specifically disclaims any liability to any party for the accuracy and/or completeness of the material or for any damages arising out of the use or non-use of any of the information contained in this document.

Director, Special Publishing: Jack Bruggeman
Acquisitions Editor: Jack Bruggeman
Senior Editorial Project Manager: Dana Battaglia
Production Editor: Johnna Hershey
Design and Composition: David Wade

ISBN: 978-1-58528-244-9

DEDICATION

This book is dedicated to the ambulatory care pharmacy leaders who helped make our current practices possible, to the many ambulatory colleagues we have worked with who constantly provide us support and inspiration, and to future ambulatory care pharmacy practitioners. May you use what we have learned to further develop an area of pharmacy practice that is essential for optimal patient care.

Mary Ann Kliethermes
Tim R. Brown

DEDICATION

I would like to dedicate this book to my family whose support and encouragement is unending and is the basis for who I am—a Mom.
Mary Ann

DEDICATION

I dedicate this book to my Mother. Although she is no longer in this world to share in both the joy and relief of completing this work, her voice has been with me throughout this process. I still hear her whispering in my ear, "You cannot learn common sense from a book." And, as always, my Mother was right! So I encourage you to use this resource to become a better pharmacy practitioner, but do so by balancing what you read with what your heart knows and feels.
Tim

Table of Contents

PREFACE

Imagine two friends who both practice in ambulatory care settings discussing the challenges of pharmacy practice and the ever changing health care world. How many times have you been one of those pharmacists? We found that we were having this conversation on multiple levels with many of our colleagues and always ending with the words, "Well, what can you do? I wish there was a guide!" It was during one of these conversations when we brainstormed a "wish list" that would make our lives easier, a resource that covered ambulatory practice from beginning to end and could be used by new practitioners as well as seasoned pharmacists. The original idea was not a book, but rather a web site that would act as a repository for materials ranging from business planning to reimbursement mechanisms to promotion of our profession. As we both decided how to have an impact, we realized our original idea of web-based materials was a good one but something more was needed such as instructional or basic information. We wanted to ensure these resources would be used by pharmacists starting an ambulatory care practice to avoid the pitfalls and errors we had made building our respective practice models.

We decided to write a book—to create an informational resource that had a traditional feel, such as a "How to" book, but coupled with a dynamic reference that could be updated such as a complementary web site outlined to follow the book's chapters. The combination of these two types of references would provide our colleagues access to material that would answer their questions, offer educational tips, and provide tools to assist in achieving their career and practice goals. For the project to be successful, however, the book and the web site would need experts who lived and worked in ambulatory care pharmacy practice and understood what it is like to search for an answer to a question that has never been asked. The nine chapters of this book are authored by pharmacists who have dedicated their professional careers to building ambulatory care practice models that allow pharmacists to provide quality care and continuity of care to their patients. Each author has provided insight, wisdom, practice tips, and everyday common sense to create a resource that will unify us, enhance the care we give our patients, and strengthen our profession as a whole.

The chapters are a sequence of steps that an ambulatory care pharmacy practitioner would use to develop or enhance his or her practice site; they build upon each other. However, each chapter can stand on its own as an informational resource for the practitioner who may only need to read about a particular topic. Within each chapter, you will find web icons ⌨ that denote additional web resources corresponding to the chapter's material and, in some cases, you may even find tools that help you achieve the goals outlined by the chapter. Each author submitted reference links, practice tools, and examples so that the chapter relates to where you are in the process of building your practice model. The web toolkit can be found at

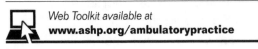

Web Toolkit available at
www.ashp.org/ambulatorypractice

(See page ix for the list of web tools and information about the toolkit.)

In addition, you will also find a case-based scenario running throughout the book depicting a pharmacist who works with a physician named Dr. Busybee. This pharmacist represents all of us! He or she is working to start and grow a practice while roadblocks, red tape, and life get in the way. We thought this was the best way for the reader to identify with what each chapter is teaching. As you read, imagine yourself as the pharmacist portrayed in the case. For some, you will find answers to a current situation or dilemma; for others, you may reflect and think this is exactly what you went through; and, for still others, you may remember an experience far worse than what we have described. This simply illustrates that no matter where you are in the evolution of your practice, you are or have been the pharmacist carving out your niche in Dr. Busybee's office.

As editors of this project, we were able to relive some of our career moments. We often wondered, "How did we ever achieve our goals and create the practice we have today?" If only there had been a book for us. But, then again, we are both surprised that a conversation between two friends yielded such an amazing collaboration among our colleagues and friends. Maybe we should have talked sooner and more often!

Mary Ann Kliethermes
Tim R. Brown

Ambulatory Care Practice: The Toolkit for Pharmacists

Overview of the Book and Toolkit

Building the Ambulatory Care Practice: A Guide for Pharmacists is a how-to guide to creating and managing an ambulatory care clinic, from building a business model to clinical practice, risk management and liability, reimbursement, marketing, and credentialing.

The toolkit was developed to work in collaboration with the book to provide more tangible tools for building the ambulatory care practice. The types of tools include sample plans, sample forms and documents, and example case studies. The toolkit is organized by the chapters in the book. Within the book chapters, tools are identified by an icon. ▣ These icons alert the reader to the tools available in the toolkit to facilitate the concepts and processes discussed in the chapter. At the end of each chapter, a QR code is inserted for smart phones.

How to Use This Toolkit

The tools included in this kit are downloadable and adaptable. To access a tool, simply click on the title of the document.

Goals are provided at the beginning of each list of tools to illustrate the purpose of the tools and organize the steps in the process.

Additional guidance to understanding the tools and how to use them is provided. For more complete information on the process and use of the tools, please refer to the designated chapter.

List of Tools by Chapter

CHAPTER 1: DEFINING THE AMBULATORY PATIENT CARE MODEL

GOAL:
• Define your practice model.

TOOLS:
Conventions Useful for Professional Networking
Example Referral Forms
    Pharmacotherapy Consult
    Generic Referral Form
Sample Collaborative Drug Therapy Management Agreements
    Collaborative Drug Therapy Management Agreement (SJRMC)
    DMG MTM Agreement
Sample Mission and Vision Statements

CHAPTER 2: PLANNING AND STEPS TO BUILDING THE AMBULATORY PRACTICE MODEL

GOAL:

- Develop a proposal for your practice model by assembling and building the key supporting data.

TOOLS:

Resource Needs Worksheet
Revenue from Reimbursement Worksheet
Sample Scope of Practice
Sample Case: Medication Therapy Management Service

CHAPTER 3: DEVELOPING A BUSINESS PLAN FOR AN AMBULATORY PRACTICE

GOAL:

- Develop a written business plan that will help you communicate the proposal, secure funding, guide the initiative, and keep the practice on track.

TOOLS:

Business Plan Template
Sample Business Plan for an Ambulatory Heart Failure Clinic

CHAPTER 4: MARKETING YOUR AMBULATORY PRACTICE

GOAL:

- Through market research, develop an appropriate marketing plan and strategy for your practice.

TOOLS:

Sample Brochures
    Brochure 1
    Brochure 2
    Brochure 3
Physician Questionnaire
Patient Survey
Marketing Plan Template

CHAPTER 5: CREATING THE AMBULATORY PATIENT CARE MODEL

GOAL:

- Use two of the four tracks to start creating the care model: Clinic Operations and Policy and Procedures.

TOOLS:

Example Referral/Order/HIPPA Consult Form
Physician Fax Form
Example of an Anticoagulation Management Face Sheet
Example Warfarin Monitoring Sheet
Work Flow Diagram
Examples of Clinic Policy and Procedure Documents
    Billing Policy Example
    Medication Management Clinic Policy and Procedure
Examples of Billing Procedure Documents
    Proposed Point-based Billing Procedure for Clinical Pharmacy Services
    Billing Incident
    -   to Physician
    Proposed Time-based Billing Procedure for Clinical Pharmacy Services
    Billing Incident
    -   to Physician
New Patient Intake Form
DM Patient Assessment
MTM Patient Note Template
Revised Initial Patient Note
Patient Education Web Resources

CHAPTER 6: COMMUNICATION AND DOCUMENTATION FOR AN AMBULATORY PRACTICE

GOALS:

* Develop efficient and comprehensive documentation for your practice: both manual and electronic.

* Develop communication techniques to manage practice quality.

TOOLS:

Chart Audit Tool
Example Documentation Elements for EMR/PMR
Examples of Community-based/Clinical Pharmacy Documentation Software
Web Sources
Example of Electronic Documentation of a Pharmacy Office Visit
Example SOAP Note and 7 Lines of Questioning
Link to AMA Web Site for Bookstore (three books on EMRs)

CHAPTER 7: QUALITY ASSURANCE FOR AMBULATORY PATIENT CARE

GOAL:

* Apply key quality principles and implement methods to the structure of your clinic or service in order to provide quality services.

TOOLS:

PDSA Worksheet
Quality Measure Feasibility Checklist
Example Case: Medication Therapy Management Clinic
Additional Selected References
Ambulatory Care Pharmacy Suggested Resource Web Sites
Resources for Information on Quality Improvement and Developed Health Care Measures

CHAPTER 8: REIMBURSEMENT FOR THE PHARMACIST IN AN AMBULATORY PRACTICE

GOAL:

- Define the appropriate reimbursement process for your practice including the necessary document and tools.

TOOLS:

Coding Reference Card Outpatient
Pharmacists' Specific Facility Fee Point Sheet
Sliding Fee Scale
Patient Intake Form
SOAP Note/Patient Case
Trinity Anticoagulation E/M Documentation Standards

CHAPTER 9: MAXIMIZING YOUR AMBULATORY PRACTICE: PLANNING FOR THE FUTURE

GOAL:

- Develop a plan for growth for your clinical services that includes future training of personnel, anticipation of health care changes, and contributions to the profession.

TOOLS:

Updated Resources and Reimbursement Form to Show Growth (Form originally introduced in Chapter 2)
Example Measures to Examine Trends in the Practice
A Tracking Tool for Non-patient Activities
Examples of eTOCs
A Sample Plan for Re-evaluating the Service

CONTRIBUTORS

Jill S. Borchert, PharmD, BCPS, FCCP
Professor & Vice Chair, Pharmacy Practice
Director, PGY1 Residency Program
Midwestern University
Chicago College of Pharmacy
Downers Grove, Illinois

Jeffrey M. Brewer, PharmD
Associate Professor, Pharmacy Practice
Albany College of Pharmacy and Health Sciences
Albany, New York

Tim R. Brown, PharmD
Director, Clinical Pharmacotherapy
Center for Family Medicine and Department of Pharmacy
Akron General Medical Center
Professor, Northeast Ohio Medical University
Akron, Ohio

Paul W. Bush, PharmD, MBA, FASHP
Chief Pharmacy Officer
Duke University Hospital
Durham, North Carolina

Michelle L. Cudnik, PharmD
Clinical Lead Pharmacist
Ambulatory Care
Summa Health System
Akron, Ohio
Associate Professor of Pharmacy Practice
NEOMED
Rootstown, Ohio

Kelly Epplen, PharmD, CACP
Assistant Professor, Clinical Pharmacy Practice and Administrative Sciences
James L. Winkle College of Pharmacy
University of Cincinnati
St. Elizabeth Family Practice Center
Cincinnati, Ohio

Kevin Charles Farmer, BSPharm, PhD
Professor, Clinical & Administrative Sciences
University of Oklahoma College of Pharmacy
Oklahoma City, Oklahoma

Seena L. Haines, PharmD, FASHP, FAPhA, BC-ADM, CDE
Associate Dean for Faculty and Professor
Palm Beach Atlantic University
Gregory School of Pharmacy
West Palm Beach, Florida

Stuart T. Haines, PharmD, FCCP, FASHP, BCPS
Professor and Vice Chair of Clinical Services
University of Maryland School of Pharmacy
Baltimore, Maryland
and
Clinical Pharmacy Specialist
West Palm Beach VAMC
West Palm Beach, Florida

Tara L. Jenkins, BSPharm, PhD
Assistant Professor
University of Kansas School of Pharmacy
Lawrence, Kansas

Mary Ann Kliethermes, BS, PharmD
Vice-Chair of Ambulatory Care, Associate Professor
Chicago College of Pharmacy
Midwestern University
Downers Grove, Illinois

Sandra Leal, PharmD, CDE
Director of Clinical Pharmacy
El Rio Health Center
Tucson, Arizona

Jeannie Kim Lee, PharmD, BCPS
Clinical Assistant Professor
Pharmacy Practice & Science, College of Pharmacy
Section of Geriatric, General & Palliative Medicine, College of Medicine
University of Arizona
Research Associate and Faculty
Arizona Center on Aging
Clinical Pharmacy Specialist - Geriatrics
Southern Arizona VA Health Care System
Tucson, Arizona

Steven M. Riddle, BSPharm, BCPS, FASHP
Vice President of Clinical Affairs
Pharmacy OneSource/Wolters Kluwer Health
Affiliate Clinical Professor
University of Washington School of Pharmacy
Seattle, Washington

Gloria P. Sachdev, BSPharm, PharmD, RPh
Clinical Assistant Professor
Purdue University College of Pharmacy
Adjunct Assistant Professor
Indiana University School of Medicine
President
Sachdev Clinical Pharmacy, Inc.
Indianapolis, Indiana

Edward P. Sheridan, PharmD
Director, PGY1 Pharmacy Residency Programs
Faculty, Family Medicine Residency Program
Director, Ambulatory Pharmacy Services
Saint Joseph Family Medicine Residency Program
South Bend, Indiana

Betsy Bryant Shilliday, PharmD, CDE, CPP
Associate Clinical Professor of Pharmacy and Medicine
University of North Carolina at Chapel Hill
Chapel Hill, North Carolina

Amy L. Stump, PharmD, BCPS
Clinical Pharmacy Specialist, Ambulatory Care
Indiana University Health Methodist Hospital
Indianapolis, Indiana

REVIEWERS

Brooke Griffin, PharmD
Associate Professor, Pharmacy Practice
Midwestern University Chicago College of Pharmacy
Downers Grove, Illinois

Kelly Lempicki, PharmD, BCPS
Assistant Professor, Pharmacy Practice
Midwestern University Chicago College of Pharmacy
Clinical Pharmacist - North Chicago VA Medical Center
Downers Grove, Illinois

Christie Schumacher, PharmD, BCPS
Assistant Professor, Pharmacy Practice
Midwestern University Chicago College of Pharmacy
Clinical Pharmacist, Advocate Health Care
Downers Grove, Illinois

Jenny A. Van Amburgh, BPharm, PharmD, CDE
Associate Clinical Professor / Residency Program Director (PGY1)
Northeastern University - Bouve College of Health Sciences - School of
Pharmacy
Boston, Massachusetts

Defining the Ambulatory Patient Care Model

Edward P. Sheridan, Jeannie Kim Lee

Chapter Outline

1. Introduction
2. Standard of Ambulatory Care Practice
3. Organization Model
4. Practice Model Settings
5. Patient Care Practice Models
6. Chapter Summary
7. References
8. Additional Selected Resources
9. Web Resources

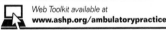

Web Toolkit available at
www.ashp.org/ambulatorypractice

Chapter Objectives

1. Define the practice of ambulatory patient care.
2. Apply the standard of practice for ambulatory care to your site.
3. Compare and contrast different practice constructs and settings.
4. Describe services provided by ambulatory care pharmacists.

Introduction

Over the past few decades, various organizations and committees have issued edicts to the profession of pharmacy: become more involved in patient care.[1,2] It was under the auspices of this challenge and factors such as the aging population, reduced hospital length of stay, and emerging pay-for-performance measures, that innovative pharmacists and health systems developed ambulatory pharmacy practice.[3]

Transcending the practice setting, the practice of ambulatory care can be defined most simply and inclusively as providing health-related services in which patients walk to seek their care.[3] This definition holds true despite the fact that ambulatory care practice, like much of health care, continues to evolve. It is interesting to note that among those who practice ambulatory care, trying to become more specific with this definition results in becoming more divisive. That is to say, you won't have the same needs, resources, collaboration, or scope of service for a practice that is based in a medical center as in a physician's office or a community pharmacy. So, although patient care services may appear to be similar, practice setting and organizational differences may affect your scope of service and the way in which those services are delivered.

Despite these inherent differences in various practice settings, enough commonality exists within the practice to define an ambulatory care standard of practice. According to Carter, "The most important aspect of developing an ambulatory practice is appropriate planning."[3] Thus, your new practice is a study of intelligent design based on the evolution of others' prior practices. Ultimately, it is your knowledge of how this ambulatory care standard of practice applies to these different settings, and in particular, your setting, that will allow successful implementation and a successful practice.

> **Key Point**
>
> Your new practice is a study of intelligent design based on the evolution of others' prior practices. Your knowledge of how this ambulatory care standard of practice applies to these different settings, and in particular, your setting, will allow successful implementation and a successful practice.

Standard of Ambulatory Care Practice

Leadership, patient care, and medication management are characteristics that exist in all ambulatory settings, contributing to the framework of an applicable standard of practice.[1,4-6] Realistically, however, these key factors exist in different degrees and complexity in different settings. This standard defines a practice with a solid foundation of each of these components and then further provides details of those attributes that exceed the standards or should be considered a "best practice." The standard of practice, then, probably contains some aspects already present in your organization or site and some aspects that will need to be initiated or further developed.

Despite the fact that ambulatory care has been a practice for the last 40 years and is growing wider in acceptance largely due to increased visibility, both in practice and in the literature, strong leadership is necessary for the success of your practice. This leadership comes in the form of profession-wide, individual practice management and personal scope.

Leadership Standard

Becoming a Leader in Ambulatory Pharmacy Practice

The practice of ambulatory care will continue to develop as those involved, perhaps you, continue to develop new and innovative practices. However, what you accomplish through leadership at your local level should also have an impact on the national practice. You must share what you have accomplished and learned along the way with others in the profession, or in other words, give back to the profession. You can accomplish this through teaching, giving presentations, or contributing to publications. Each of these venues has its own strengths. For instance, publications may reach a larger audience, be permanent, and influence national guidelines. Your precepting or clinical teaching may reach a smaller audience but give a more detailed view of the infrastructure of the practice that can live on through the next generation of ambulatory care pharmacists that you train.

Share what you have accomplished and learned along the way with others in the profession, or in other words, give back to the profession.

You should also ensure that you and your team are actively involved in local, state, and national organizations. This "active participation" is more than organizational membership; it is involvement in projects, serving on committees, and holding offices. Your participation in this manner continues to highlight ambulatory care practice. The relationship also bears benefits to all involved in the form of learning and understanding differing points of view as well as job satisfaction.

Advocacy, however, is likely the most important need for the practice. Advocacy can be accomplished at both a practice and professional level. As you build your practice, continue to advocate for it by sharing successful metrics with the stakeholders. Do not underestimate the power of patient satisfaction. Patient's word of mouth can be more powerful than facts and figures. Surely, if the patients are happy and you are getting results, physicians and other team members will be happy and likely refer more patients. Thus, the patients, physicians, health care team, and health systems are aware of your presence.

On a national level, the professional organizations have advocacy committees and training programs. Simple things such as giving information when asked, inviting government officials to your practice, and keeping up with health care reform issues can be very valuable.

Find your political voice and stay informed.

Being a Leader on Your Team

As depicted in **Table 1-1**, leadership and management roles and tasks are usually addressed separately. You need to consider both as you begin to build your practice.[7] Although a less familiar term in the pharmacy profession compared with the medical profession, practice management is literally the way you run your business of ambulatory clinical service and the way you manage your practice. You should first develop the mission and vision of what the practice should be.[8,9] As Covey states, "begin with the end in mind."[10] Developing mission and vision statements for your program or service is a good way to get started. By putting these thoughts into words, you create a powerful tool that provides a focus and guides in the creation of your service or program. The mission statement should describe the purpose of your program and why it needs to exist in a clear, concise, and informative manner. Involve all key members of your team in composing your statements so that everyone understands your program's purpose. The vision statement defines where the program and service is going, or what it wants to achieve and accomplish at some future point and time, usually at an interval of 5–10 years. The value of the service or program should be articulated in the vision statement. (Examples of mission and vision statements can be found on the web.)

Table 1-1. Leadership and Management Responsibilities[7]

Leadership	Management
Scanning	**Planning**
Identify client/stakeholder needs and priorities	Set short-term organization goals and performance objectives
Recognize trends, opportunities, risks	Develop multiyear and annual plans
Look for best practices	Allocate appropriate resources
Identify staff capacity and constraints	Anticipate and reduce risks
Know yourself, your staff, your organization values, strengths, and weaknesses	
Focusing	**Organizing**
Articulate the organization's mission and strategy	Ensure a structure that promotes accountability and delineates authority
Identify critical challenges	Ensure the systems for human resource management, finance, logistics, quality assurance, operations, information, and marketing effectively support the plan
Link goals with the overall organizational strategy	
Determine key priorities for action	Strengthen work processes to implement the plan
Create a common picture of desired results	Align staff capacities with planned activities
Aligning/Mobilizing	**Implementing**
Encourage congruence of mission, values, strategy, structure, systems, and daily activities	Integrate systems and coordinate work flow
Facilitate teamwork	Balance competing demands
Unite key stakeholders around an inspiring vision	Routinely use data to make decisions
Link goals and rewards and recognition	Coordinate activities with programs and sectors
Enlist stakeholders to commit resources	Adjust resources based on change
Inspiring	**Monitoring and Evaluating**
Match deeds to words	Monitor and reflect on progress of plans
Demonstrate honesty in interactions	Provide feedback
Show trust and confidence in staff	Identify needed changes
Provide staff with challenges, feedback, support	Improve processes, procedures, and tools
Be a model of creativity, innovation, and learning	

Once your mission and vision are determined, follow by determining your goals and strategic planning. These should closely align with your program's mission and vision. Goals are predetermined indicators for success and should be continuously and objectively measured. Those responsible for the goals should be held accountable for them. The accountability should "roll up."[11] This means that although not all of your staff may have the same goals, depending on the projects in which they are involved, you as the leader of the practice or site should be held accountable for the goals of everyone who reports to you. Chapter 7 will discuss this in more detail and proven case examples.

The team should be built with this mission/vision/goal/strategic plan in mind. Where applicable, you should incorporate peer interviewing (asking behaviorally based questions) and ranking scales (weighted, objective/subjective) to build the team. When this is done, those doing the interviewing take responsibility for the new team members. It fosters a supportive system aligned to common goals. For instance, Schneider et al. found that according to pharmacy staff, patients should (1) understand the benefits and adverse effects of their medications, (2) not experience a preventable adverse drug event, (3) receive the correct dose and medication, (4) not receive a drug to which they are known to be allergic, (5) receive medications in a timely fashion, (6) have doses individualized when necessary, and (7) receive the most effective therapy at the least cost.[12] Here, the pharmacy staff basically defined their standards for patient care, and at times the specific job descriptions can be built around these expectations.

Table 1-2 describes possible components of an ambulatory care pharmacist's job description and examples of services. Along with hiring, you must ensure fair market benefit—remuneration for associates that is fair based on what the market would bear.[13] This can be done if you have a working knowledge of or responsibility for the practice budget. You can more easily advocate for your associates if you understand the productivity and financial sustainability of the practice.

Table 1-2. Possible Job Descriptions and Examples[4,14-16]

Activity/Function	Description	Examples
Medication therapy management	Encompasses a broad range of professional activities and responsibilities within the licensed pharmacist's, or other qualified health care provider's, scope of practice. These services include but are not limited to the following, according to the individual needs of the patient:	Medication Therapy Management (MTM) Clinic; Medication Management Center
	a. Performing or obtaining necessary assessments of the patient's health status	
	b. Formulating a medication treatment plan	
	c. Selecting, initiating, modifying, or administering medication therapy	
	d. Monitoring and evaluating the patient's response to therapy, including safety and effectiveness	
	e. Performing a comprehensive medication review to identify, resolve, and prevent medication-related problems, including adverse drug events	

Table 1-2. Possible Job Descriptions and Examples[4,14-16] (cont'd)

Activity/Function	Description	Examples
	f. Documenting the care delivered and communicating essential information to the patient's other primary care providers	
	g. Providing verbal education and training designed to enhance patient understanding and appropriate use of his/her medications	
	h. Providing information, support services and resources designed to enhance patient adherence with his/her therapeutic regimens	
	i. Coordinating and integrating medication therapy management services within the broader health care–management services being provided to the patient.	
Patient care services	Establish a relationship with the patient; obtain medical and medication histories; assess the appropriateness of medication orders: identify, resolve, and prevent medication-related problems; educate patients and caregivers; and monitor patient's response to medication therapy, pertinent laboratory values, therapeutic drug levels. Also, assess patient understanding of and adherence to medication therapy and its effects and outcomes. During follow-up visits, evaluate patient progress and identify and resolve problems per scope of practice.	• Disease management clinic • Primary care clinic • Adherence clinic • Collaborative practice
Clinical care plans and disease management	As part of an interdisciplinary team, develop and implement clinical plans of care and disease management programs involving medication therapy, collaborative practice, treatment protocols, and medication error reduction.	• Clinical practice guidelines • Disease management protocols • Critical pathways
Patient encounter documentation	Document using applicable tool service provided to the patient and follow-up plans, and process appropriate encounter forms for service provision that meet the tax and insurance needs of the patient and institution.	• Electronic medical record with encounter coding • Patient chart • Superbill
Medication-use policy development	As member of a multidisciplinary team, create and implement policy derived from clinical, safety, humanistic, and economic factors that result in optimal patient care.	• Pharmacy and therapeutics committee • Non-formulary approval process
Drug information	Provide accurate, comprehensive, disease-specific and/or patient-specific drug information to patients, caregivers, and health care providers involved in the care of patient.	• Drug information service • Educational sessions • Publications
Medication provision	When appropriate, provide prospective drug review while processing prescriptions, accurately fill and verify prescriptions, and dispense to patients with proper education.	• Prescription processing • Prescription dispensing
Medication prescribing	When credentialed for prescribing privileges, order, discontinue, change prescriptions as necessitated by scope of practice.	• Prescribing under disease management protocols

Table 1-2. Possible Job Descriptions and Examples[4,14-16] (cont'd)

Activity/Function	Description	Examples
Clinic/service development	Develop, implement, and evaluate new and changing patient care services within the organization, promoting continuity of care.	• New services in clinic • New clinic settings
Committee involvement	Actively participate on committees responsible for medication use, quality improvement, performance improvement, and other aspects of patient care within the health system.	• Quality improvement committee • Peer review committee
Institutional review board	Depending on the extent of clinical and drug research, participate as voting member of the organization's institutional review board.	• Institutional review board membership
Education and training	Train new pharmacists and precept pharmacy students and/or residents to extend expertise.	• Ambulatory care specialty residency

Finally, you must discern what policies and procedures are necessary to make your practice run smoothly. Some of these may be in existence in other practice areas; however, some may need to be created from scratch. Policies and procedures should be standard enough to promote consistency but flexible enough to promote clinical judgment. Knowledge of stakeholders and accrediting organizations will guide you in compiling organizational policies and procedures in the areas of human resources, medication control, patient care, laboratory guidelines, and process management. Use Chapter 5 to help you with this process.

How to Be a Leader

In order to launch an ambulatory care practice, you and your team will be more successful if you personally possess practice experience and knowledge, an innovative or entrepreneurial spirit, and experience in building culture along with managing change. Of course, primary knowledge, as well as experience in a particular task, is an asset to any project. You can gain knowledge of successful practices through the literature. However, literature results alone may not satisfy your administrators; they may ask you for the corresponding positive return on investment. That said, successful business plans or organizational descriptions are very rarely published. Chapters 2 and 3 will help you in this regard. Also, in lieu of firsthand experience, networking can provide you with gains in this area. Experience derived in this manner may be more practical for you if it can be directly applied to your practice. The best way to get this kind of insight is to participate in national conferences in the area in which you practice. Please see the web page for a list of organizations, meetings, and meeting dates you may wish to consider attending.

Professional chat rooms, web-based professional communities, blogs, and professional organization sites such as ASHP (American Society of Health-System Pharmacists) Connect are great avenues for asking questions and getting various different points of view from those already in practice. Many practices are organization specific, so be sure to use resources within your own organization (compliance staff, billers, etc). Combine knowledge of the possibilities with the experience in other practices to create your own knowledge base.

Because ambulatory care is a diverse practice going in multiple directions, it is imperative that you or your leader has a true entrepreneurial spirit. Creativity is a must as you start to apply the knowledge and experience gleaned from others. There is no doubt that something will need to be altered to fit, that some barrier will exist to be overcome, or that someone will need to be convinced of the relevance of building or growing the practice. The key to success in many of these discussions is to listen for understanding, consider the opinions and points of view of those involved, and create a novel, better plan that more than meets everyone's needs.[10,17] During this endeavor, a leader who exhibits a spirit of innovation can provide the spark that lights the fire in others.[10,11]

Finally, you must have a leader and team who are able to deal with change while maintaining a culture of service. Even if this is not a new undertaking, your practice will continue to change as new ideas and initiatives are realized. Different metrics will need to be designed to determine the success of your practice. You must have the wherewithal to work and have others work in a rapidly changing environment while still maintaining high morale.[1,18] As shown in **Table 1-3**, communicating, empowering, and recognizing accomplishments are all ways to maintain morale.

Table 1-3. Factors Affecting Change in an Organization[18]

How to Successfully Advance Change

Establish a sense of urgency.
Form a coalition to lead the change.
Create a vision and establish strategies to achieve it.
Communicate the vision.
Empower others to act on the vision.
Plan for and create visible short-term accomplishments.
Produce more change by increased credibility.
Promote and institutionalize effective new behaviors.

A practical way to ensure that people are actively engaged and not burned-out is to talk to each person at least monthly.[11] Talking to your staff and using the questions in **Table 1-4** keeps you in touch with the practice atmosphere and needs. If this process is done sincerely, your people will feel supported and satisfied, and this translates to quality patient care. Furthermore, transparent communication to the whole group focusing on perceived problems versus reality is a proven method to allay fears and quell the rumor mill.

Table 1-4. Questions Asked During a Rounding Session[11]

Question	Comment
What is going well today?	Always start on a positive note.
What can be improved?	Make sure to have the associate focus on what can be improved with the department, not the associate's performance. Build a better process, not a better person.
Do you have the tools necessary to do your job?	Allows you to meet needs before they become critical. It is important to follow through by either getting what is needed or explaining why you can't. If not, it undermines your sincerity.

Table 1-4. Questions Asked During a Rounding Session[11] (cont'd)

Question	Comment
Is there anyone I should recognize?	Thank you notes should be written to the specified individuals. This recognizes accomplishments and rewards appropriate behaviors. It also fosters good relationship developing between the person recognized and the person who recommended the recognition.

Beyond the Leadership Standard

Everyone within your organization has a professional duty to communicate transparently with each other. Transparency, in this sense, means no hidden agendas, no grudges, no passive aggression, and clear communication and clarification of expectations. Likewise, you should disallow triangulation. As depicted in **Figure 1-1**, triangulation is the process of bringing unnecessary people into disagreement or discussion—fostering office politics. Those involved in the problem or situation must respect each other enough to confront the issue at hand, rather than involve a third party. These steps are sometimes easier said than done, and likely they become more difficult the larger the staff and the more separated, geographically, they are.

 Everyone within your organization has a professional duty to communicate transparently with each other.

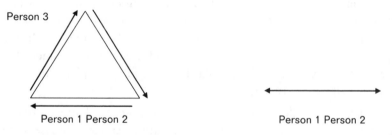

Figure 1-1. Example of Triangulation

In this triangulation, person 1 and person 2 have a conflict, and person 3 is brought into the program unnecessarily. The line on the right represents appropriate communication between two professionals.

You should encourage the development of leaders from within the practice, or site leaders from within the practice can become champions of a program or initiative, making it run smoothly.[19,20] Because these leaders are more on the "front lines," they can assist in troubleshooting or changing direction before calamity occurs. Many times you can simply foster leadership by soliciting and listening to opinions of those within the team. Another way in which to engage dormant leaders is to find and incorporate their strengths or passions into projects you would have them lead. In describing the transitions in pharmacy practice in 2000, Nimmo and Holland stated, ". . . much of what pharmacists will do or not do during a workday is driven by their professional values—by what is important and what obligations are to be met—rather than by some carefully defined list of tasks."[21]

There are no satisfied patients without satisfied clinicians. Clinicians do gain satisfaction from purposeful work.[13] However, this purposeful work must be competitively remunerated. The concept that "everyone is your competition" can also be applied to salary adjustments within the organization. When arranging the pay scale for pharmacists in your organization, is it based on like businesses or where the competition lies? Where does the competition lie? The answer is the entire profession: a pharmacist with a license could interview for any pharmacist position in any type of practice. This being the case, you must expand analysis of salary for all positions based on the entire practice of pharmacy to maintain your competitive edge.

Finally, it is imperative for you to share your systems and your "secrets" freely for the betterment of the profession, even at the local level. This could be accomplished with publications, presentations, blogs, professional electronic communities, and Twitter, to name a few. Do not let the fear of competition keep you from open and transparent communication outside of your organization. Rather, when you have done something unique or novel that positively impacts the profession or patients, tell or show others in the profession. Duplication of such a system or practice model will better establish it within the health care system and impact more patient lives. Moreover, mutual support with amicable competition results in further innovations and growth.

Patient Care Standards

Patient Care

Patient care is likely the most recognizable and defining characteristic of an ambulatory practice; you likely gravitate toward a practice in ambulatory care if you enjoy forming long-lasting relationships with patients while using your clinical skills to help them manage their various disease states and medication regimen. It is possible that this is the only part of the standard that requires implementation, as the other aspects may already exist within your system.

Patient care has been called many things over the years as pharmacy transitioned from a product to a patient-based profession: cognitive services, disease state management, pharmaceutical care, pharmacotherapy, and medication therapy management (MTM) services. Even though it existed under different names, the basic premise of pharmacy has not changed: care involves the process through which a pharmacist cooperates with a patient and other professionals in designing, implementing, and monitoring a therapeutic plan that will manage a patient's disease, eliminate or reduce a patient's symptoms, arrest or slow disease progression, or prevent a disease.[14] Moreover, these tenets apply whether your practice focuses on an individual patient or an entire patient population and whether your practice is part of a collaborative interdisciplinary team effort or a more independent venture. You should ensure that those charged with the care of another human being have appropriate training and an appropriate knowledge base, should be able to apply the knowledge base to individual patients, and exhibit empathy and compassion during patient care.

Regardless of your type of practice or practice focus, ensure that your patient care staff have appropriately trained clinically and have the ability to exhibit empathy and compassion to those in their care.

Training

Patients will assume you and your staff are appropriately trained for the position you hold simply because you hold the position.[11] It is your duty to make sure that the people on your team or those you invite to join your team are appropriately trained to take care of these patients. Since ambulatory patient care requires training and skill sets beyond that of initial pharmacy licensure, postgraduate training, pharmacy practice and specialty residency programs, or comparable experience should be considered the standard for practice.[22,23]

When considering a postgraduate-trained pharmacist, you may want to set an individual practice or organizational standard for how much time a practitioner spent in an ambulatory care setting, as residency programs differ. A residency program will assure you that your pharmacist can take care of a diverse patient population. No doubt both the new resident-trained clinicians and the established clinicians will feel slightly uncomfortable, depending on the level of experience they currently have when venturing into new practice situations; it is your responsibility to ensure that you move them from consciously incompetent to consciously competent as depicted in **Table 1-5**. It is imperative that your pharmacist should be trained appropriately for the position or patient populations with whom you would entrust them. Even though the service you offer may be very specific—anticoagulation, congestive heart failure, or diabetes management—your pharmacist will come into contact with patients with many other disease states in the context of your service. If it is a new service or program, you should ensure that a training plan is established, monitored, and completed before patient care ensues. Determining the best method to ensure competency of your staff is further discussed in Chapter 7.

 It is imperative that your pharmacist should be trained appropriately for the position or patient populations with whom you would entrust them.

Table 1-5. Stages of Competence[24]

Competence[a]	Description	How to Move to the Next Stage
Unconscious incompetence	Don't know what you don't know or happily ignorant	Listen to people who point out blind spots
Conscious incompetence	Know what you don't know or cognitive dissonance	Study and practice

Table 1-5. Stages of Competence[24] (cont'd)

Competence[a]	Description	How to Move to the Next Stage
Conscious competence	Know	You have experience
Unconscious competence	Don't know you know	You are an expert

[a] Stages of competence through which you will progress when asked to take on a new task or learn a new topic.

Application

Drawing from several references and our own ambulatory care practice experiences, we propose **Table 1-6** as the minimum standard of care for your ambulatory practice.[4-6,14,26] Patient care should be both prospective and comprehensive in nature (**Figure 1-2**).[5] Even if you have been consulted for a very specific reason, you have a duty to evaluate the whole patient, determining which things you can manage and which things need to be recommendations back to the provider based on the referral. Before you sit down in the room with the patient, you should independently gather the patient's medical information for pertinent past medical history, allergies, medications, and laboratory data.[4,6,7,14,26] Goals of therapy, including surrogate end points and patient outcomes, should be determined.

Key Point

Goals of therapy, including surrogate end points and patient outcomes, should be determined.

Table 1-6. Seven Standards of Ambulatory Patient Care[4-6,14,25]

Minimum Standards of Care for Your Ambulatory Care Practice[a]

1. Interviewing patients and caregivers to gather pertinent information for patient care
2. Assessing the legal and clinical appropriateness of medication regimen
3. Identifying, resolving, and preventing medication-related problems
4. Participating in pharmacotherapy decision making
5. Educating patients and caregivers on disease, pharmacotherapy, adherence, and preventative health
6. Monitoring the medication effects and patient's health outcomes
7. Maintaining medication profiles and other documentations

[a] For a more detailed list of standards, refer to the different domains outlined in the Board of Pharmacy Specialties' Ambulatory Care Pharmacy Specialty Certification Examination document that can be found at http://www.bpsweb.org/resources/content.cfm.

Upon reviewing this information, you should assess the current plan for appropriateness. A useful exercise is to have clinicians determine how they systematically approach patient care. If they can discover and duplicate this approach, it is less likely that issues affecting patient care will be missed. One question serves as the basis for this evaluation: are the medications appropriate based on patient-specific factors and available evidence? Applying Allen Shaughnessy's method of evaluating

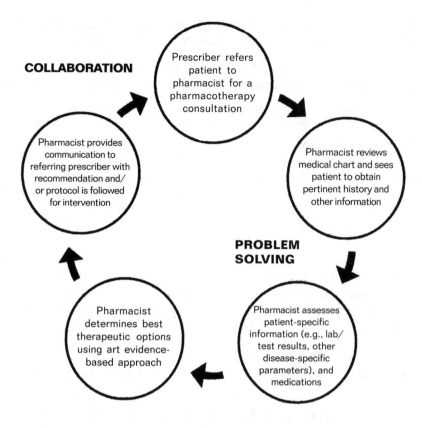

COLLABORATION

Prescriber refers patient to pharmacist for a pharmacotherapy consultation

Pharmacist provides communication to referring prescriber with recommendation and/ or protocol is followed for intervention

Pharmacist reviews medical chart and sees patient to obtain pertinent history and other information

PROBLEM SOLVING

Pharmacist determines best therapeutic options using art evidence-based approach

Pharmacist assesses patient-specific information (e.g., lab/ test results, other disease-specific parameters), and medications

Figure 1-2. Prescriber-Pharmacotherapy Specialist Relationship

(Reprinted with permission from Council on Credentialing in Pharmacy. Scope of contemporary pharmacy practice: roles, responsibilities, and functions of pharmacists and pharmacy technicians. Washington, DC: Council on Credentialing in Pharmacy; 2009.)

a specific agent—safety, tolerability, effectiveness, price, and simplicity (STEPS)— to multiple different agents for an individual patient incorporates the different aspects of many proposed standards of patient care.[27] (See **Table 1-7**.)

Table 1-7. Patient Medication Assessment: Comparison of Shaughnessy's STEPS to Other Proposed Pharmacotherapeutic Principles[27]

Author	Ambulatory Care Tenets				
Shaughnessy[27]	**Safety**	**Tolerability**	**Effectiveness**	**Price**	**Simplicity**
Carter[3]	Monitor for drug interactions	Monitor for adverse effects	Individualize drug regimen based on purpose, diseases	Consider cost	
Burke[22]	Ongoing monitoring to identify drug interactions or contraindications	Identify patient problems and potential adverse effects	Monitor therapy for appropriateness		
Hepler and Strand[14]	Decide if causing toxicity	Decide if there are any undesirable drug effects	Decide if all medications are the most effective products		Design a regimen that patient is able or willing to take

Table 1-7. Patient Medication Assessment: Comparison of Shaughnessy's STEPS to Other Proposed Pharmacotherapeutic Principles[27] (cont'd)

Author			Ambulatory Care Tenets		
Shaughnessy[27]	Safety	Tolerability	Effectiveness	Price	Simplicity
Indian Health Service[6]	Safe drug regimen	Prevent undesired effects	Evaluate regimen for efficacy	Determine cost effectiveness	Counsel for adherence
ASHP[4]	Identification of problems		Appropriateness of medications		Counsel for adherence
Residency Goals and Objectives[18]	Review for drug interactions, therapeutic duplications, and allergies	Monitor to treat or prevent adverse drug reactions	Base goals, plans, and monitoring on evidence-based medicine	Determine if problems with finances	Determine adherence

- Is the entire medication regimen safe for the patient? You must make sure that the regimen has no potential for allergic reactions, has no therapeutic duplications, and has no potential for drug-drug, drug-disease, or drug-food interactions.

- Is the patient tolerating the regimen? You must ensure that the patient is not exhibiting signs or symptoms of suffering from untoward effects from the medication.

- Is the regimen effective? Looking at patient-specific criteria, you must evaluate if the current regimen is evidence based for the diseases that the patient has. Also, you must decide if the current regimen is optimized compared to the evidence-based goals of therapy.

- Is the patient able to afford the price? Cost should always be a consideration in the choice of a regimen. Many times your patient may be ashamed to discuss financial difficulties and end up not adhering to the regimen prescribed. It is your responsibility to ensure a cost-effective regimen is provided.

- Is the regimen simple for the patient to take? Does the patient understand why and how he or she is to take the medication regimen? You must assess whether or not you think the patient could adhere to the regimen based on frequency of dosing of the different agents and plan to substitute alternatives as necessary. It is also important to form an assessment of how knowledgeable the patient may be regarding the medication therapy regimen.

On review of the patient's medication regimen, response to therapy, and medical history, you can develop a tentative pharmacotherapeutic plan going forward. Many times this may be an "if/then" scenario, not having one set plan but several courses of action plotted out. This plan should address issues unearthed during review of the patient's medical record, including modifications of the current drug regimen, suggestions for lifestyle modification, a follow-up monitoring plan, a preventative action, and a patient education plan.

Once this plan is developed, the patient interview and evaluation can take place. Initially, you should ask patients what their primary concerns are, what their understanding of the visit is, and what they hope to accomplish during the visit. This quickly sets the tone and expectations of the visit and allows the patient to start talking. You should then question the patient about symptoms of the ongoing disease processes as well as medication effects. Vital signs and laboratory data necessary for the visit should be obtained at this time. Clarification or reconciliation of the medication regimen, including differences in how the medication is prescribed versus how the patient takes or administers it, allows for a more defined pharmacotherapy plan. During the course of this conversation you can establish common goals and plans of action with the patient.

Key Point Combining your initial review of the patient's medical history with the patient interview allows you to implement or adjust your plan going forward.

This encounter should be documented in the patient's medical record.[1-6,7,14,22,26] Chapter 6 will further discuss optimal documentation.

Continuity of Care

You should ensure that care is collaborative, with steps in place to maintain continuity, in particular around medications, among all clinicians caring for a particular patient. Often the required collaboration will be defined by the collaborative drug therapy management agreement and the referral. However, collaboration goes beyond your team and may include a diverse group of providers such as the dispensing pharmacist, a hospitalist, a home nurse, etc. Not only should the ambulatory pharmacists take responsibility for medication reconciliation around all transitions of care, but it is also imperative that you have a process to communicate your patient-specific actions and plans to all providers that touch your patient so that the patient's specific plan of care is truly one coordinated plan.

Continuity assures that other appropriate laboratory and other tests are completed or that other diseases are being addressed without duplication. Most importantly, continuity measures ensure that other providers are aware of the entire patient's clinical information so that decision making at each point of care is optimal. Collaboration allows a complete management of the whole patient as a team. You have much to offer to the team when it comes to drug, dosing, interaction, cost information, adherence strategies, and beyond. Care should be taken to support the team when opportunities arise: praise efforts of other providers publicly, and question or criticize privately. This builds the patient's confidence in the whole team. Ultimately these communications should be included in the patient's medical record.

It is also important to note that once you have implemented a pharmacist-managed program, your utmost commitment to continued service should be exercised and that it should not be a sporadic service delivered only when time, resources, and staffing are plenty. It has been documented that quality of outcomes decrease when patients are discharged from a pharmacist-managed clinic or when pharmacist-delivered interventions are removed and patients have to return to the usual care. For example, even after stabilization of warfarin therapy, transition of patients from a pharmacist-managed anticoagulation clinic back to physician-managed anticoagulation care resulted in significant decrease in International Normalized Ratio (INR) control, increased medical care related to anticoagulation, and decreased patient satisfaction.[28] When a comprehensive pharmacy care program was removed from community-dwelling older patients using polypharmacy after 6 months, medication adherence returned to near-baseline levels, whereas patients who stayed with the comprehensive pharmacy care program maintained their adherence consistently above 95%, resulting in further improved blood pressure control.[29] Moreover, providing inconsistent care will compromise your credibility within the organization and among your health care team and patients.

 Key Point It is also important to note that once you have implemented a pharmacist-managed program, your utmost commitment to continued service should be exercised and that it should not be a sporadic service delivered only when time, resources, and staffing are plenty.

Patient Education

It is widely known that pharmacists are patient educators. The disease and medication knowledge you possess can be invaluable to patients and their caregivers when delivered in an effective manner. The ambulatory care setting is especially suited for educational sessions with minimal pressure of acute illness or emergent procedures. Specifically, patients being prescribed a medication for a new diagnosis, a regimen change being performed for better control of a condition, or strategies being applied to improve adherence or to alleviate a drug-related problem are golden opportunities for you to provide essential education. Patients' understanding of antibiotic resistance and appropriate antibiotic use improved following a pharmacist-initiated educational intervention in an urgent care clinic, where patients reported satisfaction with the intervention.[30] Development of a constructive and relevant relationship between you and the patient must be cultivated. Knowing the patient's condition and preferences facilitates patient encounters for education. Whenever possible, your communication strategy should be tailored to the patient's background, cultural preferences, and health literacy.[31] Pharmacists' education (primary intervention among other strategies) in a drug optimization clinic significantly improved HIV-infected patients' CD4[+] lymphocyte counts, viral loads, and drug-related toxicities.[32] Regular use of available tools to promote health communication between patients and providers should be an integrated part of your educational session.[33] However, it is important to note that education alone may not affect patient or provider behavior to a significant degree. For instance, a two-part educational intervention that consisted of academic detailing (provider-specific information) with educational materials presented to providers and educational and motivational materials given to patients resulted in only a relatively modest effect among patients with hypertension. However, multidimensional, comprehensive programs have impacted patient behavior related to medication adherence, which in turn produced significant improvements in health outcomes.[29,34] It is also important to remember that patient education needs to occur in conjunction with provider education when the pharmacist is not the prescriber of therapy for managing particular conditions.

For many chronic conditions, patient education can be provided in accordance with the available national guidelines, such as the hypertension guidelines in the seventh report of the Joint National Committee on the Detection, Evaluation, and Treatment of High Blood Pressure (JNC VII).[35] All of the disease-specific organizations (e.g., American Heart Association, American Diabetes Association, Arthritis Foundation) have specific educational information you can use. They often offer support groups and advocacy for research and clinical practice as well. Similarly, population-based organizations such as American Pediatric Society and American Geriatric Society supply educational materials tailored to the population they represent. There are various other sources as well, including pharmacy-specific online educational programs and software (e.g., MicroMedex, Thomson Reuters, Inc., Cambridge, MA) that have ready-to-use patient counseling materials. Chapter 5 will address items you need to set up your clinic, and includes a table that lists national resources and where you can access educational materials.

Compassion

As necessary as clinical competence is, compassionate competence is equally necessary to be successful in ambulatory care, meaning, you must demonstrate empathy and care when working with patients—and coworkers.[36] Despite the fact that success is being measured objectively, never forget that the patient in front of you is a person rather than a task that must be completed before you leave for the day. This is fundamental in developing a therapeutic pharmacist-patient relationship. This relationship can be as important, if not more important, than any therapeutic modality that you would recommend or manage.[4,7] This relationship is the foundation for the trust in your professional judgment and management decisions. It is one determinant in how adherent a patient will be to your established plan. Moreover, it is this relationship that will keep your patient coming back to see you. Good training material for this topic is the Heart Matters in Pharmacy Practice, a syllabus and guide developed by the University of California San Francisco, School of Pharmacy, for a course to explore "deeper human issues of patient care" with their student pharmacists, but this can be easily adopted to train practicing pharmacists.[37]

Your practice would again do well to embrace the principle that any organization providing service is the competition. This concept can be applied both to patient care as well as program operations. As stated previously, patients will assume that you and your clinicians are competent or you would not be working in this setting. The experience of the visit and interaction will influence their decision to come back. No one ever says "this looks like a great day to go see my pharmacist." The reasons for this are plentiful: they are stricken with illness, they are dealing with the health care system, they are being asked to change behavior, and they are paying for a service. However, exceeding the patients' expectations and going above and beyond to meet patients' needs will go a long way to ensure that patients are very satisfied with their care.[36] Making sure a patient gets a needed cane or walker to decrease the risk of falls, helping a patient set up a needed physician visit and assisting in transportation to that visit, securing a medication list in braille for a vision-impaired patient are some examples of going the extra mile for a patient.

Simply stated: treat your patients like people first.

Beyond the Patient Care Standard

Some concepts that would allow you to exceed the patient care standard may not be possible until the current reimbursement paradigm changes. That is to say, both the way in which you can now charge or the amount you will get reimbursed may influence the way in which you practice. You should strive to have an independent patient population that comes to the practice solely to see you. This would allow you to have more independence in the drug therapy management decisions. It also allows you to bring in an independent revenue stream into your practice and organization.

When considering hiring or training your team, you should give preference to those individuals who have taken the initiative to complete postgraduate year-2 (PGY-2) residency training or who have equivalent experience. As more pharmacists complete PGY-2 programs and as the number of available PGY-2 programs increase, this training will likely become the norm. Furthermore, you should consider those who have obtained certifications a priority, especially those requiring practice experience in the areas pertinent to the practice. Pharmacy as a profession needs a way to objectively show the increased skill and knowledge sets of residency trained clinicians, such as boards examinations.

When planning patient care, drug therapy decisions should be based as much on patient-oriented evidence, such as prevention of myocardial infarction in patients with dyslipidemia or reduction in blindness in diabetic patients, as it is the surrogate end points, such as a specific laboratory or vital sign threshold. In addition to basing drug therapy decisions on patient-oriented evidence, practices should have effectiveness measured in the same manner.[39]

You should be able to garner appropriate support personnel during the actual patient visit. A certified medical assistant could obtain a full set of vitals and laboratory data as needed, allowing you to focus on the medication management decisions. This may be more appropriate with several pharmacists operating out of the same space at the same time. If you are being plugged into an already existing clinic, such as primary care (internal medicine or family practice), you should obtain the support of the triage nursing staff as well as the front desk clerks, coders, and billers.

 You should focus on continuity of care not only with the interdisciplinary team taking care of the patient but also across the spectrum of pharmacy practices.

Should your patient require hospitalization, you should communicate the patient's regimen to the hospital clinicians: physicians and pharmacists. Should your patient require home health or visiting nursing services, you should communicate with the pharmacists in these settings. Information shared in this manner about the drug therapy can further reduce the potential for medication misadventures.

In summary, you as the ambulatory pharmacist take responsibility for all aspects of medication use for your patients. This includes the following:

- Evaluating appropriateness of therapy

- Ensuring access and adherence to medications

- Identifying and resolving drug-related problems

- Educating your patients on their drug therapy and how it relates to their conditions

- On-going monitoring of your patients

- Ensuring continuity of care with regard to patient medications and plan of care

Medication Management Standard

Medication Management

Although pharmacy is becoming more patient and less product oriented, you must remember that, at its heart, medication control is about patient safety. It is no mistake that your accrediting organization addresses medication safety and medication management directives. Moreover, it would be unusual if you did not have some element of medication control at your site, including procuring, managing inventory, prescribing, dispensing (including packaging and labeling), educating patients, administering, and disposing of medications.[4,5,26] No matter the site, if medications are present, you should be involved in leading initiatives to establish safe medication control, either through direct oversight or appropriate committee participation.

Akin to the choice of agents for a particular patient in the pharmacotherapeutic plan, and just as important, physically getting the medication to your patient can be governed by the *patient rights*: right patient, right drug, right dose, right amount, right route, and right frequency. In some settings medications may simply be stored for administration during visits. In others, patients may bring to appointments medications that are no longer necessary or that require disposal. You are likely to be more fully responsible for the entire process if you are physically dispensing a medication to the patient in your setting. In any of these circumstances, you can lessen the potential for error if you address the following interrelated variables: standardization, continuity of work flow, and patient education.

Standardization

Standardization of processes involved in medication control allows you to prevent medication misadventures caused by staff, whether they work shifts consecutively or concurrently, due to misunderstanding each other's approach to a given situation. In standardizing your processes, you improve the accuracy of medication dispensing and control processes and ensure that the medication is correctly and precisely filled; that is, you ensure the reproducibility of the correctly filled medication.[40] You can best standardize your practice by soliciting input from your staff on the rationale behind their work flow. Based on these conversations, you can devise the one best method. Then, you will need to continue to enforce standard policies, or policies quickly cease to be standard.

Continuity of Work Flow

You must maintain work flow continuity to further prevent medication errors. As noted by U.S. Phamacopeia Patient Safety CAPSLink, October 2005,[41] work flow disruption accounts for significant both potential and actual cause of medication error. In ambulatory care, disruption may come in many forms: patient care clinics, impromptu drug information questions from clinicians and patients, or practice management issues taking place during dispensing duties. For instance, if you are scheduled to be dispensing at the same time as you have clinic responsibilities, because your attention is divided you could cause mistakes in either task. You need to make sure to be protective of your time where and whenever possible. It is necessary to have the focus on the task at hand for it to be done properly. Depending on the site, you may need to separate these tasks so that two people may do the work concurrently or that one person may complete the work consecutively. However, do not set an expectation for one person to do both tasks concurrently.

Patient Education

Finally, you may catch potential medication errors simply by educating the patient regarding the medication that is being dispensed or administered. In counseling patients, not only will you decrease potential errors caused by the medication use system, but you also may decrease the chance of the patient taking the medication incorrectly. This may be done at the time of dispensing or during another medication-related situation, such as medication reconciliation or medication therapy management services.

Beyond the Medication Control Standard

A closed medication system in which a pharmacist not only sees the patient but also has the opportunity to dispense medications has strong merits. In this model, you could assess adherence simply by looking at the fill records. More information about the patient would be known in both areas. The pharmacist dispensing the medication may have a deeper understanding of why the patient is taking the medication or why changes are being made. Short of having a closed system, sharing of information between pharmacy and medical systems would have much the same outcome.

Organization Model

Organizational Structure

How a pharmacy or pharmacy service is integrated or aligned within an organization plays a large part in the scope and breadth of services provided as well as their overall acceptance. Health systems structures that affect ambulatory care generally follow two model types: a departmental model or an office model. Your site may have an organizational structure that shares some of both model types.[42,43]

The majority of departmental organizational models within a specific health system are vertically aligned but horizontally integrated. This means that you report through a set hierarchy to a pharmacy leader; however, you interact collaboratively with other disciplines at your site. The pervasiveness of pharmacy leadership differs within different organizations. In some organizations, the pharmacy leaders are found throughout, including the CEO; however, it is equally likely, if not more so, that the pharmacy director or regional manager is the highest ranking pharmacist within your chain of command. It is common for this director or regional manager to report to a chief officer of another health or business discipline. A chief pharmacy officer (CPO) position, while logical, is rare in today's organizations. Your pharmacy leader, be it director or vice president, will be responsible for deriving the mission, vision, and strategic plan for those departments that report to him or her. It is common for this pharmacy leader to have several managers, supervisors, or coordinators as direct reports, sometimes at different practice sites. These "leader reports" are responsible for assisting in executing the mission, vision, and strategic plans in the areas for which they are accountable.

In some settings, an entire section may be called an ambulatory department. However, in other areas of practice, ambulatory care may be a responsibility of the pharmacist at the site. It is not unusual to find two separate models at this level. The first model is that of an outpatient department in which the patients of the system come to one location to see the pharmacists, such as an ambulatory care department of a hospital or community pharmacy. The second model may be that in which a manager is responsible for pharmacists serving in different geographic locations, such as physician offices. In either place, leader reports manage the frontline operations and personnel. The success of this model depends on those in the system paying attention to the needs and the goals of not only the pharmacy but also the areas in which the pharmacists work (**Figure 1-3**).

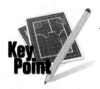

Key Point
The goals of the pharmacy and the areas in which pharmacists work should have shared initiatives.

Contrast this reporting structure with that of a clinic, office, or network of offices not integrated into the larger health system. Depending on the size of the office or network, there may or may not be an administrative hierarchy above the level of the individual clinic director. Thus there would be a mix of nursing and administration or medical personnel acting in place of a pharmacy leader. Pharmacists may not report to pharmacy leaders in these situations. Instead, pharmacists may report to a clinical manager or practice administrator at the site. In this setting, there may be a limited number of pharmacy personnel per site (**Figure 1-4**).

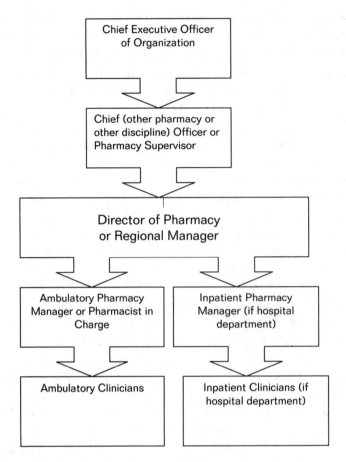

Figure 1-3. Pharmacy Department Organizational Chart

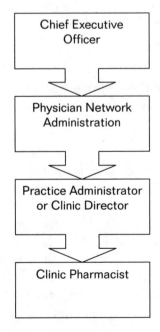

Figure 1-4. Office-Based Organizational Model

It is important to mention that because of a desire for an innovative practice but a lack of a substantiating revenue stream, many schools of pharmacy may partner with either the health system or office-based model. These situations are commonly beneficial to both the school and the practice. The school of pharmacy gets an innovative practice site in which their clinical faculty can practice and their students can learn. The patients and existing team at the sites get a practice and personnel that otherwise they would be hard-pressed to fund. That being said, this interaction creates another level of organization within the hosting organization as the faculty must report up through the school of pharmacy. In any of these situations, care and communication are keys to maintaining the strategic plan of all the stakeholders involved.

Collaborative Drug Therapy Management Agreements

Of note, the majority of state boards of pharmacy have sections of pharmacy law defining collaborative drug therapy management (CDTM) or specific instances of patient care. You should consult these regulations to make sure legal requirements or specific language is included in the agreement. CDTM has been defined as a collaborative practice agreement between one or more physicians and pharmacists wherein qualified pharmacists work within the context of professional responsibility to do the following: perform patient assessments, order drug therapy-related laboratory tests, administer drugs, and select, initiate, monitor, continue, and adjust medication regimens.[42,44,45] Ideally, you should work closely with legal counsel when developing these agreements. As you give this to potential participants, they too will give them to lawyers to review before signing. A CDTM agreement determines your relationship to the physician as well as your scope of service to the patients. (Examples of CDTM)

Depending on your strategic plan for growth, you may not want this agreement to refer to a specific service line, although it may be tempting to include them. If you are too specific in your agreement, as you open more and newer service lines you will have to create addenda to or new CDTM agreements.

Rather, build these agreements based on general actions, duties, or scope of the pharmacist.

If you need specifics for the physicians, have a section that points to other policies and procedures or guidelines. These guidelines can be service line or disease state specific. If these guidelines need to be updated because of new evidence, a new CDTM agreement need not be drafted. The CDTM agreement may also be a good place to document the mode and frequency of communication back to the physician.

Build your CDTM agreements based on general actions, duties, or scope of the pharmacist to avoid revisions and addendums.

Another consideration of the CDTM agreement is with whom the agreement is being made. Is the agreement being made between a specific practice and the pharmacy, or does it need to be specific to the individual practitioner who has referred the patient? You may decrease the complexity of the agreement if you are able to have the agreement be between the physician practice and the pharmacy practice. If your agreement is between practices rather than individuals, you allow for clinician turnover or patient responsibility coverage without additional paperwork. If it is between individuals, you can still have the same functional collaborative practice; however, you will need to ensure that all physician and pharmacist combinations have signed the agreements. Because of the potential complexity, it would be wise if you review and update your CDTMs on an annual basis as necessary.

Building a general CDTM agreement with more specific guidelines does have advantages. However, further information may be necessary to take care of an individual patient. In conjunction with the development of the CDTM agreement, a referral process should also be developed. A referral from the physician and other providers documenting treatment for a particular patient gives you further individual direction for true collaboration. (Sample Referral Form)

Practice Model Settings

Practice Settings

No matter how your practice is oriented in your organization, it should address key components of the ambulatory care standard of practice. Much has been made of the differences among practice settings and how these could potentially affect the processes and scope of ambulatory care by the pharmacist. In 2010, the ASHP Section of Ambulatory Care Practitioners conducted a survey of ambulatory care pharmacy. Of the respondents, 70% reported their ambulatory practice was associated with a hospital or health system, and 22% stated they practiced within a medical office/clinic or community health clinic. The most common clinics with pharmacist-provided services identified at each practice site included anticoagulation (73%), diabetes (68%), hypertension (67%), hyperlipidemia (61%), and smoking cessation (45%). The number and variety of clinic types, however, were wide-ranging. More than half the clinics reported having 3,000 or fewer documented patient encounters per year, yet 23% reported having more than 9,000 patient encounters per year. The results demonstrate a continued growth of ambulatory patient care pharmacy services, compared to previous surveys.[46,47] Each of the ambulatory practice settings bring with it particular strengths and weaknesses. Conducting a strengths, weaknesses, opportunities, and threats (SWOT) analysis as you choose what practice model you wish to adopt will better prepare you for the implementation stage. See **Table 1-8** for a SWOT analysis we have initiated for various practice models described in this chapter.

Office-based Practice Model

Physician Office

Pharmacists can be found practicing in the offices of many different medical specialties. In this setting, you may report up through the health system to pharmacy leaders or report to the director of the clinic. Your responsibilities will vary with the

Table 1-8. SWOT Analysis of Ambulatory Care Pharmacy Practice Models

Office Based Practice Model	Strengths	Weaknesses	Opportunities	Threats
Physician Office	Collaboration with on-site physician and team. Easy access to physicians and team to increase efficiency of patient visits. Able to bill incident to the physician via superbill. Possibly fewer hoops to jump through to initiate service.	Leadership may not understand the full scope of pharmacy. Limited patient population; may be difficult to see patients other than those who belong to practice.	No preconceived concept of what pharmacist can do; "sky is the limit." Great place to carve out physician extender practice.	May be difficult to bill other than incident to a physician. May or may not cover pharmacist's salary. Return on investment dependent on payer mix.
Community Health Centers/ Federally Qualified Health Centers	Because of the effort to reduce medication costs, pharmacists are integral to the care team.	Different levels of experience with pharmacist involvement in direct patient care depending on the area and culture.	Grants and funding for innovative pharmacy practices exist.	Medication control and access are likely as important as direct patient care and may take time away from pharmacist-run clinics.
Medical Residency Programs	Teach physicians as well as treating patients.	Constant struggle with direct or collaborative patient care and how to ensure physicians are still learning if you see their patients.	Develop unique collaborative models for teaching and treating simultaneously.	Pharmacists are not specifically required by ACGME.

Pharmacy Department-based Practice Model

Pharmacy Department-based Practice Model	Strengths	Weaknesses	Opportunities	Threats
Community Pharmacy	Prevalence and availability of different sites. Diverse patient population.	Community pharmacy ROI largely determined by prescription throughput. Limited private space, especially in older pharmacies, and the need for remodeling. Limited access to patient information other than their prescription and what they or their providers are willing to share.	MTM service in the outpatient setting could bring more business to a particular pharmacy. Large chains have the opportunity to contract with large national third-party plans for reimbursement.	Potential for competition among and with large community pharmacy chains. Large community may bill less for the service because of increased volume, thus lowering the payment rate for the rest of the profession.

Table 1-8. SWOT Analysis of Ambulatory Care Pharmacy Practice Models (cont'd)

Pharmacy Department-based Practice Model	Strengths	Weaknesses	Opportunities	Threats
Medical Center Ambulatory Clinic, or Outpatient Pharmacy	Billing and reimbursement may be counted as a facility fee rather than incident to physician. Access to inpatient information readily available to assist in continuity of care. Able to tie cost avoidance on the hospital side due to reduced admissions and emergency room visits to return on investment. Pharmacy department is likely involved in various other operations such as formulary management, QI, medication control, etc.	May be difficult to explain a fixed position to staff clinics if productivity is based on hospital census. Staffing issues can be a challenge in staffing a clinic if limited clinical staff is available for coverage. There may be more hoops to jump through in a large medical center to become credentialed as a provider.	Potentially increased clinician and patient population compared to an office practice. Opportunities abound in this setting as positive evidence of pharmacist interventions are readily available to justify various services you wish to offer. Great potential for establishing specialty practice such as a chronic disease state, anticoagulation, emergency department practice, etc.	With increased clinical function, your liability increases as well; need to be vigilant about blurred scope areas and maintain compliance with required training and authorization, such as obtaining a DEA number if needed.
Patient-centered Medical Home	Collaboration with an interdisciplinary team. Clinical information systems supporting patient registry and decision making will make your practice more efficient.	At this time, there are limited number of PCMHs in operation as health care reform is still in process. Pharmacist's role in PCMH is still being debated.	With the health care reform and aging of our population, this is a desired model of practice. With the ready access to care motto, pharmacists practicing as a physician extender will likely increase.	Information on quality and efficiency will be available to the public to compare the PCMHs, which can be a strength or threat. Pharmacists are in competition with the other physician extender clinicians.
Home-based Primary Care	Collaboration with an interdisciplinary team. Proven working models exist with performance measures already identified.	Even though quality of care has shown to be improved, cost savings are still questionable.	With the aging of our population and burden of high institutional cost to the health system, this is a desired model of practice along with the PCMH.	Home visits for certain patient population can be costly and difficult. Pharmacist home visits may or may not be billable.

ACGME - Accreditation Council for Graduate Medical Education; DEA = Drug Enforcement Agency; ROI = Return on Investment; QI = Quality Improvement.

focus of the practice but will more than likely include some aspects of practice management, medication control, direct patient care, and education. Practice management responsibilities may include performance improvement, development of practice guidelines, and patient education. Medication control may relate to medications administered at the site, medication stock, or sample medications. Whereas the focus of your specific clinic may differ depending on the specialty of your office, your role and responsibility in patient care will likely not. You will still be responsible for ensuring access to, adherence to, effectiveness of, and understanding of the medication regimen. Direct patient care services will differ with the specialty. Didactic and clinical education will depend on the type of program.

Unique to this practice setting is the amount of collaboration with the primary care provider. This may provide for an expanded scope of service, and expeditious follow-up and backup. The scope of service will have been previously defined in the CDTM; however, you may have more latitude if you are working closely with the physician. For instance, if you have a patient on anticoagulation who has not been practicing safe sex, you may be able to administer a urine pregnancy test just by walking down the hallway and discussing the case with the physician on site. Collaboration of this sort would take more time in another setting. Likewise, if you are seeing a diabetic patient who is experiencing chest pain on examination, you can discuss the case with the physicians with whom you work and obtain an EKG rather than send the patient to the emergency room. Positive evidence, such as integration of a pharmacist into an urban private physician practice resulting in significantly improving diabetes control and sustaining clinic adherence to the American Diabetes Association guidelines, may be the type of resource to use for this type of clinic.[48] Another example is an ambulatory pharmacist practice as part of a multispecialty physician group practice within a managed care environment, which has shown to positively impact clinical outcomes of patients having diabetes.[49]

Community Health Centers and Federally Qualified Health Centers

You may also practice in sites serving the underserved or underinsured patient population. Such entities include community health centers, federally qualified health centers, migrant health centers, health centers for public housing, health centers for the homeless, and HIV clinics, to name a few. Patient populations in such centers often struggle with access to medications. You can assist in obtaining drugs in these situations through various routes: 340b pricing programs, medication samples, and patient assistance programs through the pharmaceutical companies. The 340b pricing programs refer to entities that participate in the U.S. Department of Health and Human Services, Health Resources and Services Administration's (HRSA's) 340b drug discount program: certain federal grantees, federally qualified health center look-alikes, and qualified disproportionate share hospitals. You can find further information for the 340b program at HRSA's website: http://www.hrsa.gov/opa/introduction.htm. In these settings, usually your goal is to provide economically sound, efficient treatment through evidence-based medicine and formulary management. The priority or these goals likely influence the daily workload mix of patient care and medication control. Services such as medication therapy management or medication reconciliation can decrease costs and patient harm associated with medication misadventures further down the line in the health care system.

Likewise, your management of high-cost, potentially high-risk medications, such as interferon and ribavirin for hepatitis C, assures more directed appropriate monitoring of a specific medication or patient population. Federal grants are available for the development of unique practices that improve care and decrease overall patient care cost. A delivery of pharmacy services to the underserved patients at a public health department in a metropolitan area and the evolution of the pharmacy operation from a traditional dispensing function to fully integrated clinical care is described by Castro and Kummerle.[50]

Medical Residency Programs

Medical residency programs could be considered a subgroup of the physician office practice. However, as noted by Dickerson in Family Medicine Residency programs, you may encounter significant differences between the two settings.[51,52] In medical residency programs, you will find yourself having a teaching role as much as a treating role. Although two practice models are seen in medical residency programs, direct patient care versus education and consultation, it is likely you could develop a practice containing aspects of both. In this role, you need to always maintain balance between your direct patient care and the education of the resident physicians. Your direct patient care clinics can be focused on one disease state or general pharmacotherapy. Moreover, you may find yourself assisting in the care of the practice's hospitalized patients. Depending on the site, you may or may not adjust medications yourself.

You may serve as a specialty consult to assist in the management of a patient by making detailed recommendations back to the resident physician. You may also find yourself collaborating with resident physicians as patients are seen in their clinic, educating them in pharmacotherapy principles while assisting in the management of the patients. Finally, you may find yourself in a precepting faculty role. You may review the resident physicians' charts to ensure evidence-based pharmacotherapy and accuracy. You may precept resident physicians as they are seeing patients in clinic alongside the medical faculty or on pharmacotherapy rotations.[53] In this role, you not only affect the patients at your site, but through educating future physicians, impact their future patients as well.

Pharmacy Department-based Practice Model

Pharmacy Based

In the community, independent, or freestanding pharmacies, you may use point-of-service interventions to improve medication use or disease management of the patient patrons of your pharmacy. As previously hinted, incorporating clinical pharmacy practice into the dispensing operation of your pharmacy can improve effective care of patients and job satisfaction of pharmacists at the same time.[54] The most common intervention provided in this setting involves patient counseling regarding medications, especially for new prescriptions, identifying and resolving drug-related problems, and managing chronic disease for conditions that are prevalent in your patient population. The MTM program is a growing part of the pharmacy-based practice environment. You will see examples of different pharmacy-based practices here.

- Pharmaceutical care program based in community pharmacies that targeted older patients and provided education on medical conditions, implemented adherence strategies, and monitored appropriateness of drug regimen found improved adherence and evidence of cost savings.[55]

- A university-based, pharmacist-delivered diabetes management service is provided in a freestanding pharmacist clinic.[56] Three clinical pharmacists provided diabetes service with comprehensive disease state and MTM and enhanced health outcomes for the self-insured employer group members.[56]

- Twelve independent community pharmacies in Iowa participated in the 12-month demonstration project where the pharmacists used patient-reported measures of health status to identify and resolve drug-related problems in patients with musculoskeletal disorders, including osteoarthritis, rheumatoid arthritis, or low back pain.[57]

- Through collaboration between physicians and community pharmacists, a community pharmacy-based comprehensive MTM program showed improved pharmacotherapy of ambulatory patients taking multiple medications for chronic diseases.[58]

- Twenty-three community pharmacies enrolled 100 patients taking antidepressants and found that pharmacist monitoring was predictive of patient satisfaction and medication adherence in patients taking an antidepressant for the first time.[59]

- A unique practice of retail pharmacy-based ambulatory palliative care provided by consultant pharmacists with prescribing authority led to the primary care oncologists' satisfaction with pharmacists' activities, including additional time spent with patients without physician present, pain and symptom management, and psychosocial support.[60]

Medical Center Based

We see ambulatory pharmacy services affiliated with acute care hospitals or medical centers growing in numbers and scope.[61] This ambulatory pharmacy practice model is usually based in private medical centers, university-affiliated medical centers, managed care organizations, and government-run medical centers, such as those affiliated with the Veteran's Administration (VA), the Department of Defense (DoD), and public health departments. You will receive patient referrals from other health care providers, including primary care providers; however, there should also be mechanisms in place for the patients to self-refer. The flow of patient referral process and management is illustrated in **Figure 1-5**. Following are examples of medical center-based pharmacy practice that may serve as evidence for a practice you are planning to implement.

- Pharmacist clinicians having prescriptive authority and refill authorization, in a for-profit, integrated health system, provided effective pain management service for patients with chronic non-cancer–related pain.[25] A pharmacist clinician with an individual Drug Enforcement Administration number (their services were billable under New Mexico law) assumed the medication management responsibilities of the clinic.[25]

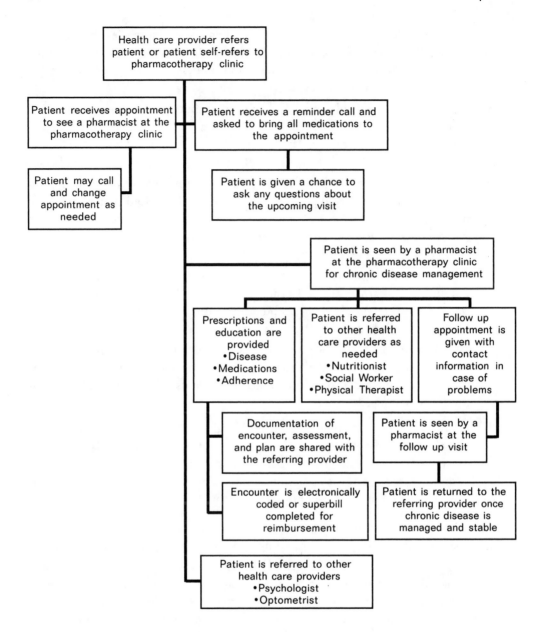

Figure 1-5. Flow of Patient Referral Process and Patient Management

- Clinical outcomes and cost avoidance were evaluated at a VA medical center's clinical pharmacy program where pharmacists' recommendations prevented patient harm in 90% of cases and resulted in mean total cost avoidance for 600 recommendations of $420,155.[62]

- Emergency department-based outpatient treatment program for venous thromboembolism disease managed by a pharmacist showed safe and effective practice that achieved a high level of patient satisfaction.[63]

- An intensive outpatient pharmacist consultation targeting the Kaiser Permanente (KP) enrollees achieved lower total mortality per new prescription filled and significantly lowered hospitalization and mortality in high-risk patient groups.[64]

- Expansion of a clinical pharmacy anticoagulation service that grew from a local monitoring service for patients of a single physician to a regional service monitoring over 3,000 patients in a group model health maintenance organization illustrates the service structure and operations in this environment.[65]

Patient-centered Medical Home

The concept of the medical home was developed over 40 years ago and aims to provide accessible, continuous, coordinated, and comprehensive patient-centered care.[66,67] The patient-centered medical home (PCMH) model provides a framework for organizing care at the practice and societal level,[66] in which all patients would have a "home" where they can receive much of their medical care and additional coordinated care as required.[67]

It is a vision of what health care should be: a setting that facilitates partnerships between individual patients and their personal health care providers and, when appropriate, the patient's family and caregivers. In 2008, the American Academy of Family Physicians stated, "A patient-centered medical home integrates patients as active participants in their own health and well-being. Patients are cared for by a physician who leads the medical team that coordinates all aspects of preventive, acute, and chronic needs of patients using the best available evidence and appropriate technology."[68] The PCMH is really meant to provide relationships that offer patients "comfort, convenience, and optimal health" within their own community, despite their disease states and throughout their lives.

You should be able to find the following features in a PCMH[66]:

1. Integrated and comprehensive primary team care

2. Clinical information systems to support decision making and patient registry

3. Ready access to care

4. Patient engagement in care and decision making

5. Patient-centered care with an emphasis on dignity and respect

6. Routing patient feedback to providers

7. Publicly available information on quality and efficiency

Some consider this model to be a pathway to excellent health care, to reclaim health professionals' role as advocates for patients and their families, and to encourage team-based care.[69] It can also channel educational opportunities and may attract health professionals to primary care. Additionally, some payers offer supplemental payments to providers that are deemed to operate a medical home practice in recognition of the coordinating role they play.[67] It is common that PCMHs have set criteria that need to be met by their enrollees. For example, you may see them seeking patients who have three or more diagnoses requiring treatment, four or more prescription medications, severe illness or chronic illness, illness requiring a visit every two months or less, or lack of insight into health care because of age or intelligence.[70] Because the PCMH is focused on quality of care and safety, and thus supports accountability, performance measures, and other similar measures, this concept is gaining support among policy makers, while the evidence bearing its practice and research continue to emerge.[67,71] Care is facilitated by registries, information technology, health information exchange, and other means to ensure that patients get the indicated care when and where they need and want it in a culturally sensitive and health literacy-sensitive manner.

> **Key Point**
> Because the PCMH is focused on quality of care and safety, and thus supports accountability, performance measures, and other similar measures, this concept is gaining support among policy makers, while the evidence bearing its practice and research continue to emerge.

As a pharmacist in this environment, you can fill the gap of too few primary care providers by playing various important roles in the PCMH, including coordinating care to enhance continuity of care after hospital discharge, managing chronic diseases, offering MTM services, and improving medication adherence.[66] In their article, "Why Pharmacists Belong in the Medical Home," Smith et al. make a good case for the benefits of a pharmacist role within this model.[72] An example would be of an ambulatory care pharmacist caring for patients with 10 or more medications within a medical home operation that uses electronic medical records to ease communication and coordination efforts.[70] This provides essential information for the pharmacist to make therapy recommendations to the physician and implement interventions for the patients.

Home-based Primary Care

In 2009, the Independence at Home Act was introduced to amend the Social Security Act to ensure high-cost Medicare beneficiaries who suffer from multiple chronic conditions get access to coordinated team care in lower cost treatment settings, such as their home. This would in turn reduce emergency room visits, hospitalizations, and admissions to long-term care facilities. Numerous health organizations, including the American Society of Consultant Pharmacists, have endorsed this act. The VA's Home-Based Primary Care (VA HBPC) program, in operation for 32 years, is given as one of the models of the Independence at Home program. The VA HBPC serves homebound patients with complex, chronic, and disabling diseases who have limited access to traditionally delivered medical care.[68] It is a comprehensive, longitudinal primary care delivered in the patient's home by an interdisciplinary team promoting independence. In general, you will find the patient population of the VA HBPC older (mean age of 76.5 years), with most having more than eight chronic conditions.[73] The mean duration of patients in VA HBPC is 315 days, with an average of 3.1 home visits per month.[73] In this model, the patient is at the center, and the interdisciplinary teams that work around them consist of, but are not limited to, physicians (often geriatricians), nurses, pharmacists, occupational or physical therapists, psychologists, and social workers. The team meets regularly and works together to develop a unified care plan for each patient with services provided during home visits.

As in PCMH model, the HBPC programs track several performance measures to ensure that patients and caregivers are receiving appropriate care, including cognitive impairment screening, diabetic monitoring, fall prevention interventions, vaccinations, care after heart attacks, medication regimen review, medication adherence, caregiver strain screening, and caregiver support as needed.[68] All documentation in this longitudinal care is done using electronic medical records in which you may enter your own pharmacy notes and participate in drafting the interdisciplinary notes. You will likely hear somewhat conflicting reports on this care model, though. The data from the interdisciplinary Geriatric Resources for Assessment and Care of Elders (GRACE) project documented improvements in care and cost savings from HBPC for frail, low-income elderly.[74] However, Berenson reported that 13 of 15 Medicare demonstration project sites showed improvement in quality of care but no cost savings.[75] A systematic review and meta-analysis of randomized controlled trials on multidimensional prevention home visit programs for community-dwelling older adults published in 2008 found a potential to reduce disability burden, but effects on nursing home admissions were heterogeneous.[76] Unfortunately, none of the 21 studies meeting the inclusion criteria of this systematic review had pharmacists as intervention personnel.[76,77] Thus this is a new practice area for pharmacists, with great potential.

Patient Care Practice Models

Primary Patient Care Services

In an attempt to fulfill the realization that pharmacy must redefine itself as a patient-centered profession, there has been an expansion of pharmacists' activities from medication-dispensing services to patient care services impacting clinical, safety, humanistic, and economic outcomes of patients.[78] Although you may not always be able to clearly distinguish them, patient care services can be broadly divided into two categories: direct care and collaborative care. Table 1-9 (page 37) lists examples of clinics or programs that have pharmacist involvement in either direct patient care or collaborative care.

Direct Patient Care

Even though a formal collaborative agreement signed by a physician champion may be required, you may provide care directly to patients as a primary care or specialty care provider. As primary care provider, you deliver "first-contact" care, positioned at the point of entry to the health care system and providing highly personalized and comprehensive care to patients.[79] Often, you will practice under the umbrella of an internal medicine or family medicine clinic. As a primary care provider, you take on an independent and continuing responsibility for your patients' chronic medical and mental problems, medication regimens, disease prevention, and health promotion and education.[79] You would also formulate a plan of care for each patient and determine process for referral or triage to secondary or tertiary level providers.[79] Direct primary care is common in the Indian Health Service, where pharmacists have been serving as certified pharmacist practitioners since 1972.[80] Pharmacist-managed primary care and involvement in general medicine clinic are also fostered in the VA and DoD medical centers where pharmacists have prescribing privileges.[81]

In contrast to primary care, specialty care pharmacists in ambulatory care clinics (e.g., cardiology, nephrology, psychiatry, neurology, etc.) provide direct patient care by managing various diseases in settings such as hypertension, diabetes, dyslipidemia, anticoagulation, and pharmacotherapy clinics.[79] As with primary care, specialty care pharmacy practice is also common in the VA and DoD medical centers, where extensive pharmacist involvement in direct patient care extends to research.[29,82-91] Numerous example practices are available for you to draw from, including a specialized pharmacotherapy clinic staffed by pharmacists, pharmacy technicians, laboratory personnel, and other appropriate staff, to which patients are referred by other health care professionals for complex drug therapy monitoring, such as pharmacokinetic consultations for drug infusion and nutrition support.[92]

Team-based Patient Care

An interdisciplinary team approach is the key to patient care where you work as a member of a patient care team.[79] In 1999, the Institute of Medicine report To Err Is Human: Building a Safer Health System recognized the need for pharmacists to be an integral part of the health care team: "because of the immense variety and complexity of medications now available, it is impossible for nurses or doctors to keep up with all of the information required for safe medication use. The pharmacist has become an essential resource . . . and thus, access to his or her expertise must be possible at all times."[93] You can make this possible in a team-based patient care setting, and the opportunities to fill the gap in quality health care is fueled by our aging population with complex comorbidities and the prevalent use of polypharmacy. Even though in this setting your independent, direct patient care activities may not be as extensive as in primary care or specialty care settings, there is professional autonomy in conjunction with mutual cooperation with the other team members.[14,79] You are not only a logical participant in such a collaborative patient care team, but you are also uniquely qualified to serve as a leader to develop and implement functional process.

Key Point As you can imagine, effective communication and interpersonal skills become critical in ambulatory care settings with team-based patient care.[94]

We now see team-based patient care being provided in diverse settings, from a private physician practice to a large multichain managed care or health system. Ambulatory care pharmacy services are also provided in collaboration with a nurse practitioner in a medically underserved rural health center setting and a practice targeting high-risk cardiovascular patients.[95,96] The degree of collaboration varies widely as well. In a clinical partners program, pharmacists, patients, and physicians partner to optimize pharmacotherapy of specific conditions, including anticoagulation, lipid management, asthma, diabetes, hypertension, hepatitis C, smoking cessation, and weight management.[12] An interdisciplinary diabetes health management program includes physicians, clinical pharmacists, registered nurses, and registered dieticians as members to provide collaborative care.[97] The clinical pharmacist provides education and comprehensive medication management through collaborative practice agreements, including prescribing functions and authority to order pertinent laboratory tests and podiatry referrals.[97]

In shared medical appointments, multiple patients having the same condition meet as a group for shared care by a multidisciplinary team. This group of patients generally comes together for a weekly shared appointment for several weeks and benefits from both the comprehensive care provided by the health care team and the peer support. This practice is flourishing in the DoD and VA treatment facilities. The conditions suggested for this practice include diabetes, smoking cessation, heart failure, hypertension, anticoagulation, mental health, depression, pain, fall prevention, erectile dysfunction, hepatitis C, end-stage renal disease, and new patient management.[83]

Prospective Patient Care Management

You may seek to provide services that revolve around a single health condition (disease state focus) or around numerous conditions patients have (patient focus), with each focus having advantages and disadvantages.

Disease State Focus

In clinics or programs that have a disease state focus, you typically concentrate on one health condition, such as diabetes, or a group of conditions involving one high-risk medication, such as warfarin therapy for anticoagulation.[98]

Strength: Having a disease state focus service can be beneficial, especially at the beginning stages of the clinic or program development, because you can focus your efforts on creating one protocol for approval, one set of outcomes to measure, more focused educational materials for use, and more concise credentialing forms to process if appropriate.[98] This is helpful when you are tasked to build the entire pharmacy clinic structure and it is a new concept to be proven at your institution. You may be able to achieve significant outcomes in a short time by focusing on one specific disease state, a group of related conditions, or one high-risk medication or drug class.[98]

Weakness: In this environment, you will not have the benefit of providing comprehensive care and therefore may need to deny certain care and refer patients to multiple different clinics or providers as a result.

Opportunities: You may create a pharmacist-run clinic that is disease specific but have broader scope and protocols to screen and manage conditions closely related to the main disease state. For example, a diabetes drug therapy management and education service provided by a clinical pharmacist targeted not only hemo-

globin A1c levels for its clinical outcome but also blood pressure, low-density lipoprotein cholesterol, high-density lipoprotein cholesterol, and triglycerides as well.[49]
Additionally, focusing on patient adherence to the American Diabetes Association
guidelines for preventative care, clinic measures also included annual eye and foot
examinations, influenza shots, and daily aspirin use.[49]

Threats: If you focus on one specific disease state where management is shared
with other health professionals, a lower-paid provider may be preferred by institutions with financial constraints. For instance, if you, a nurse, and a nutritionist (all
certified diabetes educators) apply for a position at a diabetes clinic, your salary rate
and limited feed for service billing may work against your obtaining that position.
Numerous examples of disease state focus pharmacy practices exist in the literature
(see **Table 1**-9).

Patient Focus

Ambulatory programs that have a patient focus (most often referred to as pharmacotherapy clinics) aim to provide comprehensive care for multiple conditions that
patients possess. These clinics allow you to care for patients with diverse conditions
within the same clinic structure.[98] Often, patients are referred to you due to high-
risk medication use including (1) taking at least five chronic medications, (2) taking
a complex regimen (three or more medication dosing times per day or 12 or more
doses taken per day), (3) taking high-risk medications requiring frequent monitoring, (4) having three or more concurrent chronic conditions, (5) having frequent
medication changes (four regimen changes in 1-year span), and (6) being
nonadherent to pharmacotherapy.[98]

Other patient-specific programs may concentrate on multiple conditions involving one organ system, such as psychiatric or mental health clinic, cardiovascular
clinic, and neurology clinic.[98] Additionally, you may focus on comprehensive management of a group of patients who have multiple health conditions, namely, geriatric practice and women's health practice.[55,99-102]

Strength: You can evaluate therapy and provide changes or education for multiple patient-specific diseases, such as diabetes, hypertension, dyslipidemia, anticoagulation, and polypharmacy, all during a single clinic encounter. The comprehensive medication regimen review assessing effectiveness, safety, adherence, impact
on quality of life, and cost-effectiveness becomes your focus in this environment.

Weakness: The obvious disadvantages associated with patient focus service include having to develop numerous disease management protocols, assessment tools,
and educational materials.[98] Depending on your institution's functional capacity,
credentialing procedures for multiple tasks such as prescribing and ordering laboratory tests may become cumbersome. Also, if point-of-care devices or testing machines are required for the practice, separate machines may need to be purchased or
leased, which can increase your start-up budget for the clinic.[98]

Opportunities: With this degree of comprehensive care, you can function as
physician extender or midlevel practitioner and fill the gap in the current climate of
population aging and health care reform by expanding primary care services to the
underserved patients.

Threats: With opportunity comes increased responsibility and credentialing requirements. Board certification in an ambulatory pharmacotherapy specialty is now available and will be used to help justify competence of your practice; however, liability may increase with the expanded patient care practice. Table 1-9 contains several examples of this patient care model.

Table 1-9. Examples of Pharmacist-Managed Ambulatory Care Clinics and Program[46]

Clinic or Program	Focus of Service	Clinic or Program	Focus of Service
Anticoagulation clinic Venous thromboembolic[46,62,103,104] disease treatment program[63]	Disease	Pain management clinic[25] Palliative or hospice care[60,139]	Disease
Primary care or family practice clinic[77,84,105-107]	Population based	Psychiatric or mental health clinic[59,140]	Disease
Medication therapy management[58] Pharmacotherapy clinic[29,108-111]	Medication	Nephrology, end-stage renal disease[141,142] Transplantation clinic[143,144]	Disease
Cardiovascular clinic[96,112]	Disease	Neurology clinic[145]	Disease
Hypertension clinic[82,113-115]	Disease	Liver or hepatitis C clinic[146]	Disease
Heart failure clinic[116-118]	Disease	Smoking cessation program[147,148]	Disease
Diabetes clinic[48,49,97,119-123]	Disease	Weight management program[149,150]	Disease
Dyslipidemia clinic[85,107,124-127]	Disease	Fall prevention program[151,152]	Population based
Hematology/oncology clinic[128-130]	Disease	Indigent care program[50,140,153,154]	Population based
HIV or AIDS clinic[32,131]	Disease	Immunization program[155,156]	Health and wellness
Geriatric clinic[55,86,99,100]	Population based	Emergency preparedness program[46,157,158]	Population based
Women's health clinic[101,102]	Population based	Investigational drug studies program[159,160]	Medications
Pulmonary (asthma or chronic obstructive pulmonary disease) clinic[132-135]	Disease	Substance abuse program[161]	Medication
Thyroid clinic[136]	Disease	Discharge clinic[162]	Continuity of care
Helicobacter pylori clinic[137]	Disease	Wellness and self-care[12]	Health and wellness
Alzheimer's disease collaboration[138]	Disease	Pediatric[163,164]	

Chapter Summary

You should consider the standard of ambulatory care practice as you develop or reevaluate your practice. In particular, assess your leadership, patient care, and medication control resources. You will find these criteria vary in different settings or organizations and need to be addressed accordingly. As you develop your practice, consider all settings. Investigate the opportunity for office-based practices (community health centers, physician offices), as well as department-based practices (pharmacy-based practices, medical center-based practices, outpatient medical home). You will find these settings differ in the potential they offer a new ambulatory care pharmacy practice. Once you have narrowed your focus of potential sites, you can investigate the services you wish to provide. These may be collaborative or direct patient care focused on the whole patient or a single disease. No matter what you decide, you can build successful service by matching the needs of the site with your capacity to provide the service and the capacity of the site to support that service.

References

1. Maddux MS, Dong BJ, Miller W. A vision of pharmacy's future roles, responsibilities, and manpower needs in the United States. *Pharmacotherapy*. 2000;20:991-1022.

2. American Association of Colleges of Pharmacy. An action plan for the implementation of the JCPP future vision of pharmacy practice. Available at: www.ascp.com/advocacy/coalitions/upload/JCPP-FinalReport.pdf. Accessed October 22, 2009.

3. Carter BL. Ambulatory care. In: Brown TR, ed. *Handbook of Institutional Pharmacy Practice*. 3rd ed. Bethesda, MD: American Society of Hospital Pharmacists; 1992:367-373.

4. ASHP guideline: Minimum standard for pharmaceutical services in ambulatory care. American Society of Health-System Pharmacists. *Am J Health-Syst Pharm*. 1999;56(17):1744-1753.

5. Council on Credentialing in Pharmacy. Scope of contemporary pharmacy practice: roles, responsibilities, and functions of pharmacists and pharmacy technicians. Washington, DC: Council on Credentialing in Pharmacy; 2009.

6. United States Public Health Service. Indian Health Service: Pharmacy Branch. Standards of practice. Available at: http://www.his.gov/publications/ihsmanual/part3/pt3chapt7/ma37a.htm. Accessed November 11, 2009.

7. American Society of Health-System Pharmacists. Educational outcomes, goals, and objectives for postgraduate year 2 (pgy2) ambulatory care pharmacy residency programs. Available at: www.ASHP.org. Accessed January 24, 2010.

8. Harris IM, Baker E, Berry TM, et al. Developing a business-practice model for pharmacy services in ambulatory settings. *Pharmacotherapy*. 2008;28:7e-34e.

9. Ellen K, Dusing-Wiest M, Feedlund J, et al. Stepwise approach to implementing ambulatory clinical pharmacy services. Available at: http://www.medscape.com/viewarticle/557517_print. Accessed November 12, 2009.

10. Covey S. *The Seven Habits of Highly Effective People*. 15th ed. New York, NY: Free Press; 2004.

11. Studor Q. *Hardwiring Excellence: Purpose, Worthwhile Work, Making a Difference*. 1st ed. Gulf Breeze, FA: Fire Starter Publishing; 2003 .

12. Schneider PJ, Bennett MS, Casper KA. Re-engineering an ambulatory care pharmacy practice. *Am J Health-Syst Pharm*. 2000;57(22):2091-2093.

13. Lee F. *If Disney Ran Your Hospital: 9 and ½ Things You Would Do Differently*. Bozeman, MT: Second River Healthcare Press; 2004.

14. Hepler CD, Strand LM. Opportunities and responsibilities in pharmaceutical care. *Am J Hosp Pharm.* 1990;47:533-543.

15. Kernodle SJ. Improving health care with clinical practice guidelines and critical pathways: Implications for pharmacists in ambulatory practice. *Pharm Pract Manag Q.* 1997;17(3):76-89.

16. LaCalamita S. Role of the pharmacist in developing critical pathways with warfarin therapy. *J Pharm Pract.* 1997;10(Dec):398-410.

17. MacKenzie G. *Orbiting the Giant Hairball: A Corporate Fool's Guide to Surviving with Grace.* 1st ed. New York, NY: Viking Adult; 1998.

18. Kotter J, Rathgeber H, Mueller P. *Our Iceberg is Melting.* 1st ed. New York, NY: St. Martin's Press; 2006.

19. White SJ, Tryon JE. Pharmacy leadership. In: Richardson M, Chant C, Cheng JWM, et al eds. *Pharmacotherapy Self-Assessment Program.* 6th ed. Health Promotion and Maintenance. Lenexa, KS: American College of Clinical Pharmacy; 2008:105-116.

20. White S. Leading from a staff or clinical position. *Am J Health-Syst Pharm.* 2009;66:2092-2093.

21. Nimmo CM, Holland RW. Transitions in pharmacy practice, part 5: walking the tightrope of change. *Am J Health-Syst Pharm.* 2000;57:64-72.

22. Burke JM, Miller WA, Spencer AP, et al. Clincal pharmacist competencies. *Pharmacotherapy.* 2008;28:806-815.

23. Jordan CJ, Wall GC, Lobo B, et al. Postgraduate year one pharmacy residency program equivalency. *Pharmacotherapy.* 2009;29:399e-406e.

24. Whitman N, Schwenk TL. *Residents as Teachers: A Guide to Educational Practice.* 3rd ed. Pacific Grove, CA: Whitman Associates; 2005.

25. Dole EJ, Murawski MM, Adolphe AB, et al. Provision of pain management by a pharmacist with prescribing authority. *Am J Health-Syst Pharm.* 2007;64(1):85-89.

26. The ACCP Clinical Practice Affairs Committee. Practice Guidelines for Pharmacotherapy Specialists: A positions statement of the American College of Clinical Pharmacy. *Pharmacotherapy.* 2000;20:487-490.

27. Shaughnessy AF. STEPS drugs updates. *Am Fam Phys.* Available at: http://www.aafp.org/afp/2003/1215/p2342.html. Accessed February 25, 2010.

28. Garwood CL, Dumo P, Baringhaus SN, et al. Quality of anticoagulation care in patients discharged from a pharmacist-managed anticoagulation clinic after stabilization of warfarin therapy. *Pharmacotherapy.* 2008;28(1):20-26.

29. Lee JK, Grace KA, Taylor AJ. Effect of a pharmacy care program on medication adherence and persistence, blood pressure, and low-density lipoprotein cholesterol: A randomized controlled trial. *JAMA.* 2006;296(21):2563-2571.

30. Rodis JL, Green CG, Cook SC, et al. Effects of a pharmacist-initiated educational intervention on patient knowledge about the appropriate use of antibiotics. *Am J Health-Syst Pharm.* 2004;61(13):1385-1389.

31. Oates DJ, Paasche-Orlow MK. Health literacy: Communication strategies to improve patient comprehension of cardiovascular health. *Circulation.* 2009;119(7):1049-1051.

32. March K, Mak M, Louie SG. Effects of pharmacists' interventions on patient outcomes in an HIV primary care clinic. *Am J Health-Syst Pharm.* 2007;64(24):2574-2578.

33. Miller MJ, Abrams MA, McClintock B, et al. Promoting health communication between the community-dwelling well-elderly and pharmacists: The ask me 3 program. *J Am Pharm Assoc (2003).* 2008;48(6):784-792.

34. George J, Elliott RA, Stewart DC. A systematic review of interventions to improve medication taking in elderly patients prescribed multiple medications. *Drugs Aging.* 2008;25(4):307-324.

35. Chobanian AV, Bakris GL, Black HR, et al. The Seventh Report of the Joint National Committee on Prevention, Detection, Evaluation, and Treatment of High Blood Pressure: the JNC 7 report. *JAMA.* 2003; May 21:289(19):2560-2572. Epub May 14, 2003.

36. Vachon DO [Conversation]. South Bend, IN: Saint Joseph Family Medicine Residency Program; October 2009.

37. University of California San Francisco, School of Pharmacy. Heart matters in pharmacy practice: An exploration into the deeper human issues in patient care. Available at: http://www.aacp.org/resources/education/Documents/HEART%20MATTERS%20SYL%2012-11-09%20Final.pdf. Accessed 07/28/2010.

38. Sanborn M. *The Fred Factor*. Colorado Springs, CO: WaterBrook Press; 2004.

39. Slawson DC, Shaughnessy AF, Bennett AH. Becoming a medical information master: feeling good about not knowing everything. *J Fam Pract*. 1994;38:505-513.

40. Analytical Methods Committee, AMC Technical Brief, 2003, No. 13, 'Terminology – the key to understanding analytical science. Part 1: Accuracy, precision and uncertainty'. Available on RSC website: http://www.rsc.org/. Accessed July 22, 2010.

41. US Pharmacopeia. Capslink. October 2005. http://www.usp.org/hqi/practitionerPrograms/newsletters/capsLink/. Accessed October 29, 2009.

42. Harris IM, Baker E, Berry TM, et al. Developing a business-practice model for pharmacy services in ambulatory settings. *Pharmacotherapy*. 2008;28:7e-34e.

43. Chamberlain M. The vertically integrated pharmacy department. *Am J Health-Syst Pharm*. 1998;55:666-675.

44. Hamond RW, Schwartz AH, Campbell MJ. Collaborative drug therapy management by pharmacists-2003. *Pharmacotherapy*. 2003;23:1210-1225.

45. American Society of Health-System Pharmacists. Status of collaborative drug therapy management in the United States, March 2004. *Am J Health-Syst Pharm*. 2004;61:1609-1610.

46. Knapp KK, Okamoto MP, Black BL. ASHP survey of ambulatory care pharmacy practice in health systems—2004. *Am J Health Syst Pharm*. 2005;62(3):274-284.

47. Knapp KK, Blalock SJ, O'Malley CH. ASHP survey of ambulatory care responsibilities of pharmacists in managed care and integrated health systems—1999. *Am J Health-Syst Pharm*. 1999;56(23):2431-2443.

48. Nkansah NT, Brewer JM, Connors R, et al. Clinical outcomes of patients with diabetes mellitus receiving medication management by pharmacists in an urban private physician practice. *Am J Health-Syst Pharm*. 2008;65(2):145-149.

49. McCord AD. Clinical impact of a pharmacist-managed diabetes mellitus drug therapy management service. *Pharmacotherapy*. 2006;26(2):248-253.

50. Castro CG, Kummerle DR. Evolution of ambulatory pharmacy services at a public health department. *Pharm Pract Manag Q*. 1996;15(4):44-52.

51. Dickerson LM, Denham AM, Lynch T. The state of clinical pharmacy practice in family medicine residency programs. *Fam Med*. 2002;34:653-657.

52. Ables AZ, Baughman OL. The clinical pharmacist as a preceptor in a family practice residency training program. *Fam Med*. 2002;34:658-662.

53. Bazaldua O, Ables AZ, Dickerson LM, et al. Suggested guidelines for pharmacotherapy curricula in family medicine residency training: recommendations from the society of teachers of family medicine group on pharmacotherapy. *Fam Med*. 2005;37:99-104.

54. Stuurman-Bieze AG, de Boer WO, Kokenberg ME, et al. Complex pharmaceutical care intervention in pulmonary care: Part A. The process and pharmacists' professional satisfaction. *Pharm World Sci*. 2005;27(5):376-384.

55. Sturgess IK, McElnay JC, Hughes CM, et al. Community pharmacy based provision of pharmaceutical care to older patients. *Pharm World Sci*. 2003;25(5):218-226.

56. Johnson CL, Nicholas A, Divine H, et al. Outcomes from DiabetesCARE: A pharmacist-provided diabetes management service. *J Am Pharm Assoc (2003)*. 2008;48(6):722-730.

57. Ernst ME, Doucette WR, Dedhiya SD, et al. Use of point-of-service health status assessments by community pharmacists to identify and resolve drug-related problems in patients with musculoskeletal disorders. *Pharmacotherapy.* 2001;21(8):988-997.

58. Doucette WR, McDonough RP, Klepser D, et al. Comprehensive medication therapy management: Identifying and resolving drug-related issues in a community pharmacy. *Clin Ther.* 2005;27(7):1104-1111.

59. Bultman DC, Svarstad BL. Effects of pharmacist monitoring on patient satisfaction with antidepressant medication therapy. *J Am Pharm Assoc (Wash).* 2002;42(1):36-43.

60. Atayee RS, Best BM, Daniels CE. Development of an ambulatory palliative care pharmacist practice. *J Palliat Med.* 2008;11(8):1077-1082.

61. Raehl CL, Bond CA, Pitterle ME. Ambulatory pharmacy services affiliated with acute care hospitals. *Pharmacotherapy.* 1993;13(6):618-625.

62. Lee AJ, Boro MS, Knapp KK, et al. Clinical and economic outcomes of pharmacist recommendations in a veterans affairs medical center. *Am J Health-Syst Pharm.* 2002;59(21):2070-2077.

63. Zed PJ, Filiatrault L. Clinical outcomes and patient satisfaction of a pharmacist-managed, emergency department-based outpatient treatment program for venous thromboembolic disease. *CJEM.* 2008;10(1):10-17.

64. Yuan Y, Hay JW, McCombs JS. Effects of ambulatory-care pharmacist consultation on mortality and hospitalization. *Am J Manag Care.* 2003;9(1):45-56.

65. Witt DM, Tillman DJ. Clinical pharmacy anticoagulation services in a group model health maintenance organization. *Pharm Pract Manag Q.* 1998;18(3):34-55.

66. Bates DW. Role of pharmacists in the medical home. *Am J Health-Syst Pharm.* 2009;66(12):1116-1118.

67. American Association of Diabetes Educators. AADE practice advisory medical home and its importance for the diabetes educator. Available at: http://www.diabeteseducator.org/export/sites/aade/_resources/pdf/Medical_Home_Practice_Advisory.pdf. Accessed February 10, 2010.

68. National Academies of Practice. Models of accountable, coordinated health care: A policy paper of the national academies of practice. Available at: http://nap.affiniscape.com/associations/9326/files/2009%20Forum%20Paper%20with%20cover.pdf. Accessed February 2, 2010.

69. American Academy of Family Physicians. Joint principles of the patient-centered medical home. *Del Med J.* 2008;80(1):21-22.

70. Thompson CA. Health system views pharmacist as vital to coordinated care. *Am J Health- Syst Pharm.* 2009;66(23):2067-2070.

71. Grumbach K. Redesign of the health care delivery system: A bauhaus "form follows function" approach. *JAMA.* 2009;302(21):2363-2364.

72. Smith M, Bates DW, Bodenheimer T, et al. Why pharmacists belong in the medical home. *Health Affairs.* 2010;29(5):906-913.

73. Beales JL, Edes T. Veteran's affairs home based primary care. *Clin Geriatr Med.* 2009;25(1):149-54, viii-ix.

74. Counsell SR, Callahan CM, Buttar AB, et al. Geriatric resources for assessment and care of elders (GRACE): A new model of primary care for low-income seniors. *J Am Geriatr Soc.* 2006;54(7):1136-1141.

75. Berenson RA, Hammons T, Gans DN, et al. A house is not a home: Keeping patients at the center of practice redesign. *Health Aff (Millwood).* 2008;27(5):1219-1230.

76. Huss A, Stuck AE, Rubenstein LZ, et al. Multidimensional preventive home visit programs for community-dwelling older adults: A systematic review and meta-analysis of randomized controlled trials. *J Gerontol A Biol Sci Med Sci.* 2008;63(3):298-307.

77. Davis RG, Hepfinger CA, Sauer KA, et al. Retrospective evaluation of medication appropriateness and clinical pharmacist drug therapy recommendations for home-based primary care veterans. *Am J Geriatr Pharmacother.* 2007;5(1):40-47.

78. A vision of pharmacy's future roles, responsibilities, and manpower needs in the United States. American College of Clinical Pharmacy. *Pharmacotherapy*. 2000;20(8):991-1020.

79. Establishing and evaluating clinical pharmacy services in primary care. American College of Clinical Pharmacy. *Pharmacotherapy*. 1994;14(6):743-758.

80. Copeland GP, Apgar DA. The pharmacist practitioner training program. *Drug Intell Clin Pharm*. 1980;14(2):114-119.

81. Clause S, Fudin J, Mergner A, et al. Prescribing privileges among pharmacists in Veterans Affairs medical centers. *Am J Health-Syst Pharm*. 2001;58:1143-1145.

82. Vivian EM. Improving blood pressure control in a pharmacist-managed hypertension clinic. *Pharmacotherapy*. 2002;22(12):1533-1540.

83. Cone SM, Brown MC, Stambaugh RL. Characteristics of ambulatory care clinics and pharmacists in veterans affairs medical centers: An update. *Am J Health-Syst Pharm*. 2008;65(7):631-635.

84. Carmichael JM, Alvarez A, Chaput R, et al. Establishment and outcomes of a model primary care pharmacy service system. *Am J Health-Syst Pharm*. 2004;61(5):472-482.

85. Ellis SL, Carter BL, Malone DC, et al. Clinical and economic impact of ambulatory care clinical pharmacists in management of dyslipidemia in older adults: The IMPROVE study. impact of managed pharmaceutical care on resource utilization and outcomes in veterans affairs medical centers. *Pharmacotherapy*. 2000;20(12):1508-1516.

86. Nadrash TA, Plushner SL, Delate T. Clinical pharmacists' role in improving osteoporosis treatment rates among elderly patients with untreated atraumatic fractures. *Ann Pharmacother*. 2008;42(3):334-340.

87. Ogden JE, Muniz A, Patterson AA, et al. Pharmaceutical services in the department of veterans affairs. *Am J Health-Syst Pharm*. 1997;54(7):761-765.

88. Rapoport A, Akbik H. Pharmacist-managed pain clinic at a veterans affairs medical center. *Am J Health-Syst Pharm*. 2004;61(13):1341-1343.

89. Arnold FW, McDonald LC, Newman D, et al. Improving antimicrobial use: Longitudinal assessment of an antimicrobial team including a clinical pharmacist. *J Manag Care Pharm*. 2004;10(2):152-158.

90. Cioffi ST, Caron MF, Kalus JS, et al. Glycosylated hemoglobin, cardiovascular, and renal outcomes in a pharmacist-managed clinic. *Ann Pharmacother*. 2004;38(5):771-775.

91. Schmader KE, Hanlon JT, Pieper CF, et al. Effects of geriatric evaluation and management on adverse drug reactions and suboptimal prescribing in the frail elderly. *Am J Med*. 2004;116(6):394-401.

92. Webb CE. Prescribing medications: Changing the paradigm for a changing health care system. *Am J Health-Syst Pharm*. 1995;52(15):1693-1695.

93. Muller BA, McDanel DL. Enhancing quality and safety through physician-pharmacist collaboration. *Am J Health-Syst Pharm*. 2006;63(11):996-997.

94. Carter BL. Ambulatory care. In: Brown TR, ed. *Handbook of Institutional Pharmacy Practice*. 3rd ed. Bethesda, MD: American Society of Hospital Pharmacists; 1992:367-373.

95. Andrus MR, Clark DB. Provision of pharmacotherapy services in a rural nurse practitioner clinic. *Am J Health-Syst Pharm*. 2007;64(3):294-297.

96. Reilly V, Cavanagh M. The clinical and economic impact of a secondary heart disease prevention clinic jointly implemented by a practice nurse and pharmacist. *Pharm World Sci*. 2003;25(6):294-298.

97. Brooks AD, Rihani RS, Derus CL. Pharmacist membership in a medical group's diabetes health management program. *Am J Health-Syst Pharm*. 2007;64(6):617-621.

98. Snella KA, Sachdev GP. A primer for developing pharmacist-managed clinics in the outpatient setting. *Pharmacotherapy*. 2003;23(9):1153-1166.

99. Hanlon JT, Weinberger M, Samsa GP, et al. A randomized, controlled trial of a clinical pharmacist intervention to improve inappropriate prescribing in elderly outpatients with polypharmacy. *Am J Med*. 1996;100(4):428-437.

100. Blakey SA, Hixson-Wallace JA. Clinical and economic effects of pharmacy services in geriatric ambulatory clinic. *Pharmacotherapy*. 2000;20(10):1198-1203.

101. Burt CW, Bernstein AB. Trends in use of medications associated with women's ambulatory care visits. *J Womens Health (Larchmt)*. 2003;12(3):213-217.

102. Gardner JS, Miller L, Downing DF, et al. Pharmacist prescribing of hormonal contraceptives: Results of the direct access study. *J Am Pharm Assoc (2003)*. 2008;48(2):212-21; 5 p following 221.

103. Chiquette E, Amato MG, Bussey HI. Comparison of an anticoagulation clinic with usual medical care: Anticoagulation control, patient outcomes, and health care costs. *Arch Intern Med*. 1998;158(15):1641-1647.

104. Epplen K, Dusing-Wiest M, Freedlund J, et al. Stepwise approach to implementing ambulatory clinical pharmacy services. *Am J Health-Syst Pharm*. 2007;64(9):945-951.

105. Byrd DC, Weitzel N, Herndon KC. Management of hypertension in a family medicine clinic. *ASHP Midyear Clinical Meeting*. 2003;38(DEC):P-551.

106. Irons BK, Lenz RJ, Anderson SL, et al. A retrospective cohort analysis of the clinical effectiveness of a physician-pharmacist collaborative drug therapy management diabetes clinic. *Pharmacotherapy*. 2002;22(10):1294-1300.

107. Till LT, Voris JC, Horst JB. Assessment of clinical pharmacist management of lipid-lowering therapy in a primary care setting. *J Manag Care Pharm*. 2003;9(3):269-273.

108. Kramer AD, Mitchell J, Epplen K. Urgent care pharmacotherapy clinic: A bridge between the emergency department and the primary care physician? *ASHP Midyear Clinical Meeting*. 2003;38(DEC):P-68(E).

109. Chipolle RJ, Strand LM, Morley PC. Outcomes of pharmaceutical care practice. In: Chipolle RJ, Strand LM, Morley PC, eds. *Pharmaceutical Care Practice*. 1st ed. New York, NY: McGraw-Hill Professional; 1998:205-235.

110. Singhal PK, Raisch DW, Gupchup GV. The impact of pharmaceutical services in community and ambulatory care settings: Evidence and recommendations for future research. *Ann Pharmacother*. 1999;33(12):1336-1355.

111. Strand LM, Cipolle RJ, Morley PC, et al. The impact of pharmaceutical care practice on the practitioner and the patient in the ambulatory practice setting: Twenty-five years of experience. *Curr Pharm Des*. 2004;10(31):3987-4001.

112. Ashworth RA, Kearney SE. Development of a cardiovascular wellness clinic by a clinical pharmacist practitioner in an interventional cardiologists' office. *ASHP Midyear Clinical Meeting*. 2003;38(DEC):HA10.

113. Carter BL, Ardery G, Dawson JD, et al. Physician and pharmacist collaboration to improve blood pressure control. *Arch Intern Med*. 2009;169(21):1996-2002.

114. Carter BL, Rogers M, Daly J, et al. The potency of team-based care interventions for hypertension: A meta-analysis. *Arch Intern Med*. 2009;169(19):1748-1755.

115. McKenney JM, Slining JM, Henderson HR, et al. The effect of clinical pharmacy services on patients with essential hypertension. *Circulation*. 1973;48(5):1104-1111.

116. Koshman SL, Charrois TL, Simpson SH, et al. Pharmacist care of patients with heart failure: A systematic review of randomized trials. *Arch Intern Med*. 2008;168(7):687-694.

117. Murray M, Young J, Hoke S, et al. Pharmacist intervention to improve medication adherence in heart failure - A randomized trial. *Ann Intern Med*. 2007;146(10):714-725.

118. Roughead EE, Barratt JD, Ramsay E, et al. The effectiveness of collaborative medicine reviews in delaying time to next hospitalization for patients with heart failure in the practice setting: Results of a cohort study. *Circ Heart Fail*. 2009;2(5):424-428.

119. Van Veldhuizen-Scott MK, Widmer LB, Stacey SA, et al. Developing and implementing a pharmaceutical care model in an ambulatory care setting for patients with diabetes. *Diabetes Educ*. 1995;21(2):117-123.

120. Nkansah N, Jeffrey B, Robert C, et al. Effects on clinical outcomes of diabetic patients seen by a pharmacist working in collaboration with other primary care practice providers. *ASHP Summer Meeting*. 2004;61(JUN):P-37R.

121. Morello CM, Zadvorny EB, Cording, et al. Development and clinical outcomes of pharmacist-managed diabetes care clinics. *Am J Health-Syst Pharm*. 2006;63(14):1325-1331.

122. Anaya JP, Rivera JO, Lawson K, et al. Evaluation of pharmacist-managed diabetes mellitus under a collaborative drug therapy agreement. *Am J Health-Syst Pharm.* 2008;65(19):1841-1845,1815.

123. Wubben DP, Vivian EM. Effects of pharmacist outpatient interventions on adults with diabetes mellitus: A systematic review. *Pharmacotherapy.* 2008;28(4):421-436.

124. Olson KL, Potts LA. Role of the pharmacist in the management of dyslipidemia. *J Pharm Pract.* 2006;19(2):94-102.

125. Donaldson AR, Andrus MR. Pharmacist-run lipid management program in rural Alabama. *Am J Health-Syst Pharm.* 2004;61(5):493-497.

126. Borgmann JA. Developing lipid management clinics. *ASHP Summer Meeting.* 2003;60(JUN):P1-5.

127. Bluml BM, McKenney JM, Cziraky MJ. Pharmaceutical care services and results in project ImPACT: Hyperlipidemia. *J Am Pharm Assoc (Wash).* 2000;40(2):157-165.

128. Shah S, Dowell J, Greene S. Evaluation of clinical pharmacy services in a hematology/oncology outpatient setting. *Ann Pharmacother.* 2006;40(9):1527-1533.

129. Hockel M. Ambulatory chemotherapy: Pharmaceutical care as a part of oncology service. *J Oncol Pharm Pract.* 2004;10(3):135-140.

130. Weingart SN, Cleary A, Seger A, et al. Medication reconciliation in ambulatory oncology. *Jt Comm J Qual Patient Saf.* 2007;33(12):750-757.

131. Boonchoo P, Eumkep S, Theanchairoj A. Ambulatory pharmaceutical care in AIDS patients. *Thai J Hosp Pharm.* 2005;15(2):117-123.

132. Strom BL, Hennessy S. Pharmacist care and clinical outcomes for patients with reactive airways disease. *JAMA.* 2002;288(13):1642-1643.

133. Zaiken K, McColskey W, Raval K. Implementation of a pharmacist-managed asthma clinic in a managed care organization. *ASHP Midyear Clinical Meeting.* 2004;39(DEC):P75.

134. Rupp MT, McCallian DJ, Sheth KK. Developing and marketing a community pharmacy-based asthma management program. *J Am Pharm Assoc (Wash).* 1997;NS37(6):694-699.

135. Mann R, Zaiken K. Impact of an ambulatory care pharmacist on the management of chronic obstructive pulmonary disease patients in an internal medicine department. *ASHP Midyear Clinical Meeting.* 2007;42(DEC).

136. Dong BJ. Pharmacist involvement in a thyroid clinic. *Am J Hosp Pharm.* 1990;47(2):356-361.

137. Morreale AP. Pharmacist-managed helicobacter pylori clinic. *Am J Health-Syst Pharm.* 1995;52(2):183-185.

138. Skelton JB. White paper on expanding the role of pharmacists in caring for individuals with Alzheimer's disease: APhA foundation coordinating council to improve collaboration in supporting patients with Alzheimer's disease. *J Am Pharm Assoc (2003).* 2008;48(6):715-721.

139. Akai N, Fujita-Hamabe W, Tokuyama S. Attitude survey of medical staff on the participation of community pharmacists in palliative home care. *Yakugaku Zasshi.* 2009;129(11):1393-1401.

140. Caballero J, Souffrant C, Heffernan E. Development and outcomes of a psychiatric pharmacy clinic for indigent patients. *Am J Health-Syst Pharm.* 2008;65(3):229-233.

141. Shaffer JK. Pharmacist's impact on dyslipidemia control in end stage renal disease patients. *ASHP Midyear Clinical Meeting.* 2003;38(DEC):P-61.

142. Allenet B, Chen C, Romanet T, et al. Assessing a pharmacist-run anaemia educational programme for patients with chronic renal insufficiency. *Pharm World Sci.* 2007;29(1):7-11.

143. Chisholm-Burns MA, Spivey CA, Garrett C, et al. Impact of clinical pharmacy services on renal transplant recipients' adherence and outcomes. *Patient Prefer Adherence.* 2008;2:287-292.

144. Wang HY, Chan AL, Chen MT, et al. Effects of pharmaceutical care intervention by clinical pharmacists in renal transplant clinics. *Transplant Proc.* 2008;40(7):2319-2323.

145. Kootsikas ME, Hayes G, Thompson JF, et al. Role of a pharmacist in a seizure clinic. *Am J Hosp Pharm.* 1990;47(11):2478-2482.

146. Smith JP, Dong MH, Kaunitz JD. Evaluation of a pharmacist-managed hepatitis C care clinic. *Am J Health-Syst Pharm.* 2007;64(6):632-636.

147. Marotta SE, Bajwa MK, Atlas SA. Development of a pharmacist driven outpatient smoking cessation clinic. *ASHP Midyear Clinical Meeting*. 2006;41(Dec):27.

148. Bock BC, Hudmon KS, Christian J, et al. A tailored intervention to support pharmacy-based counseling for smoking cessation. *Nicotine Tob Res*. 2010;12(3):217-225.

149. Graham MR, Landgraf CG, Lindsey CC. A comparison of orlistat use in a veteran population: A pharmacist-managed pharmacotherapy weight-loss clinic versus standard medical care. *J Pharm Technol*. 2003;19(6):343-348.

150. Malone M, Alger-Mayer SA. Pharmacist intervention enhances adherence to orlistat therapy. *Ann Pharmacother*. 2003;37(11):1598-1602.

151. Jensen J, Lundin-Olsson L, Nyberg L, et al. Fall and injury prevention in older people living in residential care facilities. A cluster randomized trial. *Ann Intern Med*. 2002;136(10):733-741.

152. Hanley A, Ali MT, Murphy J, et al. Early experience of a fall and fracture prevention clinic at mayo general hospital. *Ir J Med Sci*. 2009.

153. Brahm NC, Palmer T, Williams T, et. al. Bedlam community health clinic: A collaborative interdisciplinary health care service for the medically indigent. *J Am Pharm Assoc*. 2007;47(3):398-N_0073.

154. Miller AE, Hansen LB, Saseen JJ. Switching statin therapy using a pharmacist-managed therapeutic conversion program versus usual care conversion among indigent patients. *Pharmacotherapy*. 2008;28(5):553-561.

155. Modrzejewski KA, Provost GP. Pharmacists' involvement with vaccinations leads to preventive health care role. *Am J Health-Syst Pharm*. 2003;60(17):1724, 1726, 1728.

156. Babb VJ, Babb J. Pharmacist involvement in healthy people 2010. *J Am Pharm Assoc*. 2003;43(1):56-60.

157. Bhavsar TR, Kim HJ, Yu Y. Roles and contributions of pharmacists in regulatory affairs at the centers for disease control and prevention for public health emergency preparedness and response. *J Am Pharm Assoc (2003)*. 2010;50(2):165-168.

158. Woodard LJ, Bray BS, Williams D, et al. Call to action: Integrating student pharmacists, faculty, and pharmacy practitioners into emergency preparedness and response. *J Am Pharm Assoc (2003)*. 2010;50(2):158-164.

159. Ryan ML, Colvin CL, Tankanow RM. Development and funding of a pharmacy-based investigational drug service. *Am J Hosp Pharm*. 1987;44(5):1069-1074.

160. Sweet BV, Tamer HR, Siden R, et al. Improving investigational drug service operations through development of an innovative computer system. *Am J Health-Syst Pharm*. 2008;65(10):969-973.

161. Wiedemer NL, Harden PS, Arndt IO, et al. The opioid renewal clinic: A primary care, managed approach to opioid therapy in chronic pain patients at risk for substance abuse. *Pain Med*. 2007;8(7):573-584.

162. Dvorak SR, McCoy RA, Voss GD. Continuity of care from acute to ambulatory care setting. *Am J Health-Syst Pharm*. 1998;55(23):2500-2504.

163. Edwards R, Adams DW. Clinical pharmacy services in pediatric ambulatory care clinic. *Drug Intell Clin Pharm*. 1982;16:939-944.

164. Kalister H, Newman RD, Read L, et al. Pharmacy-based evaluation and treatment of minor illness in a culturally diverse pediatric clinic. *Arch Pediatr Adolesc Med*. 1999;153:731-735.

Additional Selected Resources

ASHP. ASHP Pharmacy Practice Model Initiative.

http://www.usp.org/hqi/practitionerPrograms/newsletters/capsLink/ Accessed July 14, 2011.

Web Resources

Conventions Useful for Professional Networking

Example Referral Forms

    Pharmacotherapy Consult

    Generic Referral Form

Sample Collaborative Drug Therapy Management Agreements

    Collaborative Drug Therapy Management Agreement (SJRMC)

    DMG MTM Agreement

Sample Mission and Vision Statements

Web Toolkit available at
www.ashp.org/ambulatorypractice

Planning and Steps to Building the Ambulatory Practice Model

Steven M. Riddle, Jeffrey M. Brewer

CHAPTER

2

Chapter Outline

1. Introduction

2. Determining How to Provide the Service

3. Evaluating the Resource Needs and Financial Impact

4. Building Support for Your Service

5. The Service Proposal or Business Plan

6. Chapter Summary

7. References

8. Additional Selected References

9. Web Resources

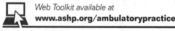
Web Toolkit available at **www.ashp.org/ambulatorypractice**

Chapter Objectives

1. Discuss the four attributes of a successful pharmacy service.

2. Determine the scope of the practice in your area.

3. Identify and determine the resources necessary to support the service.

4. Identify strategies to demonstrate financial value.

5. Propose how you will identify and engage your stakeholders.

6. Describe the key elements of a service proposal.

Introduction

The goal of this chapter is to assist you in assembling the key data that will support the proposal for your new service and lead to the creation of a successful clinical practice. The process will require pulling together a diverse array of information that will help you refine your clinical and business structures.[1] It is incumbent on the pharmacist to build high-quality clinical pharmacy services that are based on sound business principles. To ensure success, we suggest that you incorporate four key attributes into your service development: valuable, scalable, reproducible, and sustainable.

In the language of quality improvement, *value* is simply the product of the quality divided by the cost for a service or product ($V = Q/C$). Therefore, one can provide value by improving quality, decreasing cost, or both.[2] Put another way, you want to provide a needed service while using the least amount of resources. The pharmacist is the health care provider best educated and trained to identify and resolve the myriad of medication-related problems that patients and providers encounter. It is therefore critical that these services are well aligned with the unique skills and knowledge of pharmacists, they are efficiently provided, and that their value is measurable.

Your service should also be scalable. After spending quality time researching the needs of your patients, planning your service, and setting it up for success, demand will likely grow significantly. You will need to design your model to allow for growth. It is important to prepare for expected change and design your practice for expansion.

Similarly, your services should be reproducible. Within your organization, a model for an anticoagulation clinic may be replicated as a diabetes service based on common design and functionality. A practice model that is easily reproducible can also allow for recreation of your "best practice" by another practice site. Solid planning, simplicity of design, and standardized roles and processes allow models to be reproduced or transferred with minimal manipulation and can result in similar outcomes.

Finally, it is most important that your model is sustainable. The survival of your service will be a reflection of your ability to maintain the value as needs shift and resources ebb and flow. The dynamic health care environment requires continuous quality improvement and responsible resource management to maintain your model.

With these four attributes in mind, let's begin the process of developing a clinical service proposal. The key steps addressed here are determining how to provide your service, estimating your resource needs, demonstrating value, and building support. Once you have completed these steps, Chapter 3 will then make use of this information to help you finalize your business plan.

Determining How to Provide the Service

Chapter 1 helped you define the optimal ambulatory model for your service, discussed its standards, and considered the mission and vision of your organization. Once you have evaluated and prioritized your opportunities, your attention should be focused on the service that will provide the most value to your organization and patients. On the other hand, considerations such as resource limitations, political issues, and practical concerns may make the most valuable target less feasible. Therefore, selecting the opportunity that is within your reach and that ensures a positive outcome may be the wisest path. Regardless of your specific service choice, you will need to take the necessary steps to determine how to provide your service, including determining your scope of service, selecting the most appropriate care delivery model, estimating your resource requirements, performing the financial analysis, evaluating your current resource availability, and anticipating your growth.

Key Point

Selecting the opportunity within your reach that ensures a positive outcome may be the wisest path.

To help you apply the concepts, we will be introducing and discussing a case example throughout the book to illustrate how to start and assemble the aspects of your new practice model.

CASE

Dr. Busybee, a local physician, heard information about the value of having a pharmacist assist in managing patients in ambulatory clinics. He has approached you about initiating this type of service at his office-based practice site. In your evaluation of his practice and creation of the needs assessment, you determine some areas where pharmacists could provide definite value. First, Dr. Busybee appears to be at risk for losing his contract with his largest insurer based on poor performance on key disease management indicators: achievement of goal hemoglobin A1C values in diabetes and appropriate management of patients with atrial fibrillation, including international normalized ratio (INR) values in the target range for patients on warfarin anticoagulation. Dr. Busybee's patient load is also very high, which is causing delays in scheduling appointments and in attracting and retaining new patients. You are uncertain about the rules and regulations regarding pharmacist practice, particularly in physician offices, in your state (Maryland). For the necessary information you contact the Maryland Board of Pharmacy and also your state pharmacy organization to see if they can provide some practical information and perhaps connections to similar practice sites. One key item your research provides is information on a house bill in Maryland, HB781, Physicians and Pharmacists: Therapy Management Contracts, which passed in 2002 and was finalized in 2004. This law states that the protocol approved by both parties may authorize the pharmacist to modify, continue, and discontinue drug therapies included in disease state-specific protocols. Additionally, the patient must sign the protocol approving the pharmacist's involvement as part of the team on a yearly basis. This law exempts institutional facilities from the collaborative practice restrictions, which means your new community practice will need to meet the HB781 requirements, and pharmacists will not be permitted to initiate drug therapy.

Performing a Needs Assessment

A first step in planning your clinic is understanding the needs of the recipients for your proposed service. In essence, this means knowing what is desired by your customers, who include the patients, the providers, your organization, and the payers your service will affect. Determining this is called a *needs assessment* or *market analysis* and is the process for collecting the information needed to understand the gaps between the current levels of care and the level of care that is desired. Obtaining this information will allow you to optimally address how your service will fill the identified needs or gaps. This is a critical step in your business and marketing plans, both of which will be discussed in detail in Chapters 3 and 4.

In a needs assessment, there are three basic questions to ask:[3]
1. What are the needs or problems to be addressed?
2. How large is this problem, and what are the trends?
3. How well are the needs currently being addressed?

CASE

The problem with Dr. Busybee's practice is the high patient volume does not allow his patients to receive optimal care or achieve optimal outcomes. It is a significant problem for him, as he is unable to sustain and grow his practice. There is a high need for primary care physicians such as Dr. Busybee in the community. An area in which you can fill Dr. Busybee's needs is that of providing support in diabetes and atrial fibrillation management. By analyzing Dr. Busybee's panel of patients, your initial estimate for your proposed service is that 2 clinic days a week will save him at least 1 hour a day, allowing him to see an additional four patients. In support of your proposal, you have collected several published citations noting improved outcomes in similar populations when pharmacists provide these services.

Determine Your Scope of Practice

As noted in the case, you need to be aware of your particular state's regulations regarding scope of practice. *Scope of practice* is the terminology used by various professions' state licensing boards that defines the procedures, actions, and processes that are permitted for the licensed individual. The scope of practice is limited to that which the law allows for specific levels of education, experience, and demonstrated competency. For the practice of pharmacy, each state has laws, licensing bodies, and regulations that describe requirements for education and training and thus define the scope of practice. The collaborative practice laws and the use of collaborative drug therapy management (CDTM) contracts mentioned in Chapter 1 describe the range of patient care functions you can perform at your practice site or organization.[4] Your organization may also add more specific functions related to medical conditions (e.g., anticoagulation, diabetes) and populations (e.g., pediatrics). In any case, the specific allowances for managing patients' drug therapy and related care are included in these agreements, and they must stay within the scope allowed by the state. It is important that you are aware of your state's practice allowance and ensure that your service is within these legal bounds. Legal matters to consider will be discussed further in the chapters dealing with setting up your clinic, documentation, and billing (Chapters 5, 6, and 8); the related issues of credentialing and privileging will be discussed in Chapter 7.

Identify and Evaluate the Optimal Care Delivery Model

As noted in Chapter 1, the service types vary in complexity, and thus the training and experience necessary for the provider to be effective and efficient also varies. If you have not already done so, you may want to further review the published articles and trials regarding services or settings that are relevant to your initial service ideas.

Key Point

Selection of the delivery model should be based on a careful alignment of the identified care opportunity with your practice setting, your clinical strengths and expertise, and your allowed scope of practice.

Let's focus on selecting your service delivery model. The delivery model is defined by where and how you provide the service. When considering a delivery model, examine the physical setting for the service. Will it be integrated, as when the pharmacist is placed directly into the clinic or physician's office space and shares resources? Would the service location be independent or separate from the current provider service area? Will the new service be based out of the current pharmacy distribution location? Each of these models has strengths and weaknesses when applied to different settings and patient populations, as was noted in Chapter 1.

CASE

In evaluating potential service delivery models, you determine that a physician's office model makes the most sense as it provides easy access to the documentation system without having to purchase or build your own, and the electronic health record (EHR) for the office also provides access to laboratory test results and medication-prescribing software. In addition, you will be located within the office with direct lines of communication to the providers for faster decision time, and working in the physician's office will avoid any renovation costs necessary to prepare a new patient care area. Upon further discussion with the practice administrator at Dr. Busybee's office, you note that the patient care staff is uncomfortable with caring for patients on insulin and warfarin therapies due to the complexity of the treatment. The physician's office practice model will allow the pharmacists to both provide care to these patients and provide education to the staff regarding medication management.

In summary, when evaluating your care delivery model it is important to consider both current and potential needs and how you can provide value (i.e., high quality with the least amount of resources). Creativity is encouraged in matching your service to the needs of your patients, organization, and practice environment.

Evaluating the Resource Needs and Financial Impact

Once you have identified a specific service and delivery model, it is time to examine the resource and financial issues that will be a key component of your service proposal. In this section, we will discuss the essential resources for any business (i.e., people, equipment, supplies) and help you determine which you will need for your service. We will also discuss the costs related to these resource needs. Generating revenue or determining other measures of financial value will be explored as well. If finance is not one of your strengths, then we recommend that you seek a knowledgeable colleague, such as the pharmacy manager, consult your finance department, or engage an independent consultant. Additional resources on business and finance can be found through national professional organizations. We have also provided worksheets to guide you through a basic resource needs and financial assessment.

Estimating Resource Requirements

Determining Patient Volumes and Potential Demand for the Service

The most important consideration in estimating resource needs is determining the number of potential patients that may use your service. Your needs assessment should provide a rough estimate of this number. Depending on your practice setting, this type of information is often not accessible through pharmacy databases or records. A good place to locate this information is in your finance office or from someone responsible for billing at your practice site. Billing and other financial data tied to ambulatory visits will include information on the patient diagnoses (ICD coding), service provided (procedural or visit codes), insurance/payer codes, and basic demographic information. This is valuable information for determining not only patient and visit volumes but also for evaluating other aspects of your service (i.e., payer mix linked to reimbursement). Clinical data systems may also contain valuable information, such as number of persons with specific conditions or relevant laboratory data. Other persons able to assist you in finding the information related to identifying potential patients may be an administrator, clinic manager, or physician/medical director. In fact, you will likely need to collect data from various data sets and anecdotal information from physicians and other stakeholders to gain a good perspective on which patients you could help. Initiate discussions with these persons; explain your needs, and you should be able to gather the required data to create an estimate of potential patients for your service.

You will need to determine what portion of your potential patients you can capture. Consider whether your service will be a mandatory referral system (i.e., automatic transfer of care for anticoagulation services for all identified patients) or referral based on physician or patient discretion (i.e., diabetics determined to be in poor control). You are encouraged to proactively engage providers, patients, and others who are in positions that may influence the use of your service for information that will guide your workload estimates. (See the section on identifying and engagement of stakeholders later in the chapter.)

In addition, you should evaluate other factors that may impact your patient volume estimate, such as changes in the local health care market or organizational emphasis on areas of care and government policy shifts in insurance coverage or changes in your physician practice model. Another important consideration is your visit completion or "show" rate. This number can vary as widely as 40% to 75%, depending on the population served.[5] Inquire at your practice site (or an external site caring for a similar population) to determine your expected visit completion rates. You may need to consider how to manage this nonproductive time for no-shows or consider appointment strategies, such as overbooking and pre-clinic re-minder calls, aimed at maintaining capacity.

Your patient volumes will ultimately determine your total time providing direct patient care. To connect these pieces, you will need to determine the expected duration and frequency of visits. How long is a typical office visit? According to a 2001 publication, the average physician office visit ranged from 16 to 20 minutes in duration.[6] Anecdotal reports from ambulatory pharmacist practices yield similar times, with visit encounters for established patients typically lasting 15–30 minutes and initial visits with new patients taking longer, perhaps 30–60 minutes. Duration will vary with practice setting, patient treatment severity and complexity, and the efficiency of the pharmacist provider. For example, visits for defined services such as an uncomplicated anticoagulation patient may take 15 minutes, whereas patients with more complex care needs (i.e., primary care with multiple chronic conditions) may take up to 45 minutes. You will need to estimate the visit time based on your service type and population served. It is important to point out that when imple-menting a new service, all your patients could potentially be defined as "new," even if they have been cared for in the same facility. You may need to account for these longer visits in your initial visit estimates. Finally, while accuracy for this key re-source driver is preferred, if your estimates are more "guesstimates," consider using a minimum and maximum range for your patient volume estimates. You should classify your appointment types and their related duration for your service to allow for accuracy and good communication in scheduling patients and for billing purposes. We have included a basic example (below).

Example Template: Duration of Pharmacy Visits

Appointment Type	Length of Visit
New referral	30 min
Initial visit	30 min
Regular office visit	20 min
Phone visit	15 min

To create an accurate estimate of your patient volume and the time involved in providing direct care, you will need to determine the number of potential candi-dates for your service, the frequency and duration of visits, and the visit completion rates.

Key Point

Creating an accurate estimate of your patient volumes and appointments structure is critical in determining resource needs as well as the financial feasibility for your service.

Once you have determined your patient volumes and translated those into the
service visits and the time required to provide care, you can then address the major
resources required to meet these needs, such as personnel/labor, equipment, supplies, information technology, and physical plant requirements.

Expenses Related to Personnel and Labor

Personnel represents one of the largest portions of your resource needs. Your
personnel needs will depend on your practice model, setting, and the service you
provide, but most typically the needs are represented by direct-care providers
(i.e., pharmacists), support staff (i.e., pharmacy technicians, clerical staff), and
administrative support. For staffing needs and expenditures, it is important to
consider issues such as nonproductive time (i.e., educational and sick leave, vacations), benefits, and other factors. In this section and through the resource
worksheet, we will examine these personnel needs and assist you in determining
the associated costs.

When you state your personnel needs, you will want to use FTEs. The FTE, or
"full-time equivalent," is the basic unit of measure for labor, and it is most commonly
defined as the maximum number of compensable hours an individual will work in a
year, or 2,080 hours (40 hr/wk x 52 wk). Check your organizations' payroll definition, but for this chapter and the related worksheet we will consider an FTE to be
40 hours of work in a 7-day period. Determine your total FTE needs for each personnel type (i.e., pharmacist, technician, clerical). Please refer to your worksheet to
estimate the FTEs needed for direct patient care. (Resources and Reimbursement
Worksheet) 🖳

Determining Staffing Needs for Pharmacists

Direct Patient Care. In the previous section you developed an estimate of your
patient volume. We now want to determine more precisely your actual direct-care

provider needs. First, let's adjust your direct patient care time to include other necessary tasks. You will need to allow some time, perhaps 15–30 minutes per patient visit, for documentation. This number should include pre-clinic preparation, final documentation, and follow-up tasks. This time will vary significantly depending on the complexity of your patients' care, the efficiency of your documentation system, and other factors. (Refer to your worksheet for assistance in adding documentation time to your patient care time estimates.) You will also need to account for nonproductive time, such as vacation and education leave, by adding a 10% to 20% correction time to your current staffing needs estimate. At this point, the calculated value should be a good approximation of one component of your staffing requirements—your total *direct-care* provider needs.

CASE

To determine the direct-care pharmacist staffing needs for your new service, you use a resource needs worksheet. Your earlier research indicated that 95 patients are expected to use this service. Because all the patients have been receiving care in the system, you set out to determine the maintenance level of staffing needed to care for the patients with no adjustments for new visits. You will use 20 minutes as the visit duration for each patient to determine minimum needs. You walk through these steps:

Determining number of monthly visits:

- 60 patients with diabetes
    - 80% will have routine visits every 12 weeks = 48 patients every 12 weeks, or an average of 16 patient visits per 4-week intervals (roughly 17/mo).
    - 20% will need more frequent visits; we will use "every 4 weeks" for our estimate = 12 patient visits every 4 weeks (roughly 13/mo).

- 35 patients on warfarin
    - 80% will have a routine visit every 4 weeks = 28 patient visits per 4 weeks (roughly 30/mo).
    - 20% will need more frequent visits. Using 1 visit every 2 weeks, our estimate = 14 visits per 4 weeks (roughly 16/mo).

- Total percentages of visit frequency
    - 48 patients (50%) will visit every 12 weeks
    - 40 patients (42%) will visit every 4 weeks
    - 7 patients (8%) will visit every 2 weeks

- Total monthly visits = 76 (30 for diabetes and 46 for anticoagulation)

DETERMINING STAFFING NEEDS

Pharmacists' Staffing Time Related to Direct-Patient Care

- Nonadjusted staffing needs: 76 visits/mo X 20 min/visit X 1 hr/60 min = 25.3 hr/mo.

- Scheduling must account for no-shows and rescheduling of patients. The visit completion rate is 65%.

  - 76 visits/mo x 1.35 no-show correction = 103 visit slots estimated to meet demand.

  - 103 visits x 20 min/visit x 1 hr/60 min = 34.2 hr staffing/mo.

- Corrections need to be made to account for the following:

  - Documentation time, for which we will use a value of 20 minutes per completed visit
    - § 76 completed visits/wk x 20 min x 1 hr/60 min = 25.3 hr
    - § Total direct-care time = 34.2 + 25.3 = 59.5 hr every month

- Direct-care pharmacist staffing needs are roughly 59.5 hr/mo or approximately 15 hr/wk (which equates to 0.375 FTE: FTE = 15 hr/wk x 1 FTE/40 hr).

Pharmacists Staffing Needs Not Related to Direct Patient Care. Of course, not every minute of the workday is accounted for in the life of a busy clinical pharmacist! There are some other very important considerations that may impact the staffing needs of the pharmacist care providers, such as activities and possible responsibilities related to performing prescription refill authorization, reviewing laboratory results, consulting with providers, addressing external inquiries, precepting students or residents, and performing research. These activities may vary considerably between practice locations and are also somewhat difficult to estimate. Finally, we need to consider nonproductive time, which includes educational leave, sick time, and vacations. This is usually estimated to be 10% to 20% of an employee's time and salary.

CASE

Dr. Busybee's nursing staff has agreed to continue performing prescription refill authorizations for the office, and the pharmacists need only address issues related to anticoagulation and diabetes medications for the occasional patient. Thus, this time is minimal. However, pharmacists will need time to review new and pertinent laboratory results related to the patients who are receiving anticoagulation and diabetes care. After talking to Dr. Busybee, you estimate that the time related to laboratory result reviews, patient inquiries, and the resulting necessary actions for your 95 patients would require about 45 minutes per day (25 minutes for laboratory result reviews and 20 minutes for patient inquiries), based on Monday through Friday service. At this time you will not be precepting students or be involved with research.

Pharmacists' Staffing Time Related to Non-Direct Patient Care

- Laboratory result reviews, patient inquiries, and related activities

    - 45 min/day X 1 hr/60 min X 3 days/wk = 9 hr/mo

- Nonproductive time (i.e., sick time, vacation leave, education leave) adjustments 10% to 20% of staffing time

    - Based on the current estimates, we have 59.5 hr/mo for direct patient care plus 9 hr/mo for non-direct patient care time = 68.5 hr/mo.

    - Using a nonproductive time value of 10%, multiply 69.5 X 1.1 (10% correction) = 75 hr/mo for total staffing time requirements (or FTE = 0.47).

Therefore, total pharmacist staffing time is estimated to be 76 hr/mo.

Overall Pharmacists Staffing Needs—Putting It All Together. It is important that you go through the staffing needs considerations listed previously to generate a well-informed estimate of your labor cost. However, now you must determine how this estimate based on anticipated patient volumes and other activities fits into an actual clinic schedule. Also consider the other factors involved, such as patient scheduling and support staff schedules. It is wise to step back, take a practical look, and compare the detailed estimate of staffing needs to the estimated patient volumes to see if our numbers make sense. Discussions with pharmacists in actual practice indicate that, in a standard 8-hour day, they can generally accommodate 8–12 patients in disease management-style services and 15–30 patients in services with more focused care (i.e., anticoagulation). Keep this in mind as a reality check as you do the math for your direct-care provider staffing needs, and realize each practice site is different. These numbers reflect an estimate of the number of patients that may be seen in a given time span, but it may not fit all sites.

CASE

It has been determined that the total staffing needs for the pharmacists at Dr. Busybee's office is 19 hours per week. You also know you have scheduled approximately 103 visit slots every month. Using the standard 8-hour day, this would indicate there are 9.5 days of staffing for 103

visits, or 10–11 visits per day. This figure seems to be in line with the
other information you have reviewed, and you are comfortable moving
ahead with scheduling. You share information with the office manager, and
she determines that exam rooms are available for a full day every
Wednesday and possibly when needed you can expand to partial days on
Tuesday and Thursday (2–4 hours) if office scheduling allows. Working
with the schedules, you create visit "blocks" that allow for up to 12
patients in a standard 8-hour day and 6 patients on 4-hour days.

Support Staffing Needs

Let's consider labor needs for administrative and support staff functions within your
model. Examples of administrative functions include scheduling, strategic planning,
and outcomes reporting (i.e., quality and cost indicators). These will likely require
a pharmacist, but they may be handled by staff outside the service area. Also, the
time needed to complete these functions will depend greatly on the complexity of
the service, as well as the organization.

Likewise, the support staff time required in your model will depend largely on the
type of service you are planning. In an integrated model, support staff services may be
inclusive, and expenses may be covered or shared between groups (i.e., pharmacy and
the clinic operations budgets). The larger and more complex the service, the more
support staff you will need. Providing patient services such as office reception, phone
reminders, phone inquiries, and appointment scheduling are ideal roles for support
staff. Other duties may include clerical, financial, and technical functions. While teamwork is encouraged, defining roles and job descriptions will improve efficiency, decrease confusion, and be cost effective. Paying a direct-care pharmacist to pull charts
and type letters might not be the best use of time. Use your worksheet to think
through needs for support staff. There are several ways to generate cost estimates
for these employees. Using the national publications on salary estimates previously
discussed will give you a general range. For regional data, contacting your colleagues
in retail and hospital practice will give you a range for pharmacy support staff. With
these numbers and by understanding the salary scales at your organization, you will
be able to finalize fair cost estimates for your support staff.

Estimating Costs for Equipment, Supplies, and Other Resources

Creating a detailed and thorough list of your resource needs will not only ensure
that you have the equipment and supplies required to run your service but also will
allow for a more accurate financial analysis. Your practice model and service type
will determine if equipment will be an extensive resource category. You will likely
have up-front expenditures for items necessary to establish your service, such as
desks, chairs, computers and monitors, copiers, phones, fax machines, billing or
financial software, documentation systems, and laboratory or point-of-care testing
equipment. Any construction or remodeling costs for the physical space should be
included here as well. Chapter 5 will detail this for you even further.

You will also have resource needs relating to the regular operating costs of your service, and these may be directly related to your patient volumes and other workload indicators. (See **Table** 2-1 for a basic list.) Other types of operational needs could include staff training programs, marketing, mail and delivery services, and funding for recruitment and retention of staff. (Resources Worksheet to Inventory Items and Expenses) 🖥

Table 2-1. Office and Medical Supplies: An Abbreviated List

Office supplies	
	• Computers
	• Printer(s)
	• Fax machine(s)
	• Telephones
	• Software (patient scheduling, medical records, billing, communications)
	• Miscellaneous: Paper, folders, pens, staplers, etc.
	• Trash cans
Office furniture	
	• Desks (reception area, offices)
	• Chairs (reception area, offices, appointment rooms)
	• Exam table(s)
	• File cabinets
	• Lighting·Refrigerator (medical supplies)
	• Secure containers/cabinets (for drug supplies)
Medical supplies	
	• Blood pressure cuffs and stethoscopes
	• Thermometer
	• Weight scale
	• Point-of-care testing devices: INR, blood glucose, lipids
	• Sharps waste containers

Physical space needs and associated costs can vary greatly between practice settings, service structures, and delivery models. Your physical space needs include all the square footage you need for your service: patient care areas, waiting rooms, storage areas, conference and meeting rooms, Americans with Disabilities Act–compliant restrooms, etc. Include this category if you will be buying, renting, or leasing the space. Even if the space you are using is already accounted for under another budget, a responsible and thorough approach would be to include the value (dollars per square foot per time) for the space in your financial analysis. According to *Marcus & Millichap's Medical Office Research Report*, the average cost for medical office space in the third quarter of 2009 was $23.90 per square foot per year (or $2 per square foot per month).[7] Refer to your finance department or accountant for estimates on the cost or market values for this expense.

Evaluating the Available Resources

Optimally, the new service will stand on its own and bring in a profit margin that will allow the service to grow and sustain itself for many years. However, it is wise to make use of any available resources that may be at your disposal in the current environment, including personnel, equipment, physical space, and supplies. Consider reallocating resources from current services to this new service based on the relative value. Remember that reallocation will also involve spending time, effort, and political capital to move the resources to your new project. You may have to retrain the staff and reprogram the equipment, resulting in a loss of productivity from the original services.

CASE

The current pharmacists' staffing plans for the office are for 2.5 days or 20 hours per week. Dr. Busybee indicates there are no current plans to hire a new provider or expand current work flow. The medical assistants are working during those times, but they can cross-cover to assist with collecting vital signs for your patients. A discussion with your pharmacy manager reveals that two pharmacists have been expressing interest in expanding their patient care time and also have training well-aligned with your service. Your manager indicates that the department can reallocate 8 hours of service to contribute to the 20 hours of office coverage. This will meet 40% of your estimated direct-care staffing needs. This may be of value as your practice grows.

The Financial Assessment: Evaluating Expenses vs. Revenue

Estimating Expenses

Basic to any financial analysis is the comparison of expenditures and revenue. In preparing your resource needs inventory, you have accounted for much of the anticipated expenses. The top two cost areas in your financial analysis are likely personnel and durable equipment. Remember, in determining expenses related to personnel, your FTE per hour determinations for the various staff positions need to include wages as well as benefits. Benefits can account for up to 30% in additional expenses! You will likely find this information by consulting the human resources or personnel department of your organization. There are also publications from the National Association of Chain Drug Stores (NACDS) and others that document industry-wide salary data on an annual basis.[8-10] You may also take a survey of your regional pharmacy colleagues who work in similar practice settings.

Overhead is another expense category that is frequently forgotten when building a service. Overhead refers to those ongoing operating costs of running a business that cannot be immediately associated with the products and services being offered (e.g., do not directly generate profits), such as utilities, insurance, and taxes. Your sources for these expenses typically will be the practice's financial or accounting department or the supervisor or manager who oversees the area. (Resources Worksheet)🖳

When listing all your expenses, consider separating them into two major categories. In one category, capture your initial implementation costs, including your capital expenditures (big budget, long-lasting goods), remodeling or physical space costs, and necessary supplies. The second category should include your expected operating expenses (i.e., labor, office supplies, rent, overhead).

Record the estimated total expenses for your service by using the worksheet.🖳

Determining the Financial Potential of the Service

Let's turn our attention toward the financial value of your service. We will cover some basic information for your financial analysis, but for more details you may wish to consult with your organization's financial specialists. This role may vary depending on the type of your organization and its size. Your pharmacy director, a cost accountant, or a chief financial officer may be the person who can assist you in obtaining this information. Selected examples in published literature demonstrating the financial value of clinical pharmacy practices are provided in **Table 2-2**. We will discuss three general strategies for demonstrating financial value of your services: reimbursement, cost avoidance, and improved care efficiency.

Table 2-2. Data Supporting the Financial Value for Ambulatory Pharmacy Clinical Services

Title	Citation	Description
Economic evaluations of clinical pharmacy services: 2001–2005	*Pharmacotherapy.* 2008;28(11):285e-323e	Systematic review of literature for economic impact of ambulatory services.
Cost justification of a clinical pharmacist-managed anticoagulation clinic	*Drug Intell Clin Pharm.* 1985;19:575-580	Provides annual cost savings/ avoidance benefit of evidence-based, high-quality pharmacy services compared to usual care.
An economic analysis of a randomized, controlled, multicenter study of clinical pharmacist interventions for high-risk veterans; The IMPROVE study	*Pharmacotherapy.* 2000;20:1149-1158.	Provides process for patients at high risk for a medication-related event. Also provides some cost-benefit figures.
Methods to assess the economic outcomes of clinical pharmacy services	*Pharmacotherapy.* 2000;20(10 Pt 2):243S-252S.	Provides guidance on key strategies and steps in creating an economic evaluation and marketing the value of services.
A prospective trial of a clinical pharmacy intervention in a primary care practice in a capitated payment system	*Manag Care Pharm.* 2008; 14(9):831-843	Provides methods and approaches for evaluating financial outcomes in a managed care setting.
Analysis of pharmacist-provided medication therapy management (MTM) services in community pharmacies over 7 years	*J Manag Care Pharm.* 2009;15(1):18-31	Describes community pharmacy-based MTM interventions and quantifies potential MTM-related cost savings based on pharmacists' self-assessments.
Clinical and economic impact of a diabetes clinical pharmacy service program in a university and primary care-based collaboration model	*J Am Pharm Assoc.* (2003). 2009;49(2):200-208	Discusses clinical and economic outcomes related to implementation of clinical services, including overall health outcomes cost.
The Asheville Project: Long-term clinical and economic outcomes of a community pharmacy diabetes care program	*J Am Pharm Assoc.* 2003; 43:173-184	Review of seminal pharmacy project exploring health outcomes impact of public sector payer.

AACP = American College of Clinical Pharmacy; MTM = medication therapy management.

Reimbursement for clinical pharmacy services is possible in many settings. The laws of your state and the service environment may influence your ability to qualify for reimbursement, but more often than not reimbursements depend on business relationships with payers and insurers. One approach to securing reimbursement is *fee-for-service*, which can be used with contracted insurers or cash-paying customers. Another example of fee-for-service exists in outpatient pharmacies and consultant work, where payment is independent of a physician's care. *Incident-to* billing is commonly used in many community-based provider offices and hospitals with ambulatory services. In these settings, the pharmacist acts as an extension of the physician, and Current Procedural Terminology (CPT) codes may be used to generate billing claims. Some reimbursement methods involve capitated payments in which the provider assumes some risk for the patient's health and is paid a certain amount for the patient care regardless of how often the patient uses the service. Finally, any combination of the above can be used any time two parties agree on a service and reimbursement model and sign a mutually agreeable contract. (Refer to Chapter 8, which is devoted entirely to reimbursement.)

The potential for and degree of reimbursement for pharmacist's clinical services will depend to a significant degree on the insurers and payers in your practice setting. *Payer mix* refers to the number of and proportion of patients covered by different payers represented in your setting. If your payer mix reflects a high level of Medicare patients or indigent care, your potential reimbursement revenue may be less than a practice setting with a high degree of private insurance. It is also important to realize that the amount billed for a claim is usually not the amount reimbursed. In fact, depending on the contract agreements and payer mix, you may only recoup approximately 50% of your charges. You will need to consider all of this for your financial analysis. The data you requested to estimate patient visits and volume should include information on your payer mix. In any case, contacting your financial or billing representative to determine the significance of the payer mix and reimbursement for pharmacy-generated billing is a wise decision.

It is important to note that your approach to reimbursement may depend on your practice setting. For example, in a capitated model, in which reimbursement is fixed, there is clearly less focus on payment for your services and more attention on improving quality of care and outcomes with efficient resource use. That said, for most practice models payment for services will be a significant consideration.

Let's review some practical approaches to estimating your reimbursement potential. There are four important pieces of the reimbursement puzzle that you should gather: estimated number of visits, the types of visits, the payer mix, and the actual degree of reimbursement for your services. Each of these factors is discussed below. The estimated number of visits per time period (monthly or quarterly) is used not only to determine your staffing resource needs but also is the key determinant of your potential reimbursement. Refer to the resource needs section or the related worksheet to determine this value.

Breakdown of Visit Types or Levels. Visit types can be classified a variety of ways. Physician visits are classified based on time taken and complexity of care provided using CPT codes that reflect five levels of care from short and simple (level 1) visits to longer, more involved appointments (level 5). If available, obtaining billing records from the care setting in which you plan to initiate your new service may provide insight into predicting the diversity and proportion of visit types. It is important to note that if a system is already in place, you will likely need to align with current coding practices. Make sure to inquire about the current billing process and forms to assess how pharmacists will classify visits. Pharmacy visits may be defined by time and complexity, but they are often based solely on time, with initial visits and complex patient care requiring longer appointment times (i.e., level 3 or 4) and follow-up and routine visits needing less time (i.e., level 2 or 3). In some settings, simple billing forms (i.e., superbills) are used, allowing providers to quickly document care provided. Billing specialists then translate this information into the proper codes to generate claims. You should review these forms. If no previous visit classification data are available, you may need to make estimates. Determine the different visit types (i.e., how many types and how they are classified), and then estimate the percentage breakdown based on your service type(s) and the characteristics of your patient population. For example, for an anticoagulation service you may choose to designate two visit types of 15 and 30 minutes, with an expectation that 30% of visits will be new visits or complex visits requiring 30-minute appointments.

Payer Mix for Service. Visit fees or charges may be standardized across your practice. However, the amount you recover from charges is generally related to the payer contracts and your overall payer mix. We recommend contacting your billing or finance team and requesting some general numbers on the rate of reimbursement for the overall system and, perhaps, for individual payers. You should specifically inquire about reimbursement for visit types that resemble your service, such as incident-to visit codes. Ideally, you can determine what percentage of patient visits would fall into each payer and billing category and then determine the degree of reimbursement from that payer.

Payment and Reimbursement Information. Once again, you will want to contact your finance or business office to determine typical rates of reimbursement per payer or an overall rate. It is particularly important to look at charges for billing codes that most closely resemble the types pharmacists will be using (i.e., incident-to, medication therapy management [MTM]). Often, reimbursement rates are negotiated with insurers and set in the contract for a specific time period. These rates may be adequate for estimating revenue if you have difficulty obtaining billing records. Once the information is secured, you can apply the reimbursement rates against your expected charges to determine your actual revenue.

In some situations, obtaining accurate reimbursement rates is difficult due to complexity in the billing processes or to attribution issues (i.e., incident-to billing where the physician is identified as the provider, not the pharmacists or other support staff). If you are unable to determine reimbursement levels from billing records or contracts, you may need to estimate your revenue based on your actual charges. According to anecdotal information, a common range for rate of reimbursement for charges is 50% to 60%.

Figure 2-1 provides a fictional example of a basic evaluation table in which you can insert the information you collect to determine total charges based on the number of visits, type of visits, and the known charges for each visit. **Figure 2-1** estimates a visit rate of 266 visits per month for this practice site and classifies them as level 1 through 5. Visit fees were based on current nonprovider (incident-to) charges currently in place, and the reimbursement rate used was an average for all payers across all visit types for nonprovider charges. This worksheet indicates a potential reimbursement of nearly $6,000 per month for pharmacist visits.

Visit Level	Estimated No. of Total Visits per Month	Fee/Charge	Estimated Total Charges	% Collected on Charges	Total Revenue
Level 1	23	$20.22	$465	63%	$293
Level 2	55	$36.15	$1,988	63%	$1,252
Level 3	134	$41.18	$5,518	63%	$3,476
Level 4	52	$55.22	$2,871	63%	$1,809
Level 5	2	$75.66	$151	63%	$95
Totals	**266**		**$10,993**		**$5,925**

Figure 2-1. Example of Visit Analysis Table to Project Reimbursement for Clinical Services

CASE

Financial discussions with Dr. Busybee identify several options to support the pharmacy service. First, you have the option to bill incident to his practice and generate direct reimbursement. Next you consider the practice's potential financial risk and the specific dollar amount associated with loss of the performance-based payer contract. Finally, you calculate the potential increase in revenue based on increased efficiencies for the physician (e.g., less time per appointment as pharmacists handle medication-related issues) and the potential for new patients (i.e., with potentially higher reimbursement levels).

Reimbursement and payment models are continually evolving. Many pharmacist entrepreneurs are creating and delivering valuable services to the health care market and are successfully securing reimbursement. Health care organizations employ a person called a *compliance officer* who is responsible for understanding and applying the rules, laws, and regulations of the governmental guidelines and payer contracts, including policies related to reimbursement. It is important for you to contact and meet your compliance officer during the planning process for your service. He or she can assist you in understanding how your service will need to adapt to these rules. If you do not have a compliance officer, then you may want to check with your business/financial specialist or seek information via professional organizations.

Depending on your setting, it may be difficult to justify your service solely on reimbursement. Generally, you will need to find additional means of demonstrating value to support your service. Let's review some approaches.

Reimbursement opportunities for clinical pharmacy services are available in a variety of practice settings. Leveraging multiple strategies around reimbursement can strengthen support for your services.

Cost avoidance is another financial value strategy. It is sometimes referred to as "soft dollars" in that it generally produces cost savings figures based on "what didn't happen" without generating actual revenue. Cost avoidance can be described as direct or indirect. An example of direct cost avoidance would be reduction in drug expenditures. Pharmacists providing medication management services may appropriately discontinue medications or change to less-costly medications. This can be tracked for specific drugs or drug classes or for a population of patients and be reported as cost per prescription, cost per patient, cost per member, or as overall cost savings. The value and acceptance of cost-avoidance data for financial reporting can vary by practice site. In a capitated or fixed reimbursement system (i.e., managed care), where medication costs are not separately reimbursed, this may be of significant value as it reduces overall expenditures and cost of care. However, in a practice in which the payer mix is weighted toward private insurance with prescription reimbursement paid separately from the medical benefit, the value of cost avoidance may be diminished.

Let's look at an example of cost avoidance. A pharmacist manager initiates a polypharmacy service to address the problem of inappropriate prescribing and patient nonadherence to medications in a managed care facility. Patients taking more than six routine medications will now be automatically referred to the service for review of their medication regimen. One of the outcome indicators is cost savings related to a reduction in overall medication use or conversion to more cost-effective agents. To demonstrate this value the manager decides to determine the total monthly medication costs for each patient referred to the service prior to the intervention (using an average of the previous 3 months of expenditures). The team then tracks medication expenses for the patient for the next 3 months after the intervention and determines the new average monthly expenditure for medications. To demonstrate this value, you determine that most patients will remain on their new chronic illness medication regimen for 12 months. This allows extrapolation of the savings for the intervention and calculation of the potential cost avoidance (see **Figure** 2-2).

Patient	Preintervention Average Monthly Medication Expenditures	Postintervention Average Monthly Medication Expenditures	Estimated 1-year Cost Avoidance
Patient A	$330	$230	$1,200
Patient B	$540	$390	$1,800
Patient C	$240	$190	$600
Total			**$3,600**

Figure 2-2. Estimated 1-year Cost Avoidance Savings per Polypharmacy Clinic Interventions

This model can be used in a number of circumstances, including generic- and brand-prescribing initiatives, targeted high-cost medication initiatives, and elimination of unnecessary laboratory tests. Clearly, there are assumptions made in this cost-savings analysis, and this is not uncommon for cost-avoidance strategies. It is reasonable to state your assumptions and possible flaws in your methodology in your report. The challenge in using cost avoidance to support your new service is that you have to estimate the impact and resulting cost value prior to implementation. Using available data, such as percentage of generic prescribing, and identifying an achievable target, for instance 20% improvement in generic prescribing, can allow for estimation of cost savings. Generally, it is advisable to be conservative with your estimates. If there is a range of cost-avoidance savings, then the lower value may be the most appropriate for reporting.

Indirect cost avoidance includes decreases in health expenditures related to the provision of more effective or safer care. Savings result from patients who, based on the care of the pharmacist, would reasonably avoid an adverse medication event, an emergency care visit, a hospital admission, or other resource use. While these cost savings may be substantial, they can be difficult to track, document, and assign a definite cost value. It also may be difficult to attribute all of the benefit solely to the pharmacist's intervention. It is worthwhile to conduct a literature search or inquiry to locate a well-designed study that provides estimates of cost avoidance for the patient population impacted by your proposed service.

An example of indirect cost avoidance from the primary literature relates to improved safety and effectiveness in the management of anticoagulation. Chiquette et. al. reported that patients receiving care from a pharmacy-managed anticoagulation service versus the usual physician-based care demonstrated a cost savings of $900 per year.[11] In a setting where known care deficiencies exist with regard to anticoagulation management, a pharmacist interested in initiating a high-quality anticoagulation service could use this information to support their service proposal. For example, with a population of 250 eligible patients to be managed by this new service, based on the published study, converting these patients from standard care to your anticoagulation service could be argued to generate an estimated cost avoidance savings of $225,000 annually.

A third strategy used to demonstrate financial value is improved care efficiency. Ambulatory care models are becoming increasingly multidisciplinary in their efforts to optimize care (i.e., patient-centered medical home). Increasing demands for ambulatory care services combined with physician shortages can challenge site capacities in providing timely and efficient care. Patient-care services that use the pharmacist's unique education and training can streamline a provider's workflow and expand capacity. Even if the pharmacists are unable to generate significant direct revenue for services, this "physician extender" model may allow providers—who have greater billing and reimbursement potential—to generate more revenue and expand the practice site capacity.[12,13] You may want to examine the current situations in your care setting. Are physicians overbooked? Are care access issues, such as delayed appointment scheduling, a problem? Could pharmacy assistance allow providers to see new patients or schedule more visits by decreasing visit times with complex patients? Working with a clinic manager or physician leader, you may be able to estimate the financial impact of increased capacity and efficiency.

 To put your revenue analysis in perspective, in most health care models a provider will need to generate revenue at least three to four times his or her actual salary to reach a break-even point for the employer because of the numerous other costs involved in the operation of the facility.

Your service may be able to demonstrate revenue or costs savings using the strategies discussed here. While it may be difficult to accurately estimate the dollar value, a conservative estimate that shows some revenue and/or cost-savings potential is a great first step.

Evaluating the Financial Feasibility: The Pro Forma

The final step in the financial assessment is comparing your expenses to your potential revenue. First, list your service initiation expenses or start-up costs. Then, compare your estimated monthly operating expenditures to your reimbursement predictions (i.e., the solid dollars from direct care reimbursement). If your estimated monthly revenue exceeds your monthly operating costs, then determine the break-even point for the service. This is what it will take to cover your implementation costs. If your estimated monthly expenses (operating costs) trump your reimbursement, then describe the other financial strategies (i.e., cost avoidance) to demonstrate additional value.

If you would like to use a financial tool to assist you in your financial feasibility assessment for your proposed service, consider using the pro forma. This is a financial tool that helps predict the viability of your service. The tool uses the assumptions regarding the way your service will function and predicts the financial outcome of the service based on one set of assumptions. Pro forma structures vary. We have not provided a specific template, but contact your business office or accountant for more information.

Anticipating and Managing Growth

As discussed previously, it is important to anticipate and plan for growth. This expected growth should then be converted into objective metrics and preplanned time points for service evaluation. These prospectively identified evaluations are used to demonstrate the responsible management of your resources. For example, if service capacities are set at 600 patients and a visit rate of 300 patients per month, then allowance for predetermined additional staffing and supplies could be provided once these indicator levels are sustained. Alternatively, this could at least trigger the official request for resources. You may need to demonstrate financial or productivity data to ensure continued support for expansion of services. Whatever the measures, these should be included in the qualitative and quantitative outcomes that are listed in your service proposal. For additional discussions on quality measurement, see the next section of this chapter and Chapter 7, as well as Chapter 9 for information on service growth.

If resources are limited and you are not able to expand services to meet growing demands, it is important to plan how you will keep your services within your means. This plan may include limiting patient access. This is often a consideration that pharmacy services plans fail to address. Although working beyond your maximum capacity may be acceptable for short periods of time, sustaining these efforts indefinitely without plans for additional resources can undermine your service quality and lead to staff burnout. Keep in mind the attribute of a scalable service. Here are a few examples of how to maintain your service within your resource allowance:

- Limit the service to specific physicians (i.e., primary care).

- Limit the service to specific clinics (i.e., cardiology referrals).

- Develop specific inclusion or referral criteria (i.e., age, number of medications, severity of illness) to qualify patients for the service.

It is good to be on the watch for other factors that may adversely impact your growth. Examples include recruiting difficulties due to labor shortage or required training, shifts in the economic climate, and change in administrative and provider support.

Getting the Model Going: Considering the Pilot

A practical and often necessary way to approach a new service is to consider a pilot project. This approach leverages the principle of a scalable service. If resources are tight or support for the new service is weak, but the projections for the future are strong, then consideration may be given to a pilot project. The premise of the pilot is that, with a scaled-down delivery model, resources and risks are reduced significantly. Set up defined evaluation points that demonstrate outcomes (clinical, care process, financial) that can be extrapolated to the fully implemented project. It may be possible to open the service to just one physician or a small population of patients for a defined period of time. Perhaps a pharmacy resident can manage the pilot as part of their training project. In setting up the pilot, remember to set limits on the scale and timelines and, as much as possible, determine your metrics for success prior to launch.

Building Support for Your Service

In this section, you will see how building support for your service is a function that has been occurring since you first conceived of your idea. While you were gathering the data and identifying your stakeholders, you were discussing the merits and benefits of your service. For this section, we will cover two basic strategies for building support: using data and clinical evidence and identifying and engaging stakeholders.

Using Data and Evidence to Demonstrate Value

Finding Supporting Data

Your service has been designed to address a particular need. However, there are undoubtedly multiple benefits to your organization or practice site. It is critical that you consider these benefits from the perspective of all of your major stakeholders. For this you will want the most pertinent supporting evidence available to build your supporting argument. It is important that you present information that clearly supports pharmacists as the most appropriate discipline to lead this effort, especially if services are currently being provided by other personnel or staff. In this case, you want to be complimentary, but clear on why pharmacists have the right skill set and training for the job. Stay focused on the big picture question, "what is best for our patients and the organization?"

You already may have a good sense of the benefits to the organization based on your needs assessment research, your service and delivery model reviews, or from your staff's collective knowledge base. In any case, we suggest you gather the following supporting information. Collect any current pharmacy practices at your workplace that have demonstrated a history of success. Ideally, you have data supporting this as well. Second, find relevant examples of similar services provided by pharmacists in the literature or other acceptable sources that demonstrate value. The primary literature has numerous examples of pharmacy-based services. A recently completed extensive literature review was conducted demonstrating the value of pharmacists providing services in a diverse range of care settings, and this will assist you in getting started.[14,15] We have provided a list of selected literature resources and specific publications for your reference that expand and supplement those provided in Chapter 1 (**Table 2-3**). If the literature does not provide the necessary data, you may find that networking through various professional pharmacy organizations provides connections to other practice sites with similar services (**Table 2-4**). These sites will describe strategies, outcomes data, and anecdotal information that will translate well to your identified stakeholders.

Determining Your Outcome Measures

You will now want to consider how to track your program's outcomes after establishing the benefits of your new service. Demonstrating its impact will be an important component of your service proposal. The supporting evidence for pharmacy services found in your environmental scan will also provide examples of possible metrics for tracking value. It is important you consider a wide range of possible outcomes. This will allow you to determine which metrics are directly related to your services, are the most feasible to collect, and will have the most value to your stakeholders. For additional discussion on outcomes and metrics see Chapter 7. Potential financial benefits and related metrics have already been discussed earlier in the return on investment section. In this section we will discuss clinical, quality, regulatory, and humanistic outcomes.

Clinical metrics include measures of appropriateness, effectiveness, and safety regarding the care provided. Many chronic conditions have a variety of indicators for appropriate clinical care. Examples include the following:

- Achievement of blood pressure target goals for patients with hypertension
- Glycosylated hemoglobin levels below targeted levels for diabetes
- LDL-cholesterol levels below risk-stratified targets in heart disease

It is best to use clinical quality measures that have been standardized and validated

Table 2-3. Select Publications Supporting Ambulatory Clinical Pharmacy
Services

Title	Citation/Location	Description
General Pharmacy Practice Information		
The impact of pharmaceutical services in community and ambulatory care settings: Evidence and recommendations for future research	*Ann Pharmacother.* 1999;33(12):1336-1355	Article reviews and evaluates research on pharmaceutical services in community and ambulatory care pharmacy settings, specifically study designs and patient outcome measures.
Establishment and outcomes of a model primary care pharmacy service system	*Am J Health-Syst Pharm.* 2004;61:472-482	
ACCP Ambulatory Care New Practitioners Survival Guide/ Resource Manual	http://www.accp.com/(See bookstore section)	Available for purchase from ACCP, the manual contains information on clinical services and includes an extensive list of references for further study.
Assessing the structure and process for providing pharmaceutical care in Veterans Affairs medical centers	*Am J Health-Syst Pharm.* 2000;57(1):29-39	Examines the VA model for provision on clinical pharmacy services.
Service specific Information		
Anticoagulation		
Comparison of an anticoagulation clinic and usual medical care: Anticoagulation control, patient outcomes, and health care costs	*Arch Intern Med.* 1998;158:1641-1647	
Respiratory		
Pharmacist involvement in improving asthma outcomes in various healthcare settings: 1997 to present	*Ann Pharmacother.* 2009;43(1):85-97. Epub Dec 23, 2008	Evaluates pharmacists' impact on asthma management outcomes in various health care settings on the basis of updated guidelines set by the National Heart, Lung, and Blood Institute.
The BC Community Pharmacy Asthma Study: A study of clinical, economic and holistic outcomes influenced by an asthma care protocol provided by specially trained community pharmacists in British Columbia	*Can Respir J.* 2003;10(4):195-202	
Diabetes		
Pharmacist recommendations to improve the quality of diabetes care: A randomized controlled trial	*J Manag Care Pharm.* 2010;16(2):104-113	Assesses the effects of a comprehensive, pharmacist-delivered, primary care, physician-focused intervention in a large hospital-based primary care practice.
Sensitivity of patient outcomes to pharmacist interventions. Part I. Systematic review and meta-analysis in diabetes management	*Ann Pharmacother.* 2007;41(10):1569-1582. Epub Aug 21, 2007	Identifies outcomes sensitive to pharmacists' interventions and quantifies their impact through critical literature review.

Table 2-3. Select Publications Supporting Ambulatory Clinical Pharmacy Services (cont'd)

Title	Citation/Location	Description
Clinical outcomes of patients with diabetes mellitus receiving medication management by pharmacists in an urban private physicians practice	*Am J Health-Syst Pharm.* 2008;65:145-149	The noninstitutional setting provides insight in how to structure practice model and impact patient care.
Development and clinical outcomes of pharmacy-managed diabetes care clinics	*Am J Health-Syst Pharm.* 2006;63:1325-1331	Good description of service delivery model in a multidisciplinary setting.
Cardiovascular		
Assessment of clinical pharmacist management of lipid-lowering therapy in a primary care setting	*J Manag Care Pharm.* 2003;9(3):269-273	Examines the structure of the referral-based lipid clinic service and the value of pharmacy based-services compared to usual physician-based care.
Sensitivity of patient outcomes to pharmacist interventions. Part II. Systematic review and meta-analysis in hypertension management	*Ann Pharmacother.* 2007;41(11):1770-1781. Epub Oct. 9, 2007	Includes information related to intervention type, patient numbers, demographics, study characteristics, instruments used, data compared, and outcomes reported for studies of pharmacist managed hypertension.
Reduction in heart failure events by the addition of a clinical pharmacist to the heart failure management team: Results of the Pharmacist in Heart Failure Assessment Recommendation and Monitoring (PHARM) Study	*Arch Intern Med.* 1999;159(16):1939-1945	Outcomes results from adding a pharmacist to a multidisciplinary team to provide medication evaluation, therapeutic recommendations to the attending physician, patient education, and follow-up telemonitoring.
Geriatrics		
Can clinical pharmacy services have a positive impact on drug-related problems and health outcomes in community-based older adults?	*Am J Geriatr Pharmacother.* 2004;2(1):3-13	Reviews evidence from randomized controlled studies to determine whether DRPs and the related health outcomes can be modified by providing clinical pharmacy services for the elderly in community-based settings.

AACP = American College of Clinical Pharmacy; DRP = drug-related problem; VA = Veterans Affairs

Table 2-4. Pharmacy Professional Organizations and Literature Sources

Type of Information	Source	Description/Contact Information
Pharmacy organizations and advisory groups	• Academy of Managed Care Pharmacy • American Association of Colleges of Pharmacy • American Association of Pharmaceutical Scientists • American Pharmacists Association • American Society of Consultant Pharmacists • American Society of Health-System Pharmacists • European Society of Clinical Pharmacy • National Community Pharmacists Association • Society of Infectious Diseases Pharmacists • Pharmacist Services Technical Advisory Coalition (PSTAC)	Provide profession-related reviews, analysis, standards of practice, etc.
Free bibliographic/full text	PubMed	Biomedical literature from 1966 to present
Evidence-based literature review	Cochrane Library	Wide variety of clinical topics
Bibliographic/full text	International Pharmaceutical Abstracts (IPA)	Pharmaceutical information
Select bibliographic and full text	Iowa Drug Information Service (IDIS)	Over 180 medical and pharmaceutical journals on drug therapy
Disease-focused organizations	American Diabetes Association American Heart Association American Lung Association	Maintain information for professionals and patients on a variety of topic-related issues

when measuring clinical outcomes. Many medication-related and health outcomes measures are available for review through the Centers for Medicare & Medicaid Services (CMS; Physician Quality Reporting System via CMS), the Healthcare Effectiveness Data and Information Set (HEDIS), and the National Quality Measures (NQM), to name a few. For a more extensive list, see quality information in Chapter 7.

Of course, the gold standard for demonstrating quality is health outcomes measures with "hard" end points, such as myocardial infarction and death for patients being treated for cardiovascular disease. While we are not discouraging inclusion of these end points in your metric tracking, it is important to include other measures that help identify progress in shorter time frames. Examples of process measures include the percentage of patients with recorded blood pressures at each visit or proportion of patients with LDL-C levels above targeted goals who are prescribed statin therapy. These measures use medication-related problems and surrogate end points as appropriate care-measure indicators. It is important to have a variety of indicators to track different elements of the care provided, especially those which you can most influence or impact. Some pharmacy service-specific interventions may not have validated outcomes measures, such as those provided at a polypharmacy clinic (i.e., resolution of drug-related problems). In this case you will need to determine which metrics are most reflective of your service outcomes.

Health care organizations and providers are increasingly required to report quality and performance data to government organizations (i.e., CMS), regulatory and accrediting agencies (i.e., Joint Commission), and insurance plans. Public reporting and pay-for-performance are significant changes in the health care quality environment. Many of the measures necessary for these reports are medication related or tied to patient-care goals that the pharmacy service can impact. Demonstrating value by improving your organization's performance on these metrics is significant. It is possible that your organization is at risk for decreased reimbursement or loss of market share to a competitor if your relative performance does not reach targeted benchmarks. For more information on performance measures and your organization's current status, contact the person responsible for identifying and tracking these within your organization such as quality and performance improvement leaders, the medical director, or other administrators.

In most organizations, humanistic measures are frequently represented as satisfaction with the product, service, or general care provided. The last 10 years have seen a significant rise in the concept of the patient as a consumer of health care. As competition in health care escalates, the public reporting of performance data has increased. The importance of patient opinion and public perception of your organization is growing. Two examples of this type of outcome are patient satisfaction measures and provider perception.

Administrators are carefully watching patient experience data, such as Consumer Assessment of Healthcare Providers and Systems (CAHPS) scores. High-quality pharmacy services that add to patient satisfaction may be viewed favorably by certain stakeholders. Conducting your own survey of patients is an excellent metric for your new service and provides data that can be shared with administrators.

Demonstrating Value: Future Considerations

Regardless of which metrics you select, it is important to proactively determine the comparator data to demonstrate the impact of your service. Consider whether you will use a pre- and postcomparison (outcomes indicators prior to service initiation versus after), a comparator group (similar patients receiving care outside your service), or internal care and quality standards for your organization. Often services will be provided in the context of team-based, interdisciplinary care. This creates challenges when attributing value specifically to the pharmacy component of the overall care. Obtaining baseline information, securing good comparator groups, and considering other initiatives or care-process changes that may impact outcomes is important to securing the best outcomes data. If collecting comparative data from your practice site is not possible, then you may be able to benchmark your outcomes against similar organizations or services using published performance data from government, regulatory, or health plan sources.

Finally, you will want to ensure that you determine the "what, who, how, and when" for reporting your chosen measures. What data specifically will you be reporting? Who will collect, process, and report the data, and to whom will they report? (*Note:* you may have to report different types of data to different persons or stakeholders.) How will you format your reports? And, finally, how often do you need to report? How best to answer the questions raised are discussed in detail in Chapter 7.

Identification and Engagement of Stakeholders

Stakeholders are those who have a vested interest in the service. Examples of two likely stakeholders for your new service are patients and physicians. Actually, there are multiple stakeholders to consider when planning the implementation of a new patient-care service. Examples might include the medical director, administrators, risk managers, billing and compliance officers, laboratory services, pharmacists, technicians, and other providers. These individuals may be supportive, antagonistic, or initially indifferent to your proposal. Your task is to identify and proactively engage these individuals to maximize your chance of successfully implementing your service. Some stakeholders will be important for the planning of your project, such as securing equipment or providing details on key processes of care. You should engage these persons early in the process. For example, initiate a cautious discussion with those key providers or provider groups that will be the most likely source for referrals. You may want to talk with compliance and billing personnel about nonprovider billing policies and reimbursement levels. As you move through the development of the proposal, you will need to gain support from these persons of influence. It is imperative to understand that these stakeholders will likely have different perspectives on your service. Your being open to challenging perspectives will strengthen your proposal in the end. It is also important that you can package the proposal in a variety of ways. In essence, you must customize the message based on the stakeholder's areas of interest.

CASE

You have already identified and engaged some of your stakeholders. Dr. Busybee, a key stakeholder, is very interested and convinced of the potential value you will bring to his clinic. You have also engaged Dr. Busybee's finance manager, and she is concerned about the legitimacy and compliance issues related to billing for clinical pharmacy services. You collect materials that support this area of pharmacist billing and set up a meeting. At this meeting you lay out what you are trying to do, provide examples from other practice sites with similar billing models, and review specific regulations and guidance from CMS and the fiscal intermediary in your area. Additionally, you contact and receive several educational pieces

> from your national pharmacy organization as to how it views this issue. The finance and compliance people agree that moving ahead with billing for pharmacy services is an acceptable plan. However, they require several evaluation points as you move forward to manage the risk they perceive in your plan.

We have provided a list of common stakeholders for pharmacy services with descriptions of their roles and areas of interest. Consider personalizing the list to create your own site-specific stakeholder group and include contact information and specific information on relationships to the proposed service (**Table 2-5**).

It is important to realize that the credibility and success of your new service may depend greatly on how patients and providers perceive your competence to deliver quality care. If the perceived value of your services is high with providers and other prominent stakeholders, this opinion can be of great political value. Finding provider champions, particularly physician leaders, service chiefs, and the medical director, is an excellent strategy.

Key Point Research shows the three most important variables of physician collaboration with pharmacists is relationship initiation, trustworthiness, and role specification.[16]

It is important to pay particular attention to your internal stakeholders. Your pharmacy coworkers, administrators, and support staff will be some of your toughest critics. If direct patient-care services are a relatively new concept at your practice site, then you may have a mix of excitement, nervous anticipation, and significant apprehension or resistance. Gauging attitudes of staff who will play a role in the new service, and even the general culture in the pharmacy, is important. Some key questions might include the following:

1. Are your coworkers and colleagues engaged in the new service development?
2. Does your team understand, believe in, and support the service?
3. Have they experienced similar projects in the past?
4. Are your opinion leaders on board?
5. Are there any other simultaneously occurring projects?

Getting early adopters and supporters working directly with the project is a smart move. Identifying reasons for apprehension and resistance among staff is also critical.

Key Point Actively including staff members who are not supportive of the service in its planning and development is an effective strategy to diminish resistance and speed acceptance.

Table 2-5. Stakeholder Identification and Engagement Tool

Stakeholder	Role	Impact on or Interests in Service	Delivering a Targeted Message
Patients and/or family/ caregiver	Receiver of care or lay care provider.	Consumers of the service.	Engaging potential patients to determine interests or value of service. Survey past patients to determine satisfaction.
Physicians and provider staff	Patient care (top rung of ladder in care determination).	Improved patient-care outcomes, key driver of medication selection and therapy. Some will see service as threat to autonomy and income vs. welcome addition to team to decompress providers and enable improved care.	Focus on patient-care outcomes (i.e., safety, satisfaction), provision of complementary services, and possible revenue enhancement.
Administrators	Responsible for care quality and financial performance of clinic or institution.	Patient-care outcomes, improved productivity, impact on financial bottom line (i.e., new revenue vs. cost savings), return on investment, improved patient satisfaction, improved market competitiveness.	Understand key goals of administrator. What are key institutional or practice site strategic plans? Try to relate outcomes of service to these goals. Keep message and goals *very* brief and concise. Avoid clinical jargon. Know where you fit in the organizational structure, mission, vision, and goals.
Finance (billing)	Financial viability of organization or practice site.	Ability of service to save money or generate new revenue.	Must have strong financial plan/ proposal with metrics and timelines. Consider engaging low- mid-level finance staff for guidance before delivering financial data to finance director. Clinical outcomes may have value, but must have financial impact info to gain approval in most cases.
Compliance officer/ office of compliance	Designs, implements, and maintains a compliance program that supports the code of conduct and prevents, detects, and responds appropriately to violations of law and applicable health care regulations. This can include billing and regulatory processes.	Ensure care providers are acting within institutional and regulatory limits of approval. Ensure billing of services is within legal, contractual, and acceptable standards of practice (i.e., method and process for pharmacy billing of clinical services).	May approach for early guidance regarding hospital policies or payer contracts. Positions of compliance officers may be very fiscally conservative. Consider gathering legal, regulatory, and/or examples of similar models prior to initiating formal discussions or submission of proposal.

Table 2-5. Stakeholder Identification and Engagement Tool (cont'd)

Stakeholder	Role	Impact on or Interests in Service	Delivering a Targeted Message
Risk managers	Overall goal is improvement of the quality of care and to eliminate or minimize the number of accidents with an eye toward claims prevention.	Will want to ensure new service is improving care/decreasing risk and not opening possibility of new risks. May be concerned with legal claims for inappropriate care by pharmacists.	Underscore possible risk/harm reduction related to appropriate medication use and improved safety. Be able to explain communication plan with providers and patients. Understand legal boundaries of care that may be provided by pharmacists. Consider malpractice coverage.
Nurses	Primary providers of direct patient care. Patient advocates.	Nurses are often most impacted by changes in the process or structure of care. Some pharmacy services may duplicate nursing efforts and create some territorial tension. RNs may feel that aspects of their work, perhaps those they find rewarding, could be lost.	Engage nursing leaders in administration, nurse/clinic managers, and patient care nurses (in impacted areas) proactively to gain information on issues they see around current patient care. Work early and often with them to show improved outcomes for patients and to smooth out processes and define rolls.
Laboratory managers	Quality assurance related to handling of tests and assays. Patient billing for services (revenue center). Patient throughput in care cycle. Timely and accurate data dissemination. Direct patient care role with venipuncture and lab draws.	Any point of care (POC) testing by new pharmacy service may bring up issues of standardization and calibration of equipment to meet industry or institutional standards, accuracy of results (compared to lab methods and assays), pharmacy billing for services (loss of lab revenue), confusion in patient-care processes (which labs/draws done where and when?). Also, if pharmacy will need lab to complete testing (i.e., INR for anticoagulation clinic). Coordination of process for rapid results may be needed.	Engage the lab manager early on POC testing issues or any new services impact (i.e., increased demand, rapid results reporting). Be prepared to share examples of similar care processes in other sites. Offer technical specifications info on POS equipment that may be used. Discuss coordination of care issues that might arise with pharmacy service (i.e., exactly which tests and for which patients).
Quality and performance improvement managers	These persons will monitor regulatory and payer quality standards and help direct implementation of care or efficiency improvements. They often have access to the best-quality data regarding care outcomes. Roles vary among practice sites.	Quality and performance managers will know what the priority targets are for improving care. They assist with access to possible sources of data to establish or refine your targeted "need." They will likely be interested in your ideas to improve care and be good supporters and champions. These persons often have direct access to key players in the organization.	Approach these persons early. Ask questions to find out what the focus areas are for their position. Some will have more of a financial or process improvement role vs. a quality of care role. Pitch your proposal based on this area of emphasis.

Table 2-5. Stakeholder Identification and Engagement Tool (cont'd)

Stakeholder	Role	Impact on or Interests in Service	Delivering a Targeted Message
Clinic/office managers	Responsible for the smooth operation of the direct care area. Generally manage staff and processes. Track productivity data, including financial.	Depending on your specific proposal, this stakeholder may be one of the most heavily impacted. They are often gatekeepers for changes that affect processes of care and staff roles. These roles are often filled by nurses.	You will need to package your proposal to show the benefits to patient care and/or efficiency from the day-to-day running of the clinic or office. Since nurses are often the largest proportion of staff and these roles are often filled by nurses, keep that professional perspective in mind.
Medical director	The interface for the medical staff with the institutional administrators. The medical director acts as go-between for physician issues and institutional or administrative needs.	Physicians are the foremost voice for patient care, and the medical director is the ultimate physician leader. There can be no more potent voice to support your patient care proposal than the medical director.	It is important to realize that this person is in a highly political position. Approach them with the patient-care issues foremost, but they will also need to understand that you have considered the financial impact for administration. Show how you plan to work with doctors to improve care.
Payers	In most systems, insurers and payers will be a significant factor. In managed-care systems, employer payers may be more significant. Also consider cash pay in certain markets.	Clearly, payers have interests in provision of effective, efficient, high-value care. While they might not be at the table for internal decisions, your payer mix will be a significant factor in the financial assessment of your proposal.	Contracting is a vital part to gaining reimbursement with all payers. Specific criteria for billing will be needed. You will need to work with your finance/billing dept. Keep in mind the payers' perspective and what drives their business. If you are working with a PDP/Part D Medicare plan, they might not be as incentivized to pay for services that improve quality of care but increase drug use (costs).
Board of directors (BOD)	A group of directors or advisors that provide ultimate oversight for organizational direction and performance.	Recently there has been an increased drive to ensure the BOD is well-connected to critical performance indicators for health care facilities. If your project is high-level and/or serves as a model for improving care quality or efficiency, then it may be possible to get your service proposal or early results in front of this group.	The support or blessings of the BOD is a huge sign of support that will resonate throughout the organization. Don't try to inflate the value or scope of the project; simply report your plans, goals, and any outcomes. Keep in mind the board members are not all health care professionals. Match your key points to high-level organizational outcomes, mission, vision, and accreditation requirements.

INR = international normalized ratio; PDP = prescription drug plans.

The Service Proposal or Business Plan

You've done a lot of contemplating, researching, data analyzing, and networking thus far in this chapter. Now all of these elements must come together in the form of the service proposal or business plan. Check with your manager or site administrator to see if your organization uses a standard business or service plan. You can also ask for a good example of a recently used proposal. A good proposal should be an inclusive but concise document that contains the need met by the service, a description of the service, the resource requirements, the financial overview, and the benefits. This is explored further in Chapter 3.

Chapter Summary

Robust ambulatory clinical pharmacy practices tend to sprout from the launch of a successful service that provides high-quality care and delivers value to the business or organization. Once an opportunity for improving care has been identified, a strategic approach to the development of a successful service involves defining the service type and the delivery model appropriate for your practice setting. Determining the resource needs for the new service, as well as opportunities to offset expenditures through revenue generation, cost avoidance, and improved efficiencies, will build your service plan. It is possible to further demonstrate value for your service through improving patient-care outcomes and satisfaction, enhancing quality indicator performance, and ensuring compliance with regulatory requirements. Since all patient care efforts require collaboration with others, identification of key partners and stakeholders is another important step in ensuring the success of a new service. The knowledge and information gained in completing the key objectives just mentioned will serve as the key components of your service proposal.

If you have taken time to consider the key attributes—valuable, scalable, reproducible, and sustainable—then your service can be the foundation for establishing a successful clinical pharmacy practice for years to come.

References

1. Kuo GM, Buckley TE, Fitzsimmons DS, et al. Collaborative drug therapy management services and reimbursement in a family medicine clinic. *Am J Health-Syst Pharm*. 2004;61:343-354.

2. Health and Human Services homepage. U.S. Department of Health & Human Services. http://www.hhs.gov/valuedriven/index.html. Accessed November 10, 2010.

3. Chisholm-Burns MA, Vaillencourt AM, Shepherd M. *Pharmacy Management, Leadership, Marketing and Finance*. Sudbury, MA: Jones & Bartlett Publ.; 2010.

4. Advocacy. New York State Council of Health-System Pharmacists Website. http://www.nyschp.org/displaycommon.cfm?an=1&subarticlenbr=52. Accessed Aug. 2, 2010.

5. Noronha G [Conversation]. Baltimore, MD: Johns Hopkins Community Physicians at Wyman Park; May 2008.

6. Mechanic D, McAlpine DD, Rosenthal M. Are patients' office visits with physicians getting shorter? *N Engl J Med*. 2001;344(3):198-204.

7. 2009 Real estate investment outlook. Marcus & Millichap's medical office research report; Oct. 12, 2009. kippinvestmentgroup.com/upload/files/SecHalf2009_MarcusMillichap_MedicalOfficeSpecial Report.pdf. Accessed August 3, 2010.

8. 2009-2010 Chain pharmacy industry profile. National Association of Chain Drug Stores, 2009. http://nacds.org/wmspage.cfm?parm1=6264. Accessed on August 3, 2010.

9. 2010 Pharmacy compensation survey—spring edition. *Pharmacy Week.* http://www.pharmacyweek.com/job_seeker/salary/salary.asp?article_id=13026&etp=0&section=about. Accessed August 2, 2010.

10. Scott A. Pharmacists salary survey. *Drug Topics: The Newsmagazine for Pharmacists;* March 1, 2009. http://drugtopics.modernmedicine.com/pay. Accessed April 15, 2010.

11. Chiquette E, Amato MG, Bussey HI. Comparison of an anticoagulation clinic and usual medical care: Anticoagulation control, patient outcomes, and health care costs. *Arch Int Med.* 1998;158:1641-1647.

12. Chamberlain MA. The vertically integrated pharmacy department. *Am J Health-Syst Pharm.* 1998;55:669-675.

13. Nichol A, Downs GE. The pharmacist as physician extender in family medicine office practice. *J Am Pharm Assoc.* 2006;46:77-83.

14. Chisholm-Burns MA, Lee JK, Spivey CK, et. al. US pharmacists' effect as team members on patient care: Systemic review and meta-analysis. *Med Care.* 2010;48:923-933.

15. Chisholm-Burns MA, Graff Zivin JS, Lee JK, et. al. Economic effects of pharmacists on health outcomes in the United States: A systematic review. *Am J Health-Syst Pharm.* 2010;67(19):1624-1634.

16. Zillich AJ, McDonough RP, Carter BL, et al. Influential characteristics of physician/pharmacist collaborative relationships. *Ann Pharmacother.* 2004;38:764-770.

Additional Selected References

Epplen K, Dusing-Wiest M, Freedlund J, et al. Stepwise approach to implementing ambulatory clinical pharmacy services. *Am J Health-Syst Pharm.* 2007;64:945-951.

Harris MH, Baker E, Berry TM, et al. Developing a business-practice model for pharmacy services in ambulatory settings. *Pharmacotherapy.* 2008;28(2):7e-34e.

Snella KA, Sachdev GP. A primer for developing pharmacist-managed clinics in the outpatient setting. *Pharmacotherapy.* 2003;23:1153-1166.

Web Resources

Resource Needs Worksheet

Revenue from Reimbursement Worksheet

Sample Scope of Practice

Sample Case: Medication Therapy Management Service

Web Toolkit available at
www.ashp.org/ambulatorypractice

Developing a Business Plan for an Ambulatory Practice

Kelly Epplen, Paul W. Bush

CHAPTER
3

Chapter Outline

1. Introduction
2. The Business Plan Process
3. Chapter Summary
4. References
5. Additional Selected References
6. Web Resources

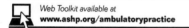
Web Toolkit available at
www.ashp.org/ambulatorypractice

Chapter Objectives

1. Recognize the importance of a sound business plan.

2. Discuss the process for developing a business plan for a new ambulatory service.

3. Apply the concepts of business plan development to a desired ambulatory clinical service area.

4. Prepare a business plan document to present to administrators.

Introduction

Creation or expansion of ambulatory clinical pharmacy services requires planning and the dedication of resources, equipment, and facilities. Whether it is for a new service, additional space, equipment, personnel, or a renovation, developing a written business plan will help you communicate the proposal, secure funding, guide the initiative, and keep it on track.

You may find it useful to use a standardized approach to allocating resources, similar to a process practiced by larger health care organizations. In such organizations, there is an annual planning process during which the organization receives requests for major new programs, projects, and equipment. These requests are cat-

egorized by type and size of the investment and then reviewed by the organization's
budget review committees and leadership.

A key to success in acquiring new resources is the ability to clearly communicate the value of the proposal to the organization. This is accomplished through
the development of a business plan. The business plan is a document with a standard
format and structure that clearly explains the what, why, when, who, and how of the
project. It is a comprehensive explanation of the opportunity the plan presents, the
people involved in it, the money required to implement it, where the money will
come from, and the plan's value, financial or otherwise, to the organization.[1]

 Clearly communicating the value of the proposal is key to
acquiring the new resources you will need.

This chapter describes the process you will need to follow to develop, write,
and present a business plan.

The Business Plan Process

There are six basic steps to the business plan process:

1. Conceptualizing the initiative

2. Researching the feasibility and details of the concept

3. Evaluating and refining the concept based on data obtained

4. Outlining the business plan

5. Preparing the business plan document

6. Presenting the plan

Step 1: Conceptualizing the Initiative

Health care and the profession of pharmacy continue to evolve in the pursuit of
improving the public's health. The many unmet health care needs and extremely
high cost of disease, linked with the important role medications play in improving
patient outcomes, results in many opportunities for the ambulatory clinical pharmacist to develop new programs and services.

For example, ambulatory pharmacists can play a vital role in the safe transition
of patients from inpatient hospitalization to the outpatient setting by implementing services that improve continuity of care. Acute and chronic conditions requiring complicated drug therapy are associated with high rates of readmission if medications are not optimally prescribed or taken appropriately. Pharmacist-managed
anticoagulation services, heart failure clinics, and diabetes management services all

have been shown to reduce costs, to improve clinical outcomes, and to be associated with high levels of patient satisfaction. Regardless of the ambulatory setting or proposed service, creation of a well-thought-out business plan will enhance the likelihood of achieving success.

Developing a business plan for a new ambulatory pharmacy service begins with a thorough understanding of your organization's current services and its ability to meet the needs of your patients. Your proposal for new or expanded services should fill the gaps in existing services and improve access or add new services. The needs assessment of your organization, conducted during the planning process (as discussed in Chapter 2), should result in identifying and prioritizing opportunities for clinical ambulatory pharmacy services. Examples of the types of opportunities you may identify include adding pharmacist staff to participate in the medication reconciliation process, establishing an ambulatory patient care practice such as anticoagulation or medication therapy management, or opening a new ambulatory pharmacy providing innovative services. Each of these proposals begins as a concept that, after you conduct your analysis, may result in a business plan and eventually a new service.

Your proposal for new or expanded services should fill the gaps in existing services.

Step 2: Researching the Feasibility and Details of the Concept

You will find developing a business plan is more a business project than a writing assignment.[2] A successful business plan will contain extensive background information and a clear and comprehensive description of the program or service you wish to create or expand. Background information is obtained by a thorough review of published literature describing similar programs or services, as discussed in Chapter 1. In many cases, new and more innovative programs may not be well-documented in the literature, so communication among pharmacy leaders and colleagues, site visits to learn about similar programs, and attendance at professional meetings are great alternatives. Another source of information on programs and services and their value are white papers or "best practice" guidelines published by national health care organizations, such as the American Society of Health-System Pharmacists, American Pharmacists Association, American College of Clinical Pharmacy, the Joint Commission, etc.

CASE

Continuing with the case introduced in Chapter 2 regarding Dr. Busybee, your next step is to create the business plan for your services. You research the published literature on ambulatory pharmacists providing services for diabetes and warfarin management for atrial fibrillation and find a number of excellent citations supporting this type of service (see Table 1-9 in Chapter 1). The background section of your business plan will be a summary of the published literature. You also speak with a colleague practicing in your state who has successfully been providing a similar service in a physician's office for approximately 1 year. You include a summary of your colleagues' services in the background material as well.

Step 3: Evaluating and Refining the Concept Based on Data Obtained

Once the research and data collection process is underway, the information gained should be used as a basis for evaluating the feasibility of the concept in your setting. Here you reassess the concept and modify it to ensure both a good fit for your organization and its success. Conducting a thorough evaluation at this stage is time and effort well invested because you may defer or eliminate concepts with no future and pursue only the initiatives you believe are viable. The key steps in performing a thorough evaluation are provided to you in Chapter 2.

Step 4: Outlining the Business Plan

The business plan is composed of several sections addressing the specifics of your proposed service. The main goal of this chapter is to allow you to use the basic components of the business plan outlined and to apply them to your particular ambulatory service proposal. Not all business plans may need to contain all components discussed here nor have the depth of detail included in the plan described below. Before writing your business plan, meet with the decision makers in your organizations to best understand what key elements they desire in your proposal. You will want to tailor your particular business plan to those elements and your organization's unique mission and vision. The plan for a new pharmacy service should include the following sections. (See the web site for a checklist of these sections and complete business plan.)

- Cover page
- Table of contents
- Executive summary
- Description of the proposed program or service
- Consistency with the organization's mission
- Market analysis
- Marketing plan
- Facility and equipment
- Management and organization
- Financial summary
- Evaluation

Step 5: Preparing the Business Plan Document

Cover Page

The first page of the business plan is the cover page. This page should include the following information: name of the plan, month and year the plan was prepared, and the name and contact information of the preparers. **Figure** 3-1 is an example of a cover sheet.

Business Plan
For
Ambulatory Heart Failure Clinic

Plan prepared March 2010

Sally G. Jones, Pharm.D.
Director of Pharmacy Services
Department of Pharmacy Services

Logo

Figure 3-1. Sample Business Plan Cover Sheet

Table of Contents

Although this section of the business plan is self-explanatory, remember this is the guide readers will use to reference your document, so it is very important that the page numbers align with the headers. It seems simplistic, but this small aspect can set the tone for your business plan and show your attention to detail.

Executive Summary

The executive summary is the most important section of your business plan. It must be clear and succinct and be written with adequate enthusiasm to compel readers to review the entire document. It is brief, one to three pages in length, and written in narrative style, drawing information from each section of the business plan. The summary should be written after the entire plan is complete. It should demonstrate that your initiative makes sense, is thoroughly planned, can be accomplished by your team, meets an organization need, and is financially viable. An example of an executive summary is included in the sample business plan. (Sample Business Plan for an Ambulatory Heart Failure Clinic) 🖳

The first major section of the plan provides an overview of the program or service you are proposing. For example, if you propose to open a new ambulatory clinic, you would describe the location, scope of services provided, benefits, staff involved, how the clinic fulfills a need not currently provided, rationale, and reference to other organizations that may provide similar clinical ambulatory pharmacy services. Completing the planning process as described in Chapters 1 and 2 should aid you in this section. If this is the first ambulatory clinic for your organization, information describing the prevalence of ambulatory pharmacy services in other similar organizations and rationale for your organization to provide this service should be included.

In this section of the plan, you should include the following information:

1. The anticipated start date and rationale for the needed time frame

2. Anticipated financial trends

3. Anticipated volume trends

4. Previous program history, if applicable

CASE

For Dr. Busybee's clinic, you do the following:

1. You anticipate that once the business plan is approved you will require 4 months to organize and set up your clinic. You will need a small build-out for space and time to order equipment and supplies, train staff, and work on policy and procedures to ensure ease of patient flow through the clinic.

2. Using your financial analysis from Chapter 2, you outline the financial plan in detail. Initially, the clinic will run at a financial loss as your only direct revenue from " incident-to" billing will not cover your costs. You then create a timeline with your calculations for anticipated revenue from improvement in performance from the performance-based payer contracts and revenue based on increased efficiencies, as well as potential new patient recruitment.

> **3. As noted in Chapter 2, you anticipate 76 visits per month based on Dr. Busybee's targeted patient population. You describe Dr. Busybee's current clinic situation of high patient load, inability to attract and retain new patients, and risk for poor performance on key disease management indicators for diabetes and atrial fibrillation.**

Consistency with Mission

This section of the business plan explains how the proposed program serves to support the mission, vision, philosophy, and strategic objectives of your organization. It is advisable to develop a mission and vision for your program that supports the larger organizations' statements. (Refer back to Chapter 1 if you need to refresh your memory on the purpose and intent of a mission and vision statement.) You should always align your proposed programs and services with the goals of your organization. Doing so improves the potential for approval.

Given the finite nature of financial resources, a major consideration for any new program development is cost of the program and return on investment (ROI). You may wish to reference ROI information found in the literature for clinical pharmacy services to help support your cause.[3] Your estimates of ROI for your particular program will be contained in the financial summary; however, you may state in this section that you expect a return on investment similar to that of other programs.

Other positive impacts on organizational performance should be clearly stated; for example, patient satisfaction may be improved with decreased wait times in Dr. Busybee's clinic. If there are ethical issues in your clinic that need to be addressed, such as providing care for unfunded patients, they should be discussed in this section of the plan. Perhaps your program facilitates access to medications for the uninsured: this could be clearly highlighted as a service that supports your mission.

The role the program may play in meeting the needs of the community or special needs of specific providers or patients should be addressed. For example, if the mission of your organization is "to provide comprehensive and compassionate care that improves the health of the people you serve," the role that the program plays to promote this mission should be clearly defined.

Market Analysis

When you decide to propose a new program, that decision is based on the premise that it would provide a service for which there is a need. The business plan should clearly identify the market (i.e., group of customers with a set of common characteristics who want to buy the service) for the new program. Examples of customers include (but are not limited to) a particular patient population, other health providers, organizational administration, third-party organizations, employees, etc. Ultimately, the consumer of the ambulatory pharmacy patient care services is the patient; however, these services actually affect a broader market as listed below.

- Physicians and other health care providers: Your proposed service can unburden these professionals by providing education, monitoring, dose titration, medication reconciliation, and other supportive services, allowing them to see more patients.

- Payers (insurers, self-ensured employers): Your service can ultimately reduce cost of care by reducing hospitalizations, emergency room visits, or long-term consequences of chronic disease.

- Health care administrators: Your service may help them meet quality initiatives, reduce costs and inappropriate utilization, such as emergency room visits or hospital readmissions, and potentially recruit more patients into your organization.

CASE

For Dr. Busybee's clinic, the proposed services will unburden the physician by providing services for diabetic and atrial fibrillation patients. The service will also improve payer-requested quality measures and allow for recruitment of more patients into the clinic.

In this section of the plan, you should discuss any barriers to market entry and projected trends of your market (is the need for your service growing or shrinking?). As you conducted your needs assessment or market analysis, you most likely identified particular barriers you anticipate or know or to exist as well the potential growth of your program. Describe how you identified these issues in the business plan, describe how you came to these conclusions, and offer solutions for how you plan to overcome any barriers. Common barriers to an ambulatory patient-care service implementation may include the following examples:

- Lack of stakeholder buy-in: Your physicians and administrators may be unfamiliar and uncomfortable with the proposed role of the pharmacist.

- Work load issues: In order for the pharmacy staff to assume this role, other personnel would need to be hired or to pick up the staff's current duties.

- Budgetary considerations: There are limited financial resources to initiate the service.

- Recruitment issues: There is a shortage of adequately trained pharmacists or pharmacists willing to expand to this type of service in your rural area of the country.

- Licensure and regulatory barriers: Your state does not allow for, or is restrictive in, its collaborative practice regulations.

- Reimbursement and pricing issues: A major payer allows only minimal reimbursement that does not cover the costs of your program.

- Staff competency: You currently do not have on your staff a pharmacist who is adequately trained in management of patients with heart failure.

A section should define the customer profile or target population of patients, health care providers, and others who may want to use your new services. Include as many of the following market analysis items that will provide the support you need for your proposed service (Table 3-1).

Table 3-1. Key Market Analysis Items: Dr. Busybee's Clinic

Market Analysis Item	Discussion
Demographics	Currently in clinic: 60 diabetic patients. 35 warfarin patients.
Primary and secondary geographic areas served	Currently serving patients in primarily one clinic. There are two other primary physician groups within the clinic complex with similar problems of patient load and meeting key performance measures.
Referral sources	Dr. Busybee, with potential to expand to other clinic physicians.
Historical and projected	Dr. Busybee 2 years ago had 30 diabetic patients market size and 15 patients on warfarin. These numbers have doubled in the past 2 years. The market demographics have changed as the population is becoming older, and there has been a growth of the Hispanic population.
Potential market growth	Community census expects both the elderly and Hispanic populations to continue to grow.
Target disease state prevalence	The incidence of diabetes is nearly double in the Hispanic population compared to a non-Hispanic population.[4] The incidence of atrial fibrillation in the elderly is 5% to 6% and doubles for those who have other cardiovascular conditions.[5]
Epidemiological information	Diabetes is a contributor to 70% of lost work days for patients in our clinic. The clinic's time within goal for INRs is 40%.
Estimated health care	20% of clinic hospital medication-related emergency utilization room visits and hospital admissions are due to warfarin complications. 10% of hospital admissions for clinic patients are due to uncontrolled diabetes.
Economic impact	Reducing hospital readmission rates for both of the targeted conditions by 10% would save an estimated $1 million in health care expenses.

Be sure to describe those key characteristics of your service that will highlight the quality level planned. Benchmarking with other similar programs, either through the literature or colleagues, can be used to measure the quality of your service. Chapter 7 will go into greater detail on how to best choose a set of quality measures for your service.

Current standards of care or clinical practice guidelines are terrific resources to help determine your level of service and the optimal goals, measures, and desired outcomes of your program. Your organization may already have quality and out-come measures it is required to (or has chosen to) collect. Aligning your measures and outcomes to support, improve, or complement your organization's measures is a good idea.

The economics of the market should be included if applicable to your proposed service. For example, a major insurer in your market is aggressively pursuing value-based insurance design for your patient population. In this payment model, attention to evidence-based therapy and procedures that improve patient outcomes is key, which your proposed program can support in an efficient and cost-effective manner. A statement on how well your pharmacist-based program can serve your market in terms of resources, strengths, and weaknesses will reinforce the proposal. Use the SWOT analysis from Chapter 1 on similar existing ambulatory clinical pharmacy programs to help you develop a specific SWOT analysis for your program.

In order for leadership in your organization to be willing to invest in your business plan, you will need to predict continued success in future years. As difficult as it is to predict, a business plan should include a discussion of the market trend over the ensuing 5 years. When thinking about the future, consider addressing it through the following four categories:

- Clinical: Current changes focusing on how health care is provided, such as quality of care and patient safety, will create new and expanded opportunities for clinical pharmacy services.

- Technology: New technology may bring new services into the marketplace that may positively or negatively affect your new program. For example, the development of point-of-care testing devices can greatly impact the efficiency of service and facilitate clinical decision making. However, costs associated with technology must be considered and accounted for in the business plan.

- Reimbursement: A breakthrough in evidence and value may turn the tide in ambulatory pharmacy reimbursement, much like what we have seen with the cognitive reimbursement rates for providing immunizations within pharmacy practice.

- Your site: Looking at the community your site services, there may be a growing number of diabetics or elderly, creating an even greater need for services your program proposes in the next 5 years.

As important as conducting your needs analysis is keeping abreast of developing changes within the health care industry (within your state and nationally) in order to understand how it is currently affecting your organization and how it may do so in the future. This may seem overwhelming; however, ready to help you are knowledgeable staff within the pharmacy organizations as well as experts from your colleges of pharmacy.

Marketing Plan

A good marketing plan is essential to business development and success.[6] If this is a foreign concept to you, as it is to many pharmacists, use the discussion in Chapter 4 to assist you with this section. You will want to inform potential customers of the new service as well as have a plan for ongoing marketing efforts. The initial focus of the marketing plan will be to introduce the new service. You will want to develop an overall strategy, but also include tactics for each key target group (patients, other health care providers, payers, etc.). Collateral materials and media should be described to provide the readers of your plan additional insight on how the new service will be promoted. Consider promotional materials such as brochures, posters, flyers, and newsletters, as well as electronic media such as web sites, mass e-mails, Twitter, and blogs to outline the service specifications. A schedule for introducing the new service and promoting it should be included, as well as a general plan for tracking results of the marketing effort. Schedule meetings with key stakeholders to promote the service, solicit their help to identify ideal candidates for your service, and explain to them your referral procedures. Examples of tracking mechanisms may include patient and staff surveys that identify what is the most effective marketing piece for your service. Questions such as "how did you hear about our service?" can be very informative and allow you to concentrate promotional material in that arena.

CASE

In Dr. Busybee's clinic, you identify the patients and clinic staff as the key initial targets for your marketing plan. Patients may not understand why they are now seeing you instead of Dr. Busybee. You will need the entire staff to understand and support this change and assist in educating patients. You plan in-services for all staff to explain your new service and how the service benefits the patients, Dr. Busybee, and the clinic in general. Your marketing plan for patients is to begin advertising and educating on the new service 30 days before your clinic opens. You will use posters and flyers outlining how this new service will help better meet their needs and that Dr. Busybee will remain completely involved in their care. For your long-term marketing plan, you describe a program that will roll out to your payers targeting the poor performance on key disease management indicators.

Facility, Technology, and Equipment

Many new pharmacy services require additional facilities or modification of existing facilities. Securing space may be as challenging as obtaining the commitment for financial resources. The plan should indicate the planned or proposed physical location for the clinic and its availability, including the required square footage and a description plus schematic of the layout. The extent of work needed and plan for construction or renovation should be discussed. Be sure to include a time frame for any construction or renovation. Include in this section office fixtures and equipment, technology such as computer software and hardware, and point-of-care diagnostic instruments you may need. Review Chapter 2, which described many of the items you may need for your clinic. The financial details, including cost of construction, will be included in the financial section of the business plan.

Management and Organization

Most new pharmacy programs or services established in health systems will report directly to the leadership of the department of pharmacy services. A pharmacy department may have divisions in one or more legal entities of the health system (i.e., not for profit or for profit, inpatient, ambulatory services, or home care divisions), and the type of new program or services may dictate in which legal entity it will reside. The business plan should clearly indicate the capabilities and expertise of the department's management team and how the new program will be overseen. The organizational structure, often termed a reporting structure, should be provided as a diagram with the new program and line of authority highlighted. If the plan calls for new managers, pharmacists, or support staff, availability of competent staff and the timing of bringing them on the payroll should be discussed. A staffing plan should be developed and included in this section of the business plan. Contractual relationships, such as contracted staffing, should be described. The impact that the new program will have on other programs and services within the department and outside the department should be discussed.

If your program will be in a physician's office or clinic, or another setting not associated with a health system, the program may report to a clinic administrator, medical director in charge of clinical services, or someone entirely different. It is most important for you to report to someone who possesses a full understanding of the type of service you will provide and all the nuances of the business plan you are proposing. In these settings, include your direct supervisor as a key stakeholder (see Chapter 2) and keep him or her completely informed of your role, the proposed program, and any changes that occur. Keeping this person in the loop will help to guarantee his or her complete support.

An implementation plan with a timetable indicating key milestones should be developed and provided in this section of the business plan. The overall size and complexity of the project and availability of funding will influence the scope and timeline of the implementation plan. Many brand new services may take from 6 to 18 months from start to finish; others that are similar to already established programs may be operational within weeks if administrative support, clinic space, and staff are already available.

Financial Summary

This section of the business plan summarizes the financial information and is commonly provided in appended tables, spreadsheets, and graphs. Guidelines to consider in preparing the financial forms to include in your business plan include the following:

- Be conservative
- Be honest
- Use standard formats and financial terms
- Be consistent and seek the advice of the financial services staff within your organization or the services of an established accountant

The actual expenses and revenues of your program will always be of primary interest to those approving your program. Chapter 2 began the discussion of various funding options, and Chapter 8 will guide you in the various options available to fund your service and address the economical barriers to your service. Include costs avoided by implementation of the program, especially if this is the optimal method to financially support your program.

The type and location of your new program will dictate which forms to include. Health system–based proposals often include the following:

- A start-up expense budget
- Staffing budget (based on the staffing plan)
- Projected payer mix
- A 3–5 year pro forma income (profit and loss) statement showing volumes, expenses and revenues, and assumptions

A pro forma, simply put, is your best estimate of anticipated expenses and revenues for your program over the next 3–5 years. Even though the tables, spreadsheets, and graphs are critical, the narrative of this section of the business plan should provide adequate detail, such that review of the financial forms is optional.

Evaluation

You should monitor the performance of the new program or service closely during the first year to make programmatic adjustments to ensure success. As you may have noticed in developing your program and business plan, many assumptions were necessary, and down the line you may need to make adjustments. Be sure to include the performance indicators in the business plan that will help you define the success of your program and include the frequency of their monitoring. Suggested indicators should include those that define success from a financial, clinical, market, and patient satisfaction perspective. Successful performance of certain indicators may be critical for program success, and you should closely monitor those chosen for a quarterly report to those above you in the reporting structure, such as the chief pharmacy officer or your organization's key administrator. The health care organization's leaders may be more supportive and willing to approve programs that include criteria for program success (and continuance).

CASE

For Dr. Busybee's clinic, your team determines the key to evaluating the success of your program is to address the issues for measurement that initiated the discussion to create your program. Therefore, the measures you choose for your business plan include the following:

- Financial
    - Reimbursement rate from performance contracts
    - Cost/revenue for your clinic
- Clinical
    - HgA1c
    - INR in range
- Market

> -   Number of new patients
> • Patient
>   -   Patient wait times in clinic
>   -   Patient satisfaction for your program's service

Step 6: Presenting the Plan

Your business plan should be a formal document that has been carefully edited and proofread by multiple reviewers. Be sure that the language is clear and the graphs and charts enhance the message. Several references are available devoted to developing business plans and providing guidance on layout design and presentation.[6] Using both black and white and color in your document will improve the presentation. You will want a polished, complete look, so consider binding the plan.

Many health care organizations have new program budget review committees that convene to hear presentation of new program requests. If your organization does not have such a process, plan a face-to-face meeting with the decision makers of your organization. A well-prepared slide presentation of the business plan is expected. Provide a copy of the business plan to each member of the committee or decision maker prior to the committee meeting. A professional, succinct, but comprehensive presentation that displays your commitment and enthusiasm for your program will go a long way.

CASE

Once your business plan is completed, Dr. Busybee places you on the agenda for the office's next administrative team meeting as well as the next physician group meeting. You provide a copy of your formal proposal to the administrative team (several key physicians, office legal representative, office accountant, office manager, and the compliance officer) 2 weeks prior to the meeting. You prepare a Power Point presentation of your business plan for presentation at both meetings, summarizing your proposed service and outlining the pros and cons identified in the plan.

Your plan and presentations were well received at both meetings and generated positive discussion. You were congratulated on the thoroughness of your preparation and receive final approval 2 weeks later.

Chapter Summary

There are many factors that contribute to acceptance of new program business plans. The organization's availability of funds and current funding preferences will be overriding factors. A well-done business plan is important and in many organizations is critical to gaining approval for programs that require significant resources.

In summary, whether you are proposing the implementation of a diabetes management service within a large health system or a medication therapy management service within a small community physician office, the process of business plan development is an essential component to your success. A thorough understanding of current services provided within your organization is required as well as an understanding of existing gaps in care that will be met by your program. The example outline provided in this chapter is intended to walk you through the essential components of the business plan from conceptualization of the initiative to presentation to organizational administration. The business plan should support and promote your organization's mission: the proposed service should be marketed as a solution to gaps in care identified in the plan. A sound business plan will estimate the economic impact of your service and potential benefits realized by the organization, patients, staff, and community.

References

1. Schumock GL, ed. *How to Develop a Business Plan for Clinical Pharmacy Services: A Guide for Managers and Clinicians.* Kansas City, KS: American College of Clinical Pharmacy; 2001.

2. Abrams R, ed. *The Successful Business Plan: Secrets and Strategies.* Palo Alto, CA: The Planning Shop; 2003, 13.

3. Perez A, Doloresco F, Hoffman JM, et al. Economic evaluations of clinical pharmacy services: 2001-2005. *Pharmacotherapy.* 2008;28:285e-323e.

4. CDC. Fact Sheet. The prevalence of diabetes among Hispanics in six U.S. geographical regions. http://www.cdc.gov/diabetes/pubs/pdf/hispanic.pdf. Accessed 4/28/2011.

5. Furberg CD, Psaty BM, Manolio TA, et al. Prevalence of atrial fibrillation in elderly subjects (the Cardiovascular Health Study). *Am J Cardiol.* 1994;74:236-241.

6. U.S. Small Business Administration. *How to Write a Business Plan.* http://www.sba.gov/smallbusinessplanner/plan/writeabusinessplan/index.html. Accessed March 19, 2010.

Additional Selected References

Epplen K, Dusing-Wiest M, Freedland J, et al. Stepwise approach to implementing ambulatory clinical pharmacy services. *Am J Health-Syst Pharm.* 2007;64:945-951.

Web Resources

Business Plan Template

Sample Business Plan for an Ambulatory Heart Failure Clinic

Web Toolkit available at
www.ashp.org/ambulatorypractice

Marketing Your Ambulatory Practice

Mary Ann Kliethermes, Tim R. Brown,
Tara L. Jenkins, Kevin Charles Farmer

CHAPTER

4

Chapter Outline

1. Introduction
2. Understanding Consumer Behavior
3. Conducting Market Research
4. Creating the Marketing Plan
5. Chapter Summary
6. References
7. Web Resources

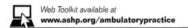
Web Toolkit available at
www.ashp.org/ambulatorypractice

Chapter Objectives

1. Identify the phases a consumer goes through during the decision-making process.

2. Recognize service characteristics that increase marketing difficulty and identify strategies to overcome the barriers.

3. Compare and contrast different methods for conducting market research.

4. Plan and execute an appropriate marketing strategy.

Introduction

An ambulatory care pharmacy practice, like any other type of business, requires marketing in order to be successful. Without it, a patient may not be aware that your service exists, a health care provider may not refer patients to you, an administrator may not include you in organizational plans, or a payer might not consider providing reimbursement for your services. Each of these scenarios decreases the likelihood of continued viability for your ambulatory care practice model.

Marketing is commonly mistaken as simply promoting an existing product or service, but according to the American Marketing Association, marketing is the "...processes for creating, communicating, delivering, and exchanging offerings that have value for customers, clients, partners, and society at large."[1] A definition that may resonate more with you as a clinician is provided by Hillestad and Berkowitz in their book on health care marketing: "Marketing is the process of understanding your customers' wants and needs, listening to those wants and needs and then, to whatever extent possible, designing appropriate programs and services to meet those wants and needs in a timely, cost-effective, competitive fashion. It is the process of molding your services to the market, rather than convincing the market your services are what they need."[2] There are several key concepts in both of these definitions. First is the word, *value*. You, as an ambulatory care pharmacist, may feel that the service you provide, no matter what its setting, has the ability to help patients achieve better health outcomes, but this does not necessarily equate to value for others. It is the buyers who need to feel your service is beneficial so they will exchange their offering of value: money. Second, you may have been trained in your residency to provide a diabetes-related service, but in the patient population you are planning to service, diabetes may be well controlled due to other providers or payer incentives already in place. Although it may be ideal and easier to create a service in which you are experienced, this may not be the need in the clinic in which you are proposing your service. If you do not understand your customers' needs, your attempts to add another cog into a currently well-oiled wheel may not work. Rather, you need to use those same skills to build a service that will meet something your customers are not currently doing well.

Key Point Marketing requires an understanding of the wants and needs of the consumers of your service and a plan or marketing strategy that successfully promotes and delivers your service at an acceptable cost, ultimately resulting in a satisfied customer.

Unlike other industries where there are one or, at most, two types of customers, an ambulatory care pharmacist is unique in that there are three to four target groups. Of course, as an ambulatory care pharmacist your primary customers are your patients, as they are the direct recipient of your services. Other health care providers, primarily physicians, who refer patients and with whom you will collaborate, are indirect consumers in that your services support their work and responsibilities in patient care. The patient usually does not pay for your service; therefore, payers or insurers are third-party customers with significant influence on how you will be reimbursed for your services. Most ambulatory care pharmacists will practice in larger organizations or a newer health care model, such as accountable care organizations, which add administrators as a fourth consumer. Administrators have the responsibility to keep the organization viable while providing quality health care services. They need to understand and determine which providers are best suited, considering licensing, knowledge, efficiency, and cost, to execute the business of patient care services within your organization. Administrators are customers in that you need to demonstrate that your pharmacy services fit as the best provider for a set of services provided or to be provided by the organization.

When marketing clinical services and understanding your customer or consumer behaviors, you need to consider and target all potential target groups.

Successful marketing for your ambulatory care clinic requires three steps. The first step is the basic understanding of your customers' behavior and the connection to the inherent characteristics associated with your services. It is essential to understand why and when a person makes a decision to fulfill an unmet need or want so that you know what information a person needs and when that person needs it in order to determine if your service offers something of value. It is also crucial to be aware of service characteristics that make it difficult for a buyer to determine value. In particular, there are several barriers to overcome when getting target groups to value a newer health care service such as pharmacist-provided services in an ambulatory clinic. After the first step of background knowledge is complete, the second step is conducting market research to understand target groups' wants and needs, as well to identify your potential competitors, and then determining how you can better meet the wants and needs of potential partners. Armed with all of this information, the third step is crafting the message that will convey your value to all groups and determining how you can most efficiently relay and deliver that message. This chapter provides the background information necessary to successfully complete each of these steps and provides useful tips and examples for how to incorporate the presented concepts into marketing your ambulatory care pharmacy model.

Understanding Consumer Behavior

Consumer behavior is the psychological processes individuals go through in recognizing needs and finding products or services that will meet those specific needs.[3] Of the numerous models proposed by marketers over the years, seemingly the most popular divides the consumer decision-making process into three stages.[4] In the pre-purchase phase, a consumer recognizes a need and searches for ways to meet that particular need. During consumption, the consumer chooses and procures a product or service. After this has occurred, a consumer will evaluate his or her experience. The reality of the post-purchase experience is compared to the expectations held prior to consumption.

Pre-purchase Phase

A model for buyer behavior is every stimulus engenders a response. This is where the consumer's decision-making journey begins: a stimulus that brings awareness to an individual's need. For a patient, especially with a chronic disease such as heart failure, this can be as simple as experiencing shortness of breath or leg swelling and desiring relief from those symptoms. For a diabetic patient, the stimulus could be the results of physician-ordered lab work, HgA1c levels, and the recognition that something must change if the patient wants to maintain or improve his or her current level of health. A physician may recognize that a large number of patients in the practice are not at therapeutic goals and need more intense education and monitoring regarding medications or diseases, and the physician does not have time to provide it. An administrator may note decreased pay for performance revenue due to the organization not achieving benchmarks for patient or disease state outcomes and thus is looking for effective cost-efficient changes in the processes to improve performance measures. A payer may note a certain population, such as heart failure patients, exceeding average yearly costs due to a high rate of rehospitalizations and be in search of a program that will effectively help control these costs. Each of these consumers may not have considered or sought out pharmacist-provided ambulatory patient care services, but each may find, if informed, that these services address his or her current health stimuli. As you think of marketing, how do you as an individual practitioner ensure that you are considered a potential solution to each of these customers' needs?

CASE

Dr. Busybee realized he was going to lose one of his biggest payers if he did not find a way to decrease patients' HgbA1c levels as well as increase the percentage of time their INRs were in target range. His administrators prompted him to research what would be needed to meet the payer's treatment goals. This research led him to conclude that the clinical pharmacy services you plan to provide will help him with his patient care goals. You both meet with the office administrative team to present your business plan and get the approval for you to join the practice. Administration personnel are unclear about the value you bring to their operations, as they have never witnessed this type of pharmacy practice and are concerned about the potential cost of the program. After reviewing your business plan, however, they are enlightened regarding the possibilities of this service and would like to see it, not just for Dr. Busybee's patients, but expanded to his partners' patients in the practice setting. They have noted that this physician group is performing below other local physician groups on health outcomes for several of their payers, and this is negatively affecting revenue. Using your services is an attractive option, and they request that you work with Dr. Busybee to determine the best plan for your integration and collaboration with all the physicians of the practice. They inform you they are in negotiations to secure preferred provider status with an additional payer. They ask you to identify how your services may benefit them in these negotiations.

Consumer Stimuli

To better understand the external forces involved, consumer stimuli are usually divided into three categories: commercial, social, and physical.

Commercial Stimuli

Television, radio, and Internet advertisements constantly bombard consumers about products and services, including those associated with health care. Are we sleeping enough? Do we feel tired all of the time? Are we anxious? Are we sore? Do we need life to just slow down a little? In our medical world, we witness constantly the marketing of new medications, services, and equipment from salespeople in our institutions, offices, and meetings. These types of advertisements are considered commercial stimuli. (Sample MTMS Brochure and MTMS Patient Brochure)

CASE

Knowing that expansion of your practice to include collaboration with all physicians of the group will take time, you initiate the marketing process by targeting Dr. Busybee and his patients. Your first step is to read a book entitled *Building a Successful Ambulatory Care Practice: A Complete Guide for Pharmacists*, then you start brainstorming not only how to create a marketing plan for your current practice implementation but also for expansion of your practice over the next 1 to 5 years. The use of commercial stimuli is one strategy suggested to reach the physicians and their patients. You would like to model the pharmaceutical sales approach and use written material such as a brochure with an appealing message and title. You think about some catchy lines, such as "Can't seem to get that patient's HgA1c levels below 7?" or "Warfarin management putting you over the edge?", and plan to follow them with information on your service and patient referral. You are also thinking of planning an in-service at a physicians' meeting, as well as placing the brochure electronically as a link on the organization's intranet web site. You are also considering developing an easy-to-use flyer placed visibly in all physicians' exam rooms and nursing stations to remind them to refer patients appropriate for your service and guide them through the process.

You anticipate that when Dr. Busybee's patients are referred to you they will have a poor understanding of why they should see you and what you can offer them. Realizing you need a plan for this target group, to explain your service you develop a brochure with another catchy title, "Why Does My Physician Want Me to See a Pharmacist?", written in terms and phrases easily understood by patients. In that brochure, you address the services you will provide and explain how they will help patients manage their disease states.

Additionally, you will need to address the administrators' request to identify how your services can benefit the payer negotiations. This task

> has you overwhelmed, and at this point you are not quite sure what that plan should entail.

Social Stimuli

Social stimuli can also initiate the consumer decision-making process. This can occur when a friend or colleague recommends a product or service, or in some instances, the stimulus is an individual's desire to be more like someone he or she admires or envies. Social stimuli can be particularly important for clinical service providers because an individual experience with the first clinical ambulatory pharmacist they encounter will shape his or her perceived value of that service. This is particularly true for patients and their providers. A satisfied patient or physician may provide a positive word-of-mouth referral to a friend, thus initiating a social stimulus and awareness of need. Since health care decisions often involve a weighing of both emotional and practical factors, this reference may serve as the deciding factor about whether or not your primary customers will use your service.

Do not discount this method for administrators and payers. As medication therapy management continues to evolve into health care legislation and payer initiatives, and experiences with pharmacist ambulatory services reach these groups through publications and meetings, they may have already heard about such services. The presentation of your business plan with your services may align well with their social stimuli and be the impetus to gain support or achieve final approval for your services. Coming armed with support for ambulatory pharmacist-type services from material found in each customer's social or professional base can be one way to optimally use this concept. Have the publications or organizations for your administrator's peers addressed your type of services?

> ## CASE
>
> Knowing that Dr. Busybee understands your proposed services well and is well liked and respected by his peers, you ask and he agrees to be part of your campaign to inform his partners of your new services. He agrees to share the impact you are having on his patients' care with his partners to stimulate referrals to your service.

Physical Stimuli

The final way that consumers become aware of needs is by experiencing physical stimuli. If a patient experiences an adverse reaction to a new medication, he or she will seek ways to alleviate the pain and discomfort of that situation. Someone who is experiencing bleeding with their anticoagulant will call the physician's office. A need you can fulfill is to lighten the load of your triage nurse by accepting those calls in your service. The example of an unexpectedly disconcerting lab or test result could also be classified as a physical stimulus. A patient may have a HgA1c greater than 10 or new atrial fibrillation on EKG at a physician's visit; this stimuli can be used for an automatic referral to your services. If your payer or organization has financial attribution for rehospitalization for certain conditions, those patients may be automatically referred to you for a visit upon discharge as an effort to control those costs.

CASE

Physical stimuli could really help jump start your referrals. With the support of administration and Dr. Busybee, a report is generated identifying all of his patients with HgA1c levels greater than 10, as well as those patients with poor time in therapeutic range for their INRs. Dr. Busybee's partners are informed that these are the types of patients he is referring to your service. They will be provided with the names of their patients that fall into these categories as potential patients they may refer to pharmacist services.

How to Address the Need

After a consumer becomes aware of his or her need, the next step in the prepurchase phase involves a search for ways to address that need. This search can occur either internally or externally, but often one leads to another.

CASE

In Chapter 2 Dr. Busybee was a potential customer for your service. However, before he contacted you he may have investigated resources currently within his practice to address the large number of patients with HgA1c levels greater than 10 and those with INR out of the target range. His office may have another practitioner such as a certified diabetic educator or a nurse practitioner that could help him manage these poorly controlled patient populations. For example, he may recall that one of his nurses had worked previously in an endocrinologist office and may have some base knowledge in diabetic management to provide additional education needed by his patients.

This would be classified as an internal search. If the experience with the nurse practitioner or diabetic educator is positive and patients' HgA1c and INR levels are improving, there is a strong likelihood that Dr. Busybee's search for alternatives will end here. However, if Dr. Busybee is facing a need that has not been previously realized or experienced, or if past methods to fulfill this need have proved unsuccessful, such as having no personnel in his office who could take on these populations, then an external search for alternatives becomes necessary.

During the external search process, Dr. Busybee seeks information from outside sources. These sources might still include recommendations from colleagues, professional journal articles, advice from administration, or even a search of the Internet. At this point, the information gathered is unprocessed by Dr Busybee, who is the customer. The level of effort put forth in this search will vary and will be affected by numerous factors, including an individual's attention span, perceived seriousness of the need, or the amount of information available to the searcher. Sometimes an overabundance of available information can be overwhelming to a customer and can be just as detrimental as a lack of information.

At some point, the customer will reach his or her own threshold for information gathering; then the evaluation process begins. All potential methods for fulfilling the customer's need that were identified during the internal and external searches will now be compared and contrasted with one another. Weighing the pros and cons of each alternative can be a fairly analytical process; it is not uncommon for emotional factors to influence these decisions as well. The price of a service may be an important element for Dr. Busybee to consider, but a clinician's availability and reputation for service and results may elevate Dr. Busybee's estimated value of this service. In our case, Dr. Busybee's external search found you! He may have considered other options, such as a higher level and more expensive service provided by hiring a part-time endocrinologist. He could consider hiring a nurse or a diabetic educator. If the cost of services is comparable to yours, but one is less available or lacking an equally positive endorsement from colleagues, then the customer, Dr. Busybee, can decide what is his best choice. How well you positioned yourself and promoted yourself to meet Dr. Busybee's needs are key in his choice.

Consumption Phase

After identifying and considering the various ways to fulfill their need, customers ultimately make a choice about what services to consume. When they do, they enter the consumption phase of the customer decision-making process. This involves not only the consumption of the product or service itself, but also the way it is utilized. From a clinical services standpoint, this phase would include the patient and his or her choice to visit your practice site and the degree to which he or she utilized the services offered. For the physician or other health care provider it will be how beneficial they find your service and their resulting willingness to continue or increase your patient referrals. Administrators and payers will be evaluating the value of your services from their perspective or how well you meet their quality and cost measures as noted in Chapter 7.

Post-purchase Evaluation

The final stage of the consumer decision-making process is the post-purchase evaluation phase. How does the reality of the purchase compare with the consumer's expectations? Did the purchase adequately fulfill the consumer's needs? Did the experience disappoint or exceed expectations?

With the benefit of hindsight, a consumer can now evaluate his or her own decision-making process. Were the trade-offs of another patient visit, choice of you as a clinical pharmacist versus another provider, and cost of your service justified by the level of services rendered and patient health care outcomes you impacted? How heavily did emotional or political versus practical factors weigh on this decision? Was it the correct decision?

If cost was a concern during the decision-making process, it is not uncommon for consumers to begin to doubt their own choices. To override such concerns for your pharmacy service, your value proposition has to be well balanced between cost, worth, and quality of your service to patients and referring providers and the resulting patient health outcomes.

The following are some tips for incorporating the consumer behavior principles into your marketing activities.

1. Consumers routinely seek out information to satisfy needs, so be a visible source to all your potential customers. Make sure each customer has heard about ambulatory pharmacy services, including patients, physicians, administrators, and payers.

2. One-to-one interactions with your target consumers to inform them of how you can meet their needs with your services is always an effective strategy. Be persistent in securing the face-to-face time, which allows the potential customers to associate the service with a person and that person's vision.

3. Have pertinent written information readily available for all types of customers. The information should address their needs and how your services can and will meet them. Think about your business plan from Chapters 2 and 3.

Characteristics of Services

Product versus service is the defining comparison for what you do as a clinical pharmacist compared with those who sell a physical product. Promoting a service creates a significant challenge for marketers.

Key Point

Unlike tangible objects that can be seen, touched, felt, weighed, or measured at any time to determine their usefulness and value, services are moments-in-time experiences, and their unique characteristics make assigning value a bit of a challenge.[5]

As already noted, the first characteristic of a service is its intangibility. It doesn't exist before it is delivered.[5] In a clinical setting, you bring your specialized knowledge to interactions with patients and other health care providers. As a pharmacist, you educate, provide advice, and monitor. For each encounter, whether with a patient or provider, your service is unique and provided in the moment. The personal nature of these experiences makes them difficult to explain and understand, especially when you are marketing your services to someone who has never experienced what a pharmacist can do in terms of direct patient care. Consider someone telling a friend about the new sports car he or she just purchased; "it's red with racing stripes, dual exhaust, leather sporty seats with a great stereo." It is easy to visualize the car being described in exact detail. Now think about the same person telling a friend about the medication evaluation session a pharmacist just conducted for him or her; "well, the pharmacist looked at the computer, asked me some questions, wrote something down, spoke with my doctor, and then I ended up with a different medicine, directions, and things I am supposed to do." The acquaintance has a very difficult time visualizing what their friend just "bought" at the visit with the ambulatory care pharmacist. However, there are visual clues that indicate what type of services may be offered or expected. The professional nature of your brochures, how well and professionally you communicate, the professional appearance of both you as a provider and your practice setting all leave visual impressions. These visuals paint a picture that can be relayed. People conveying their experience can add that the pharmacist was very attentive to their needs and really helped them manage their condition by answering all questions in a manner laypersons can understand. Other visuals, such as a busy or noisy office with minimal privacy, do not readily convey that personal or comprehensive clinical services will be provided. A practice site that provides a comfortable, professional waiting area with private consultation or exam rooms indicates that professional services are being provided.

As you can see, the clinical skills used by a health care provider are not always evident to a patient. This is also true of other health care providers, administrators, and payers. If physicians have not had experience with pharmacist-provided, direct patient care services, they may have difficulty understanding and differentiating what you do versus what they—or other providers such nurse practitioners—do. Administrators and payers may not even consider clinical pharmacist services in their internal or external searches, as they have never had knowledge or experience with such services.

In choosing you to provide services, your customers have to have some measure of confidence that you can provide the services. Knowing this means that you need to examine your proposed practice from the consumer point of view. In other words, if you were in their position, what would you need to know about your services for you to be comfortable with a decision to use your services? Your marketing plan should address why you as a clinical ambulatory pharmacist are qualified and skilled to provide the services that will meet each customer's needs. Marketing your qualifications includes communicating your degrees, licenses, residency, or fellowship training, in addition to any other training certificates you may have, such being qualified to administer adult immunizations. This type of marketing will help provide "physical" evidence of your clinical expertise.

Of course that leads to another challenge in marketing clinical services, and that is the services you provide are variable and are meant to adapt to individual patient needs and those particular characteristics of the patients in your community. Services are unique interactions between you and a patient, provider, administrator, and payer and therefore can be quite variable. The service you provide one patient or physician may differ from that provided the next patient or physician you encounter as each individual and that person's respective needs are different. This variability means that your customers may perceive varying levels of service from visit to visit. As all human encounters, one may go exceedingly well and another very poorly. Your customers and even you may have unrealistic expectations about what can be achieved by a pharmacist clinical visit. If the reality of the experience does not match up with these predetermined ideas, your customers may develop a low opinion of your service and not see the value.[6] Your marketing plan has to address the breadth and depth of your patient care roles and define your service so others have a clear understanding of what you are offering, yet understand the inherent variability of patient care services.

Services also differ from products in that services are both produced and consumed simultaneously.[5] In marketing terminology, services are referred to as *perishable*. Your patient–pharmacist or provider–pharmacist interactions cannot be stored for later use. They happen in real time, and the experience is only beneficial if both parties are actively involved in the transaction. Your workload can negatively affect your ability to be available for a patient, and conversely, an inattentive or unwilling patient can result in a fruitless interaction. Likewise, if a physician is too busy or unwilling to carve out time for his or her necessary role in your provision of patient services, you may find yourself ineffective. In such cases, your service is lost and cannot be stored for later use.

This directs you to the final point in differentiating products and services. Because what you do as an ambulatory patient care pharmacist is an interactive service experience, you as the provider, your consumer (patient, physician, etc), and the service are inseparable.[5] Each of your target groups has just as much of a role as you do in determining the success of an encounter. If the service you provide during a patient interaction is to help achieve better control of blood glucose levels or to reach a target INR, you can offer education, monitoring services, and collaboration on medication therapy selection as well as reinforce lifestyle modifications. However, if the patient is not an active, willing participant in this process or the physician elects not to follow your clinical management plan, then the encounter will ultimately be a failure. This failure is just as important as the successes. Just because you, the ambulatory pharmacist, have joined the team, not every goal you set will be successful. As with any other health care professional, your impact depends on many factors, including willingness of other members of the team to participate and work collaboratively with you. To increase the chance of receiving buy in, remember you are always marketing yourself each time you interact with your customers. Persistence, positivity, and a realistic expectation of the time and effort it may take, depending on the culture of your organization and the acceptance of your patients and physicians, are important characteristics for you to realize and uphold.

> **CASE**
>
> Realizing that you will need to gain the trust and acceptance of Dr. Busybee's patients, you make time in your schedule to review each referred patient's chart prior to the office visit. One advantage you have at this time relates to the fact that you know why the patient has been referred to you, which allows you to create a tentative management plan based on the management of the patient in the past. In other words, why has the patient not reached the HgA1c goal with the treatment choices made by Dr. Busybee? Does the patient need more attention in the office? Does he or she understand the role of the medications? Is administering insulin problematic? These are all questions you can address with patients during the office visit, complementing the care they are receiving from Dr. Busybee.

Specific Barriers for Ambulatory Care Pharmacist Services

One of the challenges for an ambulatory care pharmacist is associating what you do clinically with the practice of pharmacy. Clinical ambulatory pharmacy services are still relatively young services. For the average person in each of your target groups, direct patient care is not something traditionally expected from pharmacists. These patients' pharmacy experiences most likely have been the historic retail pharmacy model where they have received a physical product, like a prescription drug, and minimal if any recommendations on managing medical conditions and resulting medication-related therapy.

When your customers initiate the decision-making process to address their patient care needs, if they are not aware of the availability of the clinical services provided by a pharmacist, then you will not be a factor during the internal or external search phase. Fortunately, increasing numbers of pharmacists are practicing in this capacity, and health care reform will help make this unawareness less and less the case. You must continue to promote yourself and ambulatory pharmacy services and approach the many barriers you will encounter not as obstacles to which to succumb, but as challenges that you can overcome. Doing so may take time and require patience. All target groups should be educated about the clinical skills a pharmacist possesses and shown how they and the organization can benefit from these services. You are a valuable resource that can help patients achieve positive health outcomes through monitoring, consultation, and collaboration.

The following are some tips for incorporating service characteristics into your marketing activities.

1. Clinical services are intangible and more difficult for customers to perceive than physical products; therefore, your customers require some measure of confidence in your abilities. The professionalism of every aspect of your service, from your written material and personnel behavior to the look and

atmosphere of your clinic, will help consumers visualize that you offer specialized quality services. Promote your credentials and experience and display licenses, certificates, and evidence of additional training.

2. Services can be quite variable and depend on the unique needs of your patients. Experiences among your customers and their view of your services can be quite different. Therefore, patients and other health care providers need to know and understand what they are going to receive in return when using your services. Clearly define, display, and promote the full array of services you are able to provide.

3. Your services are consumed as they are produced and cannot be stored for later use. Therefore, each encounter reflects you and the service you provide. Maintain continued professionalism and a personal standard level of service regardless of the situation.

4. You cannot separate yourself from your service or the process of how it is provided and how your customer receives it. All have major input into your ability to successfully provide your service. Persistence, positivity, time, and patience are often needed as you cannot control all three variables for long-term success.

Conducting Market Research

Now that we have you thinking about the many issues you may need to address in your marketing plan, let's focus on a marketing plan's basic steps. Effective marketing always begins with planning and a purpose. Marketing planning should emanate from the research and thought you put into your business plan that was discussed in a previous chapter. The marketing plan covers everything, including aligning with your mission statement, understanding the needs of your customers, and identifying your competitive edge and how you are going to get your message to your customers such that you are their first choice for services. Start with reviewing your mission statement, which defines who you are and what you want to accomplish. Your job is to marry your mission with the needs of your customer to create a service that benefits both you and your customers.

Determining What Customers Want

A first step, which has been previously emphasized, is understanding your target group members' needs.

Efficient and successful exchanges occur when suppliers (you) offer a good or service of value (ambulatory patient care services) that a buyer (patients, physicians, administrators, and payers) desires and is therefore willing to exchange something of value (continued visits, continued referrals, and payment) in order to get.

CASE

Dr. Busybee has been through the internal and external search process and concluded adding a pharmacist to his practice is the best choice to help him achieve his goals and continue to be reimbursed by one of his payers. The administrators and payers are won over by your business plan and the impact you can have within Dr. Busybee's practice. They also ask how your service will assist them in current negotiations to secure preferred provider status with an additional payer. This request is overwhelming initially, and then you realize the administrator has just provided you with the future value of your proposed service. While the request is daunting, you realize that by creating a marketing plan you are working to secure your services at the practice site.

Without adequate information regarding who are potential consumers, what their specific needs are, and how you can address those needs, promotion or just stating that ambulatory clinical pharmacy services are available will be unsuccessful in creating an efficient exchange. You will not get takers for your service, and you will not establish a value proposition. Successful marketing plans and promotional activities are by-products of marketing research. In today's environment, health care leaders rely on significant research and analysis before making major decisions.[7] Good marketing research and analysis will result in informed decisions about the services included in your array of skills and scope of practice that will benefit your organization. However, the process of marketing research requires time and planning and should be performed proactively not retroactively.

Decisions regarding the design and delivery of health service provider services such as yours are generally made by professionals providing the service or product, not the consumers.[8] This professional domination of decision making in lieu of a consumer-oriented philosophy used by non-health care consumer products organizations leads to products and services not necessarily responsive to consumer needs. The concept of pharmaceutical care (the medication-related relationship between the pharmacist and the patient) was developed by academicians.[9] Medication therapy management (MTM) was introduced in 2003 by the federal government's Centers for Medicare & Medicaid Services (CMS) to identify and describe a service for which CMS would reimburse health care providers (including pharmacists) when providing such services to Medicare part D patients.[10] Although pharmaceutical care and MTM are significant developments in describing patient-oriented pharmacy services, the concept is difficult for those outside the profession of pharmacy to understand or see how it directly addresses current health care needs. Research has noted that patients may not perceive the role of medication manager for pharmacists and may not see the pharmacist as someone who can help in this process based on prior interactions with pharmacists.[11,12]

Marketing research is the process of gathering and analyzing information for use in the market planning process, which is the method used to solidify the specifics of your customers' needs. A number of tools or processes can be used to collect relevant information regarding your potential customers: who they are, how many there are, their current perceptions, and what their unmet needs are. There are two basic types of information that can be collected and analyzed: qualitative information and quantitative information. Refer to **Table 4-1** for specific examples of each type of data and the tools used to generate needed data.

Table 4-1. Marketing Research: Types of Information Resources

	Qualitative Data	**Quantitative Data**
Type of Information Needed	Identify scope of problem	National/state/local:
	Generate questions	• Population data
	Challenge assumptions	• Demographic information
	Investigate customer	• Disease prevalence
	perceptions	• Patient satisfaction
Tools	Focus groups	Census data
	Individual in-depth interviews	State health department data
		County/local data
		Pharmacy computer data
		Survey/questionnaire data

Qualitative Research

Qualitative research aims to gather in-depth information regarding behavior and the reasons that govern behavior. This type of research will better help you understand your customers' pre-purchase phase and their stimuli used in decision making for your services. Qualitative research relies on subjective responses that focus on words and themes instead of easily quantified numerical data. Qualitative information is extremely useful early in the planning process, as much can be learned from your customers regarding their perceptions, opinions, and reasoning. One of the most common qualitative techniques used is that of focus groups. The focus group is a small number of representative people (i.e., patients or a group of physicians) in an interactive environment, generally managed by a moderator who generates discussion by asking a number of focusing questions to stimulate discussion and emotional responses. Participants are free to talk with other group members, and experiences are shared and explored further. Focus groups should be repeated with different individuals until a full range of opinions is collected. Your target groups' perceptions may be very different from the assumptions held by you regarding the value and utility of clinical services offered.

You will find examples of focus group evaluations in the literature, although most have concentrated more on the retail setting versus the office- or clinic-based practice site. In the retail setting, it was found that consumers did have a number of medication-related concerns and wanted more information about their medications.[13] For patients, there are needs and wants in this area. Participants in the focus group appreciated when pharmacists worked as "problem solvers." However, they also felt that pharmacists were busy, and they indicated they had minimal or no interaction with their current pharmacists and generally did not experience counseling in the retail setting. In this case, patients indicated medication-related needs, but saw pharmacists as very busy and had little if any prior experience with pharmacists in non-dispensing roles and activities. This type of information gleaned from focus groups or interviews may be the impetus to create a marketing plan to approach administrators, payers, and other health care providers to illustrate what patients are not receiving in the outpatient setting and how you can correct this oversight by offering ambulatory pharmacy services in your setting.

CASE

The administrators of your organization, Dr. Busybee, and you meet to discuss the feedback. Since the administrators would like you to offer your service to all physicians within Dr. Busybee's practice, you suggest conducting a focus group meeting with Dr. Busybee and his partners during one of their routine meetings. The goal is to understand the physicians' perceptions of your service and determine what areas they perceive as patient care needs where you may have an impact. Dr. Busybee thinks this is a sound plan. Your office manager agrees to be the focus group facilitator. You help design the questions for the physicians' focus group. With the results, you discover that the physicians agree that additional assistance, especially with anticoagulation, would help them. They are more hesitant with diabetes management because they are not currently comfortable with your ability to manage these complex patients. They are willing to try a small number of their patients, but would want any medication changes to be approved by them first. New out of the session is a need for medication reconciliation during transitions of care. This is perceived as a major problem that no one currently in their practice (i.e., medical assistants or office nurses) has been able to adequately solve. The results of the session are very interesting to you, and the idea of providing medication reconciliation is something you are interested in and willing to pursue. (Physician Questionnaire)

Another qualitative technique is the use of the individual in-depth interview, which is useful as a follow-up tool to further explore or refine topics discovered in focus groups. These interviews can also be used in place of focus groups if the topic is awkward or uncomfortable when discussed in a group environment.

CASE

To better understand what patients in Dr. Busybee's practice may desire from such services, Dr. Busybee and you identify five patients who have appointments in the next 2 weeks. You plan on interviewing these patients to discover their needs and desires regarding their medications and their willingness to use your type of services. After the interviews, you discover that the patients have a large knowledge deficit with regard to dietary issues surrounding diabetes and anticoagulation. You also discover that the patients are struggling with self-management of their disease and medications. The patients also tell you that they do not want to have another health care provider visit. You understand that for patients to come to you, they must feel that their medication and health care issues are addressed. As you think about your marketing plan geared toward patients, you will need to build a process to educate on diet and home self-management plans for patients.

Quantitative Research

Once problems and general questions have been refined (using qualitative methods), quantitative methods can be used to define, refine, and analyze data relevant to the question or problem at hand. Secondary sources of data can be quite useful in this endeavor. These sources can include census data, public health data, county records, electronic pharmacy prescription files, or even metrics or outcomes collected from paper or electronic chart reviews. For example, the Agency for Healthcare Quality and Research (AHRQ) provides state snapshots on quality of health care yearly for the purpose of understanding needs and disparities in health care in your state.[14] You may note in the report that your state is very weak on diabetes care and has even declined since the baseline was established. Such data may be helpful in your marketing plan to payers with a large presence in your state or to state Medicaid plans. Demographic information such as age, gender, ethnicity, income level, education level, and historic trends can help identify targets or niche markets.

CASE

Using information from your focus group and in-depth patient interviews, you can develop a questionnaire or survey instrument to further define specific patient needs, interest in such programs, and willingness to pay for such services, depending on what source is being targeted to gather information. Caution should be used with survey responses, however, as a lack of understanding or prior experience with the topic can influence responses.

> You are comfortable with the information you received from your focus group with Dr. Busybee's physician colleagues. You are not sure, however, that the in-depth interviews with the five patients helped you understand the patient needs in Dr. Busybee's office population. Using your questions from the in-depth interview, you develop a survey to give potential patients as they wait in the physicians' visit rooms. You decide to survey 20–30 patients. (Example Patient Survey)
>
> You are pleased with the results of these techniques and decide to use an in-depth interview with your administrator and solicit help to develop a survey for your payers in order to gain perspective on these two customers: administrator and payers.

Marketing research does not stop with implementation of the new program or service. Research is also an essential feedback and evaluation mechanism. Many new questions arise once a service is in place: Is the service reaching the target market? What is consumer acceptance? What is the satisfaction with the new service? Marketing research is a key ingredient throughout the planning process and after. Periodically, you should reevaluate your impact on the practice, patient care, and outcome measures for administrations. This is all part of the balanced scorecard of quality measurement discussed in Chapter 7.

To receive feedback from your target groups for your services, consider the following

1. Conduct an informal focus group.

   a. For patients, are their health and medication needs being met?

   b. For other customers, are their patient care and organizational management needs being met?

   c. What information or services would they like, but don't receive?

2. Survey your target groups for satisfaction and unmet needs.

3. Conduct one-to-one interviews to receive feedback from your target groups on how they may perceive the service you are providing.

4. Check patient health care data from your practice as well as local and state health departments for recent report cards and public health statistics.

Creating the Marketing Plan

There are four key steps for you to address when creating your marketing plan.

Step 1: Identify your practice model (the ambulatory pharmacist patient care practice model).

Step 2: Analyze the situation.

Step 3: Lay the groundwork for your marketing strategy.

Step 4: Create and implement your marketing plan.

Step 1: Identify Your Practice Model

Through your research, you are comfortable that you understand your target groups' needs and have identified opportunities for your services to fill those needs. The next step is matching the type of practice you want to provide, both now and in the future, with your target groups' needs. This is not an easy task. For example, companies that manufacture cellular phones are not in the phone business, but in the communication business. The phone is simply a conduit for communicating with other people, places, and things (i.e., the Internet). Big box retailers such as Wal-Mart are in the business of providing a wide variety of consumer goods at a very low price. Wal-Mart's stated mission is "saving people money so they can live better." As a clinical ambulatory pharmacist providing patient care, you should have a clear understanding of your practice model identification: who you are and what you want to do. Think back to your mission statement, and it should help you. Marketing does not stop once you see your first patient or provide your first report to administrators, physicians, or payers. You must continually assess your practice model and continue to tweak as necessary your long-term plan. A great example is a pharmacist who has had an anticoagulation practice for 15 years and is now faced with new products that do not require INR monitoring. What does this pharmacist see as the future practice model for the practice? Should the pharmacist shift to broader disease state management? Is continuing to care for anticoagulation patients a viable option? Will the services today continue to meet the needs of customers in the future? The point is to clearly identify and continue to review what you do, your purpose, and your goals.

Step 2: Analyze the Situation

The third step is to know the environment or climate in which you will roll out your marketing plan. This includes a review of the business and economic environment combined with a review of your organization's assets available to use in your marketing plan. Components of your business plan will aid you in this section. A review of the business environment includes evaluation of the state of the current and local economy, political and legal variables, technological variables and advancements, and social and cultural variables that can affect demand (**Table** 4-2). These factors can have a significant impact on the success of your marketing plan. For example, the recession in the United States beginning in 2007 significantly affected the ability of businesses to borrow money from banks for new projects or initiatives. Capital became more difficult to obtain. Ability to pay for your marketing plan may be affected by such economic factors and how they affect your organization. However, from an opportunity standpoint, technological advances such as smart phones, Twitter, text messaging, and electronic adherence reminders create the opportunity for you to communicate with patients on a more frequent and intimate basis for drug therapy monitoring. Should this be part of your marketing plan in Dr. Busybee's clinic? Having patients do home INR monitoring would allow more office time to see diabetes patients.

Your organization may have assets that will be helpful to you in developing your marketing plan. Larger organizations may have marketing departments or other resources that you can tap into, such as a graphics department to assist in designing any written material you create. Your organization may already have a brand or look that they wish to use on all material. Investigating what resources are available in your organization can provide you with professional expertise and save you time and energy in preparing your plan.

Table 4-2. Situation Analysis Environment Review

Federal Health Care Legislation and Rules
- Health care reform, such as accountable care organization or patient-centered medical home
- Meaningful use criteria for information technology
- CMS payment policies and rules

State Pharmacy Practice Legislation
- Collaborative practice
- Scopes of practice

Pharmacy Profession Initiatives and Standards
- Pharmacy Practice Model Initiative
- Professional practice standards

Technology Factors
- Smart phones
- Internet and personal computer access
- Home video conferencing and Skype

Cultural and Societal Changes
- Personal health records

Step 3: Lay the Groundwork for Your Marketing Strategy

Concurrent to the situation analysis, you need to begin to lay the groundwork for building your marketing strategy. Information gleaned from the qualitative and quantitative research phases should be instrumental in this process. Particularly in the case of new pharmacy services, knowledge regarding how your target groups make decisions and the motivations for seeking pharmacy services by patients and other health care providers is crucial to designing your strategy. In your business plan you identified goals, objectives, and competitors, and completed a SWOT analysis. You will want to review this information as you develop a marketing strategy so that a reasonable person may choose your services over competitors or conclude that yours is a service they must have. This is brainstorming time where you pull all that you have learned together to create your marketing plan.

Before constructing your marketing plan, consider the following tips.

1. Start with your business plan.

2. Determine how to marry your mission statement to your customers' needs.

3. Determine the available resources you will need.

4. Evaluate the current business and practice environment and how it will affect your marketing plan.

5. Build your marketing strategy

Step 4: Create and Implement Your Marketing Plan

The marketing plan includes strategies and tactics for putting all the pieces from your marketing research and preparation into an executable plan. Basic to marketing principles are the traditional framework of a marketing plan, or the four Ps of (P)roduct, (P)rice, (P)lace, and (P)romotion. Because services have intangible attributes that are very different from physical products, marketers of service products have expanded this framework to include an additional three Ps: (P)eople, (P)ackaging, and (P)rocess.[15,16] Focusing on the seven elements of the marketing "mix" for a service product will help you achieve the goals of your marketing plan, and to create the elements needed to deliver your product/service to your customers with maximum satisfaction. (Marketing Plan Template) 🖼

Key Point The traditional framework of a marketing plan includes the four Ps of (P)roduct, (P)rice, (P)lace, and (P)romotion. Service products have expanded this framework to include an additional three Ps: (P)eople, (P)ackaging, and (P)rocess.[15,16]

The Seven Ps
PRODUCT

Your products are the services you intend to offer that meet the needs of each of your identified target groups. You will need to outline and discuss each of your target groups and clearly define the services you will be providing them. An outline for Dr. Busybee's clinic may look like the following:

Services provided to clinic patients

Anticoagulation Patients

• Disease state and medication therapy monitoring through history and INR testing

• Anticoagulation education on diet and drug therapy

• Patient education on self-management and provision of written self-management plans.

Diabetic Patients

- Disease state and medication therapy monitoring for not-at-goal patients

- Education on diet and drug therapy

Services provided to clinic physicians

- Assistance in management of high-risk patients on anticoagulation through collaborative practice agreement

- Assistance in management of diabetic patients above target goals through education and knowledge assessment, intensive education on self-management, and monitoring for therapy efficacy and medication-related problems

- Assistance with medication reconciliation at transitions of care to identify medication-related problems or issues that need to be resolved and generation of adequate medication lists

Services provided to clinic administration

- Quarterly reports on number of patients seen and identified workload measures

- Quarterly reports on hospitalization rates, adverse drug event rates, and secondary outcomes measures such as HgA1c, FBS, and time in therapeutic range

Services provided to payers

- Yearly report on clinical and economic outcomes derived from administration reports

As you discuss the services or product you plan to deliver, be sure and connect it to your market research and the needs you have identified for each of your target groups. You will need to address how your services are distinguishable from those offered by any competitors you have identified.[16] The goal of this section of your marketing plan is to make a persuasive argument that your services provide the best value to meet your target groups' needs.

PRICE

Price is the amount "paid" to you for your service, and it should reflect the value your target groups place on your service. This is a tough one for clinical ambulatory pharmacists because of the influence of third-party payers in determining if the pharmacist will be reimbursed and the reimbursement price for any particular service (discussed further in Chapter 8). One way to address price is to think about the cost/benefit equation for each of your customers.[17] A review of the financial assessment section in Chapter 2 will also help as you determine pricing strategy in your marketing plan. In your deliberations, consider the demand for your service, current and potential number or market size of each of your target groups, and the cost to provide your service.

Pricing policy is not just about prices being less than a competitor's. If you are competing on the basis of performance and delivering a high-quality service, the price should be commensurate with the quality of the service. If your service does a superior job of meeting consumers' needs and expectations, it will be highly valued by your customer and there is no need to compete on price. Your customer may be willing to pay more if the value in the long run provides an overall benefit. Defend this extra cost in your marketing plan by defining your high level of service and its anticipated value.

Organizations commonly make a number of mistakes when considering pricing policy.[18] Do not let this be you. Some of these mistakes include thinking as follows: Nothing we do deserves a premium price. Average pricing seems fair. Cost-based pricing is easier to explain. Everyone does it that way. Our work is driven by volume not value. Don't make waves or offend. The customer will tell you the price. All of these common mistakes demonstrate poor pricing policy and a lack of coordination with your business plan. Your business plan and the environmental scan on health care billing should guide pricing policy. Organizations whose goal it is to compete on price should do so. Clinical ambulatory pharmacists fall into the category of those whose goal is to offer high-quality professional services and should price the services accordingly with the value the consumer expects to receive from those services.

PLACE

Place in the marketing mix is a consideration of access to and availability of your service to your target groups. It is where and how your services are delivered. Similar to the five rights of drug therapy, your services must be available at the right place at the right time and in the right quantity.[17] Clinical pharmacy services are perishable and can happen only when the provider and patient or other health care provider interact. Therefore, time is very important to you, the provider, and to your patients, physicians, administrators, and payers. If patients do not show up for appointments, time and money is lost; some providers charge for appointment no-shows. Conversely, if patients or a physician cannot reach or meet with you in a timely fashion, they will seek services elsewhere. How accessible will you be? What are the backup plans during off hours or when you are not in the clinic? Do not let an inability to maintain an expected level of service when you are unavailable undermine the success of your practice.

Location is important. Can your customers find you, and are you visible to them? If the physicians do not see you in clinic, will they think about your service when meeting with a patient that may be an appropriate referral? Is your phone number easy to remember? In summary, your marketing plan needs to include your goals of how to place yourself physically and strategically into your organization and how you plan to be accessible to all your target groups.

PROMOTION

Promotion is a diverse set of activities used to communicate, educate, and persuade your target groups regarding the merits of your services, with an end result of those services being purchased or used. Promotional activities include direct interaction such as personal (face-to-face) selling, advertising in the media (television, radio, newspaper, etc.), sales promotions and events, and public relations. Promotion of clinical pharmacy services must be professional; it should gain your customers' attention, be appealing, and tell a consistent message. Most of all, it must give your customers a reason to choose you.[17] Your promotional material should not just state the features of your service but also communicate the benefits your target groups can expect from using your service.

Word-of-mouth is a great place to start, and it is free. Encourage your patients to share their experiences of your visit with others, including their other health care providers. Talk to those responsible for public relations in your organization and ask them to create a piece on your available services, both for internal and external promotion. Make sure your services are placed on your organization's web sites. Include testimonials from your customers on how your clinic helped support them in their self-care or their work.

Depending on your budget, you can create various advertising pieces such as brochures, folders, or information sheets. Remember that once they are printed, information on them is fixed, so if your services are dynamic and evolving, you may want to consider this in your financial investment in and quantity of this type of promotion. Whatever the method you choose for promotion to your target groups, it must grab their attention. Testing your promotion plan on your marketing research groups can provide you with valuable information before you spend your marketing budget. (DMG Example of a Brochure)

Many service-oriented organizations use the traditional promotional techniques of advertising, such as television, newspapers, radio, outdoor billboards, and direct mail. They remain very important tools in reaching target audiences. The correct mix and frequency of use depend on the goals developed in your strategic marketing plan. Hiring a marketing consultant may be valuable in selecting the correct media to best deliver your promotional message to the target audience, if such funds are available. Although technological advances have created several new avenues of communicating with customers, you should not overlook traditional means of promotion. Research involving an urgent care center found that outdoor advertising using billboards was well accepted by consumers and was effective as a promotional tool.[21] The majority of patients surveyed (72%) visiting the care center noticed the billboards, which included 65% of first-time patients.

Technological advances have created new opportunities to interact and communicate with current and potential consumers. Over 160 million people in the United States use the Internet as a source of health information.[22] Pharmacists using this type of media can help meet the needs of patients and providers as sources of medical and drug information, in addition to accessing patient medical information in a secure manner. Patient satisfaction can be enhanced by allowing patients access to information and the ability to forward questions at any time. Personal e-mail can also be used to communicate important information to patients and providers regarding questions they may have. Social media such as Facebook and Twitter are now being used routinely by consumers and marketers to communicate.[23] MD Anderson Cancer Center and the Mayo Clinic both use YouTube and have Facebook pages, and the Mayo Clinic has a news blog. These venues can also be used as effective feedback mechanisms to see what patients are saying about the organization. Potential drawbacks to these new electronic tools include the expertise needed to develop good, functional, secure sites and the required money to support them. Although these tools can enhance communication and relationships with consumers, they should not be used in lieu of face-to-face communication. When promoting services, nothing can replace the one-on-one relationship.

PEOPLE

People in the service-marketing model are those individuals who come in contact directly or indirectly with customers. Health care is a "people" business and deals with services and care that is most treasured in our culture: the length and quality of life. When service is the product, customers usually cannot separate the service from the person who provides it. People skills are very important for every team member associated with your service. Choosing the right people with the right attitude and communication skills to perform the services and providing them with correct training are musts in your marketing plan. A review of Chapter 7, which discusses qualifications for personnel providing clinical ambulatory pharmacy services, may be helpful. You will inevitably depend on a well-trained and motivated staff to provide services that are superior to those of competitors and that create a favorable image in the eyes of your customers.

PACKAGING

Packaging is the experience your customers get from the environment or atmosphere during the provision of your services. Consumers seek out tangible cues to help them understand the nature and quality of the service experience; therefore, the image of your clinic communicates what your services provide. It is expected that you provide your services in a pleasant, functional environment with adequate space and privacy. Your customers will desire a sense of well-being, competence, and support during your interactions.[16] Tangible packaging includes clean, neat, professional, and comfortable clinic space. Intangible packaging includes how welcome patients feel at your clinic, how at ease they are during the visit, and how responsive you are to their needs.

PROCESS

A service cannot be delivered without an efficient process. The process and procedure for receiving the service should be understandable to your target groups. The quality of your services will be judged by your target groups by what they experience before, during, and after acquiring the service. Your customers are less interested in the details of how your clinic runs. What matters to them is that it works.[17] Waiting excessively long times, feeling ignored, or being treated in an unprofessional manner by anyone they come in contact with will dictate a negative experience and adversely affect your marketing endeavors. This emphasizes the importance of Chapter 5 in this book, which addresses clinic procedures.

Relationship Marketing

The concept of relationship marketing has also evolved to assist in marketing services. Relationship marketing focuses on building and developing relationships with your target groups well beyond just purchasing the service. In the context of your practice, this can be defined as all marketing activities performed to attract, enhance, and maintain the relationships with your target groups that benefit both you and your customers.[19] Relationship marketing is more targeted at the individual level, whereas most promotional efforts attempt to hit as many people in the target market as possible. In this effort, personal selling becomes a more important tool in building relationships with individuals within your target groups: your patients, the physicians that refer to you, the administrator you directly report to, and a particular contact with a payer.[20] Relationship marketing also takes on a long-term approach to these relationships, focusing on retaining your customers for continued and lasting positive experiences. Building trust and the working relationship with patients, other health care providers, etc., takes considerable time and effort on your part. Personal selling is an important component of relationship development for successful patient care. Include your personal touch and demonstrate your passion for your work in interactions with your target groups as this will aid you in building trust, answering questions, and discussing mutual objectives for improving patient care. Your goals are to collaborate with your target groups and not compete against them. In relationship marketing, advertising or pamphlets are no substitute for one-on-one interactions.

Consider the following useful tips for incorporating the marketing mix presented above into the marketing plan for your practice.

1. Make sure to include the seven Ps of product, price, place, promotion people, packaging, and process related to services in your marketing plan.

2. Develop an appropriate pricing policy consistent with service quality.

3. Use relationship marketing principles when interacting with your target groups.

4. Do not overlook new and developing technologies when promoting your services.

Chapter Summary

Marketing an ambulatory care pharmacy practice requires implementation of a well-thought out marketing plan developed in conjunction with your business plan and your organization's strategic direction. A thorough plan will include understanding consumer behavior regarding health needs and identifying those needs and how your new pharmacy service can address them. This is achieved by conducting appropriate marketing research, which may include both qualitative and quantitative research tools. Bringing together all the information gathered helps you develop your marketing plan. Using the seven Ps, which constitute the marketing mix, provides the tools you will need to execute your plan. The time and energy spent in this process will be a key factor in the success of your new service.

References

1. American Marketing Association web site. Definition of marketing. http://www.marketingpower.com/aboutama/pages/definitionofmarketing.aspx. Accessed February 8, 2010.

2. Hillestad SG, Berkowitz EN. *Health Care Marketing Plans: From Strategy to Action.* Homewood, IL: Dow Jones-Irwin; 1984.

3. Consumer Psychologist web site. http://www.consumerpsychologist.com/intro_Consumer _Behavior.html. Accessed March 6, 2010.

4. Engel JF, Blackwell RD, Miniard PW. *Consumer Behavior.* Fort Worth, TX: Dryden Press; 1993.

5. Zeithaml VA, Bitner M, Gremler D. *Services Marketing.* New York, NY: McGraw-Hill; 2005.

6. Chewning B, Schommer JC. Increasing clients' knowledge of community pharmacists' roles. *Pharm Res.* 1996;13(9):1299-1304.

7. Mass P, Martin E. Hatching a new identity. *Marketing Health Services.* 2009;Spring:8-13.

8. Flexner WA, Berkowitz EN. Marketing research in health services planning: A model. *Public Health Rep.* 1979:94(6);503-513.

9. Hepler CS, Strand LM. Opportunities and responsibilities in pharmaceutical care. *Am J Hosp Pharm.* 1990:47;533-543.

10. Centers for Medicare & Medicaid Services. Medicare Prescription Drug, Improvement, and Modernization Act of 2003. http://www.ssa.gov/OP_Home/comp2/F108-173.html. Accessed June 1, 2010.

11. Law AV, Ray MD, Knapp KK, et al. Unmet needs in the medication use process: Perceptions of physicians, pharmacists, and patients. *J Am Pharm Assoc.* 2003;43:394-402.

12. Nau DP, Ried D, Lipowski E. What makes patients think that their pharmacists' services are of value? *J Am Pharm Assoc.* 2003;43:424-434.

13. Garcia GM, Snyder ME, Harriman McGrath S, et al. Generating demand for pharmacist-provided medication therapy management: Identifying patient-preferred marketing strategies. *J Am Pharm Assoc.* 2009;49(5):611-616.

14. AHRQ. 2010 State Snapshots. http://statesnapshots.ahrq.gov/snaps10/index.jsp. Accessed September 18, 2011.

15. Nzekwue N. Developing the right marketing mix to promote pharmacy services. *Pharm J.* 2008;(280) March 22: 337-340.

16. Smith MC. Marketing pharmaceutical services. In: Brown, TR, ed. *Handbook of Institutional Pharmacy Practice.* 4th ed. Bethesda, MD: American Society of Health-System Pharmacists; 2006.

17. The Chartered Institute of Marketing. Marketing and the 7 Ps: A Brief Summary of Marketing and How It Works; 2009. www.cim.co.ui/marketingresources. Accessed September 18, 2011.

18. Cespedes FV, Ross EB, Shapiro BP. *The Wall Street Journal.* May 24, 2010.

19. Doucette WR, McDonough RP. Beyond the 4 Ps: Using relationship marketing to build value and demand for pharmacy services. *J Am Pharm Assoc.* 2002;42(2):183-194.

20. McDonough RP, Doucette WR. Using personal selling skills to promote pharmacy services. *J Am Pharm Assoc.* 2003;43(3):363-374.

21. Fortenberry JL, Elrod JK, McGoldrick PJ. Is billboard advertising beneficial for healthcare organizations? An investigation of efficacy and acceptability to patients. *J Healthc Manag.* 2010;55(2):81-96.

22. DeTora G, Linkon N. The new age of healthcare communications: Why developing a patient portal should be part of your strategy. *Mark Health Serv.* 2009; Fall:23-27.

23. Morarity LD. Whisper to a scream: Healthcare enters the brave new world of social media. *Mark Health Serv.* 2009; Summer:9-13.

Web Resources

Sample Brochures
    Brochure 1
    Brochure 2
    Brochure 3
Physician Questionnaire
Patient Survey
Marketing Plan Template

 Web Toolkit available at
www.ashp.org/ambulatorypractice

Creating the Ambulatory Patient Care Model

Gloria P. Sachdev, Michelle L. Cudnik

CHAPTER

5

Chapter Outline

1. Introduction
2. Clinic Operations
3. Policy and Procedures
4. Chapter Summary
5. References
6. Web Resources

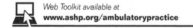
Web Toolkit available at
www.ashp.org/ambulatorypractice

Chapter Objectives

1. List at least four clinic operation considerations that should be pursued when creating a new pharmacist service.

2. Discuss the various clinic policy and procedure documents that are required rather than optional.

3. Discuss the purpose and recommended content for a billing procedure document.

Introduction

Congratulations on getting approval to start a new clinical pharmacy service! There are numerous next steps, and with thoughtful planning you will be on your way to seeing your first patient in a few months. We have attempted to categorize the many next steps into four tracks: clinic operations, policy and procedures, legal, and billing. The first two tracks are discussed in this chapter, and the latter two are discussed in Chapter 8. The goal is to pursue all four tracks simultaneously to optimize efficiency and effectiveness.

Clinic operation considerations include everything from getting your exam room set up to developing the process for how patients flow through your clinic.[1,2] The key when traveling down this track is to use your organization's resources and procedures that already exist. In a physician's office, as in our Dr. Busybee sample case, develop clinic operations that mimic the processes of your referring physicians. To maintain your service efficiency, it is important to use existing clinic support staff in the same manner and in the same roles as the clinic physicians use them. If this is done from the beginning as an expectation, the road ahead will be much smoother. Clinic operation considerations in a community pharmacy setting vary significantly and depend primarily upon space and ancillary staff options available.

The point remains the same: try to use already established processes and current staff roles as much as possible.

Policy and procedure considerations involve developing required and recommended processes and paperwork. Often, developing policy and procedures is the easiest and least time consuming of the four tracks to complete. You may find policy and procedures to be the most tedious of activities; however, in the end you will be thankful that you spent the time developing them. Policy and procedures maintain a standard of quality, help in training new personnel, and keep everyone on the same page with regard to processes and services, which is especially important as you grow. Usually, policy and procedures can be addressed near the end of your program development, such as for a small private physician-based clinic. However this may not be the best strategy in a large organization such as a community chain pharmacy-based clinic or a hospital-based clinic. In these latter practice settings, the process for getting policy and procedure documents approved may be time-consuming. For this reason, we recommend that you at least become familiar with what is both required and recommended early on so that there are no surprises at the end that delay your grand opening.

Clinic Operations

Clinic operations involve addressing tasks that impact the proposed clinical service on a day-to-day basis at the practice site. This includes (1) office space considerations, (2) clinic scheduling, (3) clinic work flow, and (4) training and credentialing.[3-6]

Office Space Considerations

It is imperative that the practice site at which you are intending to establish services has office and exam room space for you. To protect patient privacy, finding space away from other patients, health care providers, and the public is imperative because waiting rooms, counters, and front windows are not considered ideal locations for patient visits to occur. Flexibility is needed. For instance, the situation may indicate that an extra exam room is available on Wednesdays and Fridays or that a rotating exam room is available 2 days a week. In most ambulatory patient care settings, space availability is a premium commodity and depends on the patient load of other clinic providers. You may also find space currently not being used that could be converted into an exam room (for example, a medical records room that is being vacated due to practice's conversion to an electronic medical record system). It is essential for you to see the space to ensure it will meet your needs. Remember, if you plan to have pharmacy students, residents, or fellows at your practice site, plan for the additional space they will need.

CASE

After all the background work and approval of your business plan, you are now ready to get started seeing patients in the new setting. First, however, you must secure adequate space to see the different types of patients Dr. Busybee and you have agreed to serve. Dr. Busybee and you meet with the office manager and decide that Wednesday mornings and afternoons would be the best initial time to add you to the rotation for seeing patients. This day is not as busy in the clinic since several of the physicians take the day off. The office manager suggests that you be treated just like all other practitioners in the office and follow the same rooming procedure used for the physicians and the nurse practitioner. Two exam rooms are allocated, one for anticoagulation management checks and another for medication therapy management (MTM), where you will first focus on diabetes management.

If the office and exam space that you are going to be using is already in an established physician's office, the items noted in Table 5-1 (page 130) will already be in place. If it is not, work with the office manager to arrange the purchase of these supplies and add them to the existing space. If you are establishing your clinic in a new location or a community pharmacy, you will need to work with architects who may create blueprints of your exam room (see **Figure 5-1** as an example). Be sure that your space is large enough to accommodate all needed equipment and supplies listed and that the entrance can accommodate a wheelchair. If you are lucky enough to be directly involved in creating your clinic space, be sure to consider the efficiency of your visits in terms of space. In a community pharmacy, you may want to consider when patients would see you in clinic, that is, before they pick up their prescriptions, while prescriptions are being filled, or afterward. Each time frame has its unique benefits: beforehand allows you to resolve any medication problems that may result in a change of medication before the filling process; during filling is efficient use of patient wait time; and afterward allows you to focus on tying filled medications to the education you are providing. Your decision will depend on the unique characteristics of your patient population and their needs, wants, or desires.

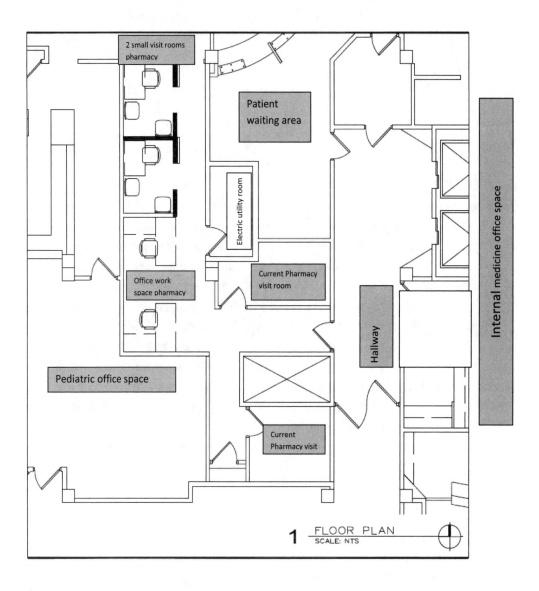

Figure 5-1. Blueprints of an Exam Room

Blueprint reproduced courtesy of Eckenhoff Saunders Architects, 700 S Clinton, Suite 200, Chicago, IL 60607. www.esadesign.com

Finally, if you are establishing a new service in a hospital-based clinic and space is going to be built for you, consider the location as it relates to the collaborating physicians' group. If you wish to use incident-to billing for Medicare patients in a physician-based outpatient office setting, your space must be in the same suite or location as the supervising physician.[7] The supervising health care provider (usually a physician, but it may also be a nurse practitioner or physician assistant) cannot be in a separate building. For more information refer to Chapter 8 for the rules for using this type of billing.

A requirement of using incident-to billing for Medicare patients is that auxiliary personnel, including pharmacists, must meet the direct supervision requirements. What defines direct supervision depends on where your service is located. If it is in a hospital-based outpatient practice, direct supervision is defined in the Hospital Outpatient Prospective Payment System (HOPPS).[8] If it is in a physician-based outpatient clinic, what constitutes direct supervision is noted in the *Federal Register.*[9] You cannot bill incident-to from within a community pharmacy setting unless a section of that setting is designated as provider office space where a recognized provider such as a physician, nurse practitioner, physician's assistant, or any other professional designated as an independent practitioner by the Centers for Medicare and Medicaid Services (CMS) sees patients and your service provides care "incident-to" this practitioner.

Most third-party payers follow CMS guidelines. In those areas of the country where Medicare Part D plans, Medicaid, or other payers allow you to bill as a pharmacist provider using MTM CPT codes or other qualified codes, be sure to check for any specific supervision or space requirements in the particular rules and regulations.

Additional office space considerations may also include a receptionist area for check-in and check-out and waiting room space.

Once office space has been addressed, consider what additional supplies you may need (**Table 5-1**). This may include office items such as a desktop or laptop computer, phone, and a file cabinet to store patient education material and paper, pens, and notepads. Consider if any additional physical exam equipment may be needed, such as a pulse oximeter; monofilament; peak flow meter; tape measure; pill boxes and point-of-care (POC) laboratory testing devices for assessing PT/INR, blood glucose levels, or fasting lipid profiles. In some cases, the POC device cartridges must be kept in a refrigerator that is separated from an employee refrigerator and maintained in the clinical area. A temperature log of the refrigerator needs to be maintained according to the requirements of the College of American Pathologist laboratory guidelines.[10] Many of these decisions are based on the type of clinic and service you will be providing. The key is to anticipate your needs ahead of time and plan for procurement, storage, and disposal (needle containers) of your needed supplies.

Clinic Scheduling Processes

Set up a patient scheduling system that is managed by clerical staff who directly schedule patients. The most important rule to remember when setting up your space is integrate, integrate, integrate.[3-5] Often when starting a new service, clinical pharmacists do not wish to disturb the harmony of work flow by adding additional work

Table 5-1. Essential Items Every Space Will Need

1. Chairs with durable vinyl coverings (not cloth due to difficulty in cleaning) and armrests for ease of getting into and out of the chair. Depending on your patient population, consider purchasing bariatric chairs that accommodate larger body weights. Consider obtaining at least two chairs, one for the patient and one for a friend, significant other, or child.

2. Exam room table with paper table covers if a physical exam will be part of the visits. Consider whether the table will need to rise and lower based on the age and dexterity of your patient population.

3. Desk or countertop to set chart or computer on during visits.

4. Desk chair or stool for clinician to use during visit.

5. Wall-mounted or portable sphygmomanometer with appropriate-size blood pressure cuffs (based on population of patients—pediatric, adult, large adults). Based on the service provided, you may consider obtaining an otoscope, ophthalmoscope, and thermometer to be added to the wall mount or in a portable basket.

6. Other equipment such as weight scales, microfilament probes, measuring tapes, and thermometer (see Chapter 2).

7. Clock with second hand for monitoring patients' heart rate.

8. Latex-free exam gloves in multiple sizes.

9. Wall-mounted shelf to place educational materials.

10. Sharps containers if you are performing any lab draws, point-of-care testing, or injecting medication (immunizations for example).

11. Hand soap if the space has a sink. A hand sanitizer dispenser may also be considered.

12. With regard to technology, if using an electronic medical record or other electronic documentation system, you will need to assess how many computers are preferred. In addition, if patient documents or educational material will be printed, consider whether multiple printers are needed or if a network printer is a more suitable option.

for other staff. However, the more clerical work you take on, the more inefficient your service will be, and thus revenue generation potential will be impacted. The support staff is there so you can be productive. It is highly recommended that you set up your practice from the beginning using the model that meets your long-term needs.

 Integration is the key to getting your practice up and running quickly and efficiently.

CASE

It is fortunate that you are entering an office space already set up for patient care. The next step is to prepare the exam rooms, and you ask that the exam room used for anticoagulation management be rearranged so that it includes a work surface for the INR machine as well as supplies for finger pricks. You request that lancets, alcohol pads, gauze squares, and adhesive bandages all be assembled in a small tote basket for easy access. You also realize you will need to have access to the office's electronic medical record (EMR), so you can request a laptop from the office supply and spend time setting up the electronic documentation templates to ensure each visit will flow smoothly and work within the current office documentation system.

A common mistake is for pharmacists to assume all the clerical responsibilities in the beginning because their office hours are not fully booked. However, once established, you will thus continue to schedule patients, pull your own charts, and perform your own vitals. It is highly unlikely the support staff will ever take on these responsibilities in the future. A major premise of health care reform and the new models of care are for all health care providers, including pharmacists, to spend the majority of their time practicing at the top of their skill level. Doing so will greatly contribute to a more cost-effective health care system.

 Clinical pharmacists should engage primarily in tasks commensurate with their skills in direct patient care.

Integrating your service into the norm of clinic flow brings overall efficiency to the clinic as well. Oftentimes, each clinician's schedule is reviewed electronically or printed as part of the process used to determine the workload for the support staff, including nurses, medical assistants, and technicians. Clinicians' schedules are also reviewed to assist in managing patients who no-show for appointments.

In order for the office manager or assistant to begin developing your schedule, also known as "building your books," he or she will need to know what days you wish to see patients, what times each day you are available, how long each new patient visit should last, how many new patient visit slots you want available per day, and how long follow-up visits will be on average.[11] If you are developing a service that involves significant time spent identifying patient barriers to compliance and encouraging lifestyle modifications such as conducting cardiovascular risk reduction clinics (CVRRC), or managing diseases such as diabetes, hypertension, hyperlipidemia, congestive heart failure (CHF), chronic obstructive pulmonary disease (COPD), or asthma, it is recommended that 45–60 minutes be allowed for new patient visits and 30 minutes for follow-up visits as a starting point.[12-14] You may need to adjust the time in the future depending on the clinic or patient nuances.

CASE

In Dr. Busybee's clinic, your service would be open for patient visits all day Wednesdays. To be patient centered, you build flexibility into your schedule, with new patient appointments designed for 30-minute slots and

20 minutes for follow-up appointments. You set a maximum of 12 patient
visits for days in clinic. You build in 20-minute slots around patient visits to
use for any needed post-visit work, phone calls, and documentation.

To embrace the patient centeredness of the new care models, it is best to be as
flexible as permitted by the nuances of your organization. More progressive practice management systems permit you to define the parameters in general terms, thus
offering more flexibility. If you are developing a new service that is medication-
monitoring focused, such as an anticoagulation clinic, chronic pain management
service, or GI management for patients receiving chemotherapy, maintain new patient visits at 45–60 minutes and have follow-up visits at 15–20 minutes. Remember
to focus your services on the best balance between best care and efficiency to
maximize patient outcomes and the reimbursement potential.

Billing Processes

If you are billing incident-to and would like to keep track of your workload, patient
diagnoses, and revenue of your service, have the billing department assign you an
internal provider number. This internal provider number is often called a performing provider number (PPN) and is an efficient option for assessing what the ancillary staff is engaged in. The PPN is not a billable provider number; however, it can
be placed on a charge document along with a billing provider number (BPN). The
BPN is assigned only to providers who have been authorized to bill a given payer.
Thus, if you are billing incident-to a physician, you may note a PPN and BPN on
the charge document. If you are a recognized provider for only one payer, for
instance, for Medicaid, then you would use your assigned BPN on the charge document when seeing these patients, and for other patients you would use your assigned PPN along with another clinician's BPN on the charge document. The PPN
could be designated as your national provider identifier (NPI), but more often than
not it is just an in-house number that is provided by the billing department.[15] See
Chapter 8 for details regarding NPI and which provider's BPN to place on your
charge document when billing incident-to a physician.

Referral Process

The next step is to develop a referral process for your new service. Considerations
include *which* providers are permitted to refer patients to your service, *if* patients
may self-refer, *how* the referral will be made (i.e., electronically entered by the
provider, handwritten/faxed order in the provider progress note to be followed up
by support staff to complete a referral form, or handwritten/faxed referral form completed by provider), and once the referral form is completed, *who* is responsible for
actually scheduling the patient into your office hours. These referral forms should
be kept for reasons discussed in greater detail later in this chapter. It is best that you
implement the same referral process that already exists within the practice setting.
If the physician practice group uses an electronic referral system, then have your
clinic name added to the list of profile options, which means your service name will
appear under the same consult tab where all other consult options appear. In such a
scenario, typically a customizable referral form is available. (Referral Form Example)

If a paper referral process exists for other services, then try to adopt this same form as it will be challenging for providers to remember to use a unique pharmacy referral form. Disadvantages of developing a new referral form include educating all staff on how to complete a new form, noting that it is located in a spot different from the regular referral forms, and keeping this special form stocked in all exam rooms (or central area). The goal is to integrate all your processes into the existing clinic processes.

Follow-up Process

Two other processes that need to be developed involve managing urgent patient care issues that arise in your clinic and implementing follow-up for consultations that you initiate with other services. Many times an urgent patient care issue is discovered for which you need a supervising physician to evaluate the patient immediately, later the same day, or the next day. If there is no existing protocol, invite key stakeholders such as the office manager or nursing and clerical staff to provide recommendations regarding how to best manage this situation. Similarly, invite such staff to educate you about the process to address consultations, as permitted, to other services. For example, if you are seeing a patient in your diabetes clinic and your collaborative drug therapy management protocol permits delegated authority to write orders for consultations, you could send this patient to ophthalmology, podiatry, social work, or dietary services, as appropriate. The existing staff will be instrumental in helping you navigate the consulting process in your practice setting.

Access to Patient Information

If your practice site is in a community pharmacy, then you will likely need to develop a new process or obtain access to the providers' EMR, or at a minimum, acquire basic medical information to perform your services. Currently under development nationally is the certification for the functionality of developing a pharmacy/pharmacist-EMR (PP-EMR). This would permit bidirectional electronic communication with clinic practice sites whose EMRs recognize the PP-EMR. Additional information regarding PP-EMRs can be found at the Pharmacy e-HIT Collaborative web site (www.PharmacyE-HIT.org). Another option is to request virtual private network (VPN) access to each providers' EMR for which you have established a collaborative practice agreement. VPN connectivity permits remote users access to local networks. This is a routine, well-established practice that practitioners implement to access their own EMRs from home, and with proper security you can be given access to the patient medical records. This would permit you to directly access progress notes and lab results as well as to add your progress note into the EMR. This is an exciting prospect that decreases faxing notes and lab results to the physician's office. This also helps resolve the problem of pharmacists' progress notes sent via fax or mail not making it into the patient's medical record. To be fair, some physicians' offices are able to keep track of loose filing and to scan all records so that there is an electronic copy; however, it is not uncommon to see a stack of documents pending scanning in an office, which means there could be a delay with your documentation being signed off and placed in the EMR. This could lead to a host of problems, with the most evident being oversight in patient care. If communication via fax is your best option, then consider developing a fax form that is well organized and stands out as a progress note.

CASE

Dr. Busybee completes documentation for each patient visit within the practice's EMR in which special templates were created and added for a pharmacy visit. Dr. Busybee and you worked with the IT department to facilitate this process prior to seeing patients. Once you complete your documentation, your SOAP note is sent electronically to Dr. Busybee for review and sign off. You are aware that in your home state it is required that referring physicians sign off on every note within 48 hours of the time you saw the patient, so you complete your documentation after each visit to minimize any delays in the process.

Clinic Work Flow Processes

Another task to consider when addressing clinic operations is clinic work flow.[3] Clinic work flow involves all processes of how the patient moves through your service from first entering the building to leaving it. This process ideally would appear seamless to the patient. The patient at no time should backtrack through the space or have the opportunity to get lost. If the service is in a physician's office, work flow should mimic that of the other providers by using the same clinic staff as the referring and ordering providers. If it is in a community pharmacy setting, new processes may need to be developed. Considerations include the following.

> **Patient check in.** Who will check in your patients? What paperwork (if any) is printed and where is it placed? Where will the patients be waiting (general waiting room or a special designated area)? Standard paperwork usually given to patients when they check in includes the demographics form that patients review to ensure the clinic has the proper address and insurance information for billing, the HIPAA form that indicates what information the patient authorizes you to share and with whom, and possibly a consent form to participate in a collaborative practice agreement with a pharmacist and physician. The latter is required by some state laws, so check your state to see if the patient has to sign a contract/agreement in order to participate in clinical pharmacy services. (Other forms that may be given to the patient include a medication list to verify and an initial medical assessment form.)

Clinic work flow involves all processes regarding how the patient moves through your service from first entering the building to leaving it and should appear seamless to the patient.

> **Vital signs.** Who will do vital signs—you or medical assistant or LPN? How will staff be notified that patients have arrived? Where will the vital signs be

documented (handwritten on sticky note, progress note, or EMR)? Where will the patient be placed after vitals are completed (back in the waiting room or in your exam room)? How will you be notified that the patient is ready for consultation? The key is to develop a process that is considered the standard of care for each visit. You may wish to solicit the support of the clerical and nursing staff to develop and take ownership of the various steps in the process. If you are in a physician's office, pattern your process on what is established as the standard of care for other providers.

Schedule follow-up appointments and manage no-shows. What staff will be assigned to manage this process? How will you follow up to ensure accuracy? If you have the resources, this task should be delegated to support staff. For an efficient, cost-effective service, the majority of your time should be spent practicing and providing services at the top level of your skill set.

Clinic visit documentation. How will you document the patient visit (handwrite or type in an EMR)? When do you document (during patient visit, immediately after a patient visit, or at the end of the day)? Where do you document (clinic pod, hallway, or exam room)? Ideally, all documentation would be done during the visit or immediately afterward to ensure that all necessary information was captured. If this is not possible, all documentation should be completed within 24 hours to ensure that nothing is missed and that billing can be completed. In a hospital setting, you will need to check with your billing department, as duration for completion is standard across the system. Dictation is an option, but it is fairly expensive and not as common as other types of documentation. The service may be used by physicians as an in-house or contracted service for which they pay per line or page. These charges typically show up on the cost reports for each department, so before you use an existing dictation service, note the potential costs in your financial projections. If you are in a community setting, dictation is often too expensive, leaving paper or electronic progress notes as good options. Chapter 6 will explore documentation standards and options to help you decide the optimal path for your clinic.

Legal Issues with Documentation

Maintaining additional clinical documentation beyond your patient progress notes may be required by state law or may be a personal preference. Laws vary from one state to the next regarding this topic, thus it is recommended that you familiarize yourself with your particular state law regarding what clinical documentation is required. In addition, each state board of pharmacy has the authority to develop rules or regulations that further define existing law. Thus, if your state law notes that clinical documentation is required, your state board may develop rules and regulations that specify the types of documents (i.e., referral or order forms with a physician's signature), what is considered to be acceptable storage (i.e., hard copy or electronic copy), and duration of storage (i.e., 5 years). Many states do not have any specific documentation requirements, and should this be the case in your situation, it is then your preference regarding what, where, and how long you wish to store clinical documents.

The purpose for going through this effort and for following all other legal considerations, as noted in Chapters 6 and 8, is for one reason: to show due diligence in case you are involved in a law suit. You do not have to be negligent to be sued. We live in a litigious society, and if a patient has an adverse reaction due to a medication that you adjusted; even though it is a potentially known risk that was discussed and documented, you could be sued by the patient or family member for malpractice. Should this occur, a jury comprised of lay members of your community will decide if you were negligent. In most states, the average lay member is likely not to have heard of a pharmacist adjusting a patient's drug therapy regimen per protocol. Their personal experience with a pharmacist may be limited to a traditional dispensing role only. Opposing legal counsel will ensure that there are no health care clinicians on the jury and will scrutinize every aspect of your clinic's protocol and collaborative drug therapy management agreement, documentation, and state law to assess if you were negligent in any way. Hence, it is critical that your service is developed within the boundaries of your state law and board's rules and regulations. Now that we have thoroughly scared you and your heart is beating 110 bpm, we would like to point out that no known clinical pharmacist, at the time of this book's publication, has been sued. That being said, as pharmacy practice progresses down the path of provider status, we assume the same attributed practice risks.

 You do not have to be negligent to be sued.

If you are required or choose to maintain hard copy documents, two options are a referral binder or a shadow chart. A referral binder contains hard copies of all provider referrals, orders, and consultations that are sent to your clinic. If not otherwise specified by law, it is recommended that the referral form include, at a minimum, the patient's name, patient's medical record number, date, provider's signature (hard or electronic), and the diagnosis code (ICD-9 code) that designates reason for referral. (ICD-9/ICD-10 codes - Note: The United States will be converting over to the ICD-10 codes starting in 2012 and this system will become mandatory for Medicare on October 1, 2013.) It is important to have the ICD-9 code noted, especially if you plan to bill incident-to a physician for your services (refer to Chapter 8 for further billing discussion). Pharmacists who do not have provider status should not be construed as diagnosing, but rather as assisting in managing an already diagnosed condition. Thus, in this case, it is important when billing for services that you note exactly the same ICD-9/ICD-10 code(s) that the referring provider uses. Referral binders may be of assistance to you if internal regulatory compliance auditors (i.e., compliance officer, billing auditor, etc.) or external regulatory auditors (i.e., board of pharmacy, payers, etc.) wish for you to produce a quick list of all the patients you have been authorized to see. The purpose of maintaining a referral binder is primarily for ease of regulatory-based audits. (Chapter 8 will explain further the need and reason for audits.) (Referral Form)

Even if all your progress notes are available on an EMR or electronic health record (EHR), what happens if your system is "down" when you are audited. At the very least, you have documentation of all of your patients' names and documentation of the physicians who refer to your practice. Some states require that you maintain such a list and be able to produce it immediately. Some EMRs and EHRs are able to sort all progress notes by author or clinical service name; however, many are not, as they simply list all entries by date with limited sorting capabilities. In your consideration for what documents you wish to maintain as hard copies, separate from the official medical record, familiarize yourself with how sophisticated your electronic record system is and how often it goes "down." If your electronic or written medical chart is not well organized and consistently accessible, you may wish to maintain hard copies of all your progress notes in a shadow chart. A separate shadow chart is developed for each patient and can be a very handy tool if portability is desired, if there is limited access to EMRs/EHRs in the clinic, if the written medical chart is difficult to locate, or if you have students and residents who could benefit from quickly reviewing your previous notes without gaining access to an additional computer or have time to review the patient's medical record. The shadow chart can contain any patient-specific material you wish as it is not considered a legal document, as is the official patient medical record. In addition to your copies of your progress notes (your original is in the patient medical record), you may wish to include copies of progress notes of other providers, procedure results, and/ or a summary form to succinctly record changes in specific lab values or dosing recommendations, for instance, an anticoagulation management chart.

If you choose to use the referral binder or shadow chart, remember the contents contain personal health information (PHI) and must be kept in a secure location. HIPPA PHI regulations are updated frequently, thus it is recommended that you review them to ensure that you are familiar with current requirements, as needed.[16]

Work Flow

It can take several weeks to months for all the work flow issues to be resolved. We recommend that you develop a work-flow diagram to be shared with all stakeholders.[3] In addition, for each staff member you may wish to put in writing specific agreed-upon responsibilities to facilitate mutual understanding of what each staff member's specific role is for the new service. This can be a frustrating time for you and all stakeholders; however, do your best to be patient, sympathetic, and kind to all staff during this process, as in the end, you need their full cooperation to be successful as a team. Remember you and your organization desire patient satisfaction and have as a mutual goal that patients easily understand how they move through a typical appointment with you in your practice setting. (Work-flow Diagram)

Training and Credentialing

The last primary task to consider under operations is what credentialing and training is needed for various entities. If practicing in a hospital-based outpatient clinic, you may need to seek credentialing for clinical privileges from the hospital credentialing board. Hospital credentialing is required for all recognized providers. If you are in a physician-based outpatient clinic or community pharmacy, credentialing is typically verified and documented by administrators.

Separately, training and credentialing may need to occur for use of the EMR and POC devices. It may be an organizational requirement that you are certified in basic life support. In addition, you may need to ascertain if the Clinical Laboratory Improvement Amendments (CLIA) waivers need to be applied for, if staff POC device training should be pursued, and who will perform the required quality assurance tests for the POC devices.[17]

Additional training or certification may be a requirement by the state board of pharmacy, a payer such as Medicaid, or by the physician practice group. These typically involve participation in a national or state-recognized condition or disease management program by completion of a course or exam. Such certification may be required for diabetes management, smoking cessation management, immunization administration, and anticoagulation management. If the pharmacist has completed a specialty residency, then this may take the place of such certifications. However, some organizations may require national board certification for practicing in their respective specialties. Refer to Chapter 7 for more details about credentialing and training.

CASE

Since Dr. Busybee and you took the time to meet with both receptionist and the nursing staff, you were able to ask questions about their laboratory requirements and certification process. The clinical nurse manager explained the process to integrate the INR machine into their office setting and what would be required for CLIA. You were asked by Dr. Busybee to show the margin of error was within acceptable standards per the office policy. This was done by first checking the patient's INR in the office and then sending the patient to the lab on the same day to see if the result coincided. Of course, you used this opportunity to solicit patient referrals from the physicians in the office and to also establish relationships with 10–20 current patients in the practice. In addition to certifying the machine, you did have to undergo technique training in order to use the INR machine per CLIA. All of the steps were facilitated by the clinical nurse manager since she was in charge of laboratory compliance for the practice site.

Patient Education

Other operation tasks that should be addressed involve choosing appropriate patient-education material and devices that you wish to have readily available. This can be a time-consuming task, and therefore you may wish to solicit clerical staff or students, if available, to help with this step. Clerical staff or students can be trained to identify the patient population's specific health literacy needs, maintain educational materials in the office space and exam room, and be in charge of tracking a borrowing system for patients to check out videos and books available in English and other languages, as needed.

Having various ways of providing educational material to patients will enhance the success of your education efforts. If you have a printer in your office space or exam room, then you may wish to develop electronic files of patient education material organized by condition or disease state, literacy level, and language. The advantage is that this material can be customized by the pharmacist to meet patient-specific needs. If a printer is not easily accessible, then contemplate which materials you wish to maintain as hard copies. For most ambulatory care practices today, high-quality materials are available for purchase or obtained at no charge from a variety of organizations. See **Appendix 5-1** as a starting point of web resources for patient-education material. If you choose to create your own materials, start by developing a template of what key points you wish to include.

Research the Internet for organizations relevant to the disease states and conditions you are managing. For example, if establishing a diabetes clinic, one place to start looking for material is the American Diabetes Association web site, which has a consumer section to assist in creating personalized patient-education material. Additional sources include various state organizations, national organizations, and pharmaceutical organizations that often have handouts provided at no charge. The latter can be a great source; however, careful scrutiny should be given to branded patient-education material as this can be particularly confusing if the patient is not on the medication seen on the sponsored educational material.

Should you wish to pursue evaluating material from pharmaceutical companies, begin by contacting your local pharmaceutical representatives or using the company web site. If choosing this route, you will need to spend time evaluating all the available options as they often have many different versions of similar products. When choosing what educational material to use, consider forming a committee that includes a pharmacist, clerical staff, and a physician to review the material. Through the perspective of the clerical staff, you can glean the potential impact and issues from the patient's perspective. If you are in a community pharmacy setting, review the material with other pharmacists and consider showing the material to your referring providers to ensure that everyone agrees regarding the patient education being provided.

Similar considerations should be given to obtaining patient demonstration devices such as inhalers; peak flow meters; insulin injection pens, vials, and pumps; low-molecular-weight heparin syringes; glucometers, home blood pressure devices; and tobacco cessation products. If you have access to a television and VCR/DVD player, you may wish to obtain videos/DVDs for those patients who may appreciate visual learning. This may require an initial investment if such a player is not already available at your practice site. A wheeled cart makes the TV portable between exam rooms. One advantage of a cart is that it eliminates the need for an education room, if space is limited.

Miscellaneous

Additional common considerations include

- obtaining your identification badge,

- having office keys made,

- ordering a pager and lab coat,

- securing photocopier pass code,

- ordering business and appointment cards,

- setting up phone, fax, and voice mail, and

- ordering a copier, fax, and scanning machine, as needed.

It is vital that all employees working in your clinic are properly identified by name and title on an ID badge. This adds value by clearly identifying who you and your staff are and invites patients to approach you. The title indicates each person's role in the patient's care. Business and appointment cards contribute to success as they provide patients permission to call you with questions, a separate number to call if they need to reschedule an appointment, and perhaps even a third number to call in case of an emergency.

Patients will also need to be educated regarding how to contact you after clinic hours, if you and your service are available. Regarding the latter, consider what mode works best for you: paging the pharmacist on call, calling a paging service, leaving a message on voice mail, or e-mailing or texting a specific address or number. For example, patients in an anticoagulation clinic will need to be educated regarding the person(s) to contact if they have general questions, are immediately concerned about a new medication that they have been prescribed, or develop bleeding issues. Ultimately, addressing these fine details from the beginning are what facilitate patient satisfaction and an effective practice.

Maintaining security of your office space is important, especially if you have computers or PHI stored there. You will need to decide who will have access to your exam room after hours and during clinic. In a hospital setting, often this decision is not yours, but if equipment or data go awry, it is important to understand who has access.

Lastly, when you are close to your "go-live date," start preparing an introductory presentation. The purpose of this presentation is to kick off your new service to all staff members, including all providers and nursing, clerical, and lab staff. It provides an open forum for staff to ask questions and for your provider-champion to show support. Begin by explaining the educational path for a pharmacist and what your particular educational path has been, and then elaborate on what services you will provide. Spend time discussing what a typical new patient and follow-up patient visit would entail. Food is always appreciated, so bring coffee and bagels or other treats for all staff to let them know you are excited to be part of the team.

Policy and Procedures

Having policy and procedure (P&P) documents is the standard of practice. We

develop various P&Ps to ensure quality of care and consistency in processes. Depending on your practice site, there are national accrediting organizations that
require certain processes be clearly delineated in a practice P&P document. Each
organization will have a specific format for how P&P documents should be formatted. If your practice site is in a physician's office, review the current P&P manual of
your referring physicians. If you are in a community pharmacy setting, then begin
by reviewing the P&P manual in the pharmacy to see what the existing format is and
if it is conducive to your practice. Reviewing existing P&Ps provides general information regarding the preferred format, level of detail expected, and who, if anyone,
should sign off. In this section we discuss what is typically contained in various P&P
documents, including clinic policy and procedure, laboratory policy and procedure, and billing procedure documents. It is recommended that you address these
topics with a brief bullet point or sentence.

Key Point
It is prudent to have your office manager and compliance
officer review your P&Ps to ensure that organizational
standards are met.

Policy and Procedure Document

The required content of P&P depends on the practice setting, namely hospital-
based outpatient clinic, physician-based outpatient clinic, or community pharmacy.
The compliance department or officer at your facility should be familiar with these
requirements and should be able to provide you with a document template and an
example of what is preferred.

   For hospital-based outpatient clinics and numerous other ambulatory care sites,
the Joint Commission, a standards-setting national accrediting organization, publishes a manual for ambulatory care sites yearly that should guide your P&P. The
Joint Commission also publishes the National Patient Safety Goals for a variety of
practice settings, including one called ambulatory health care. A number of resources from the Joint Commission can be accessed on the Internet at
www.jointcommission.org.

   In a physician-based ambulatory clinic, check with your compliance officer for
any state, payer, or other requirements that may affect your P&Ps for your new service. The Accreditation Association for Ambulatory Health Care (AAAHC;
www.aaahc.org) is an accrediting body for ambulatory organizations through which
your office may choose to seek certification. A number of organizations have established patient-centered medical home accreditation programs, including the following:

- National Committee for Quality Assurance (NCQA): www.ncqa.org
- The Joint Commission (JC): www.jointcommission.org
- Accreditation Association for Ambulatory Health Care (AAAHC):
  www.aaahc.org
- Utilization Review Accreditation Commission (URAC): www.urac.org

In a community practice setting, there are several national accrediting bodies your organization may choose to use, including the Community Health Accreditation Program (www.chapinc.org) and the National Association of Boards of Pharmacy Accreditation Program. Bear in mind the potential for new entities to enter into this arena and new requirements as standards and quality become a greater focus in our health care system. It is best to set up your procedures to meet the highest standards available as this will help you ensure that you are providing a high-quality service.

Your local department or practice site may have additional requirements regarding P&P content, so consider collecting examples from similar services, as appropriate, prior to initiating the process. In most cases, the content is not specified, thus the following list, though not exhaustive, does provide reasonable content from which to begin. (See **Table 5-2.**) (Examples of P&P Content)

When writing this P&P document, you need only write one or two sentences or bullet points to convey the intent of each policy and process. The document is not meant to be detailed, but rather to acknowledge that each task has been given consideration and a defined process to maintain quality and consistency of care. You want your P&P to be clear and easy to follow.

Table 5-2. Policy and Procedure Document Content

1. General title, such as Clinical Pharmacy Services or Medication Therapy Management used to cover all clinical pharmacy services provided if the content of the P&P applies to all services; if not, consider developing separate P&P documents for each unique clinical pharmacy service

2. Required credentials and preferred experience for all clinical pharmacist staff (i.e., PharmD required with 2 years of experience in primary care preferred)

3. Clinic job descriptions, including duties and responsibilities

4. Practice site location (i.e., hospital-based outpatient clinic located at XYZ clinic in Indianapolis, IN)

5. Hours of operation and off-hours coverage (i.e., 9–5, Mon–Fri, with off-hour coverage by clinical pharmacy staff who carry pagers for which the after-hours service operator has the number)

6. Referral and order process used for providers to send patients to your service and identification of type of patient for referral

7. Referral process for clinical pharmacist to manage urgent consults back to the supervising or ordering provider

8. Patient consent, as applicable (i.e., HIPAA, service consent, sharing personal health information, patient rights and responsibilities)

9. Patient scheduling process into your clinic

10. Length of new and follow-up patient visits

11. Description of direct supervision, as appropriate (i.e., will be provided by supervising clinic physician)

12. Standard and method(s) of clinic visit documentation (i.e., handwritten in patient's medical record, in patient's EMR, in shadow chart)

13. Location clinic visit notes will be stored (i.e., clinic medical records department, clinic EMR, pharmacy office)

14. Access by the referring or ordering provider and other providers to your visit progress notes and documentation, noting the time frame in which you will have your notes accessible as part of general continuity of care or communication process (i.e., within 24

hours)

15. Recommended follow-up intervals for patient and patient visits

16. Managing of urgent and emergent patient care issues (such as acute infection/distress, evaluation of DNR status, code blue, and when to call 911 versus taking patient to the emergency department if in a hospital outpatient practice setting)

17. Process by which to produce a list of patients seen and your progress notes, as may be required for state board of pharmacy (i.e., patient's hard-copy medical record, patient's EMR as can be sorted by your name, referral binder noting patient's medical record number that permits accessing progress notes in EMR)

18. Clinic billing process (i.e., subcontracted billing specialist from XYZ will perform billing or physician clinic billing staff will be used to process claims for this service)

19. Discharge or transfer from service and no-show policy (i.e., if patient no-shows for three consecutive visits, they will be discharged from this service back to the referring or ordering provider)

20. Point-of-care testing (if applicable)

21. Data to be collected both prospectively and retrospectively noting purpose and methodology, as appropriate (i.e., the named labs will be collected in an clinic database prospectively for the purposes of maintaining continuous quality control)

22. Clinical privileges included (i.e., per physician-signed collaborative drug therapy management protocol, delegated authority has been granted to provide the named service)

23. Continuous quality improvement of clinical service

24. Patient-education procedures (tools used for patient education and their procurement, education requirements for each visit, updated medication list, self-plan of care)

25. Continuing education requirements or options for staff

26. Assessment of staff

Laboratory Policy and Procedure Document for Point-of-Care Testing

The Centers for Medicare & Medicaid Services (CMS) administers all clinic laboratory testing requirements through the Clinical Laboratory Improvement Amendments (CLIA) passed by the U.S. Congress in 1988.[17,18] To receive a certificate of waiver under CLIA, a lab must perform only tests that the Food and Drug Administration and the Centers for Disease Control and Prevention have determined to be so simple that there is little risk of error. An active list of the labs that may qualify for waived status is maintained on the CMS website, www.cms.gov/clia. Clinics that wish to have such laboratory status simply complete an application online and pay the required fees.

Although having a CLIA-waived laboratory status precludes you from receiving routine inspections, CMS maintains the authority to conduct inspections at any time. In April 2002, CMS initiated on-site visits to approximately 2% of laboratories that had been issued a CLIA-waived certificate. This was the first time that CMS conducted visits in all 50 states, although smaller scale visits had been implemented. The purpose for these surveyors was to ensure that personnel conduct quality lab testing in a manner that protects patient safety and to determine laboratories' regulatory compliance. Waived laboratories must meet only the following requirements under CLIA:

- Enroll in the CLIA program
- Pay applicable certificate fees biennially
- Follow manufacturers' test instructions

If you are planning on maintaining any CLIA-waived devices, which includes most of the POC devices used in clinical pharmacy programs, then you will need to ensure that all devices are in compliance with CMS regulations. A worthwhile document to review is the *Good Laboratory Practices*, published in 2005 by CMS (www.cdc.gov/mmwr/preview/mmwrhtml/rr5413a1.htm).

If your practice setting already has a laboratory in it, and you plan to use its POC devices, then you are not responsible for maintaining CMS regulations for CLIA-waived devices, but rather the laboratory personnel is responsible. You would be required to develop a laboratory P&P only if your service is maintaining the POC devices used. Document content would include ensuring instrumentation validation, quality assurance, and proficiency testing of staff. For all CLIA-waived tests, users are required to follow the manufacturer's instructions for use. These include instructions for method limitations, intended use, and performing quality control.

Billing Procedure Document

A billing procedure document notes the specific criteria used to determine what CPTs, current procedural terminology, you plan to bill for your services. Even if you will only be billing using one CPT code, you are required in a hospital-based outpatient clinic to develop a billing procedure document.[9] See the web site for examples.📇 If you are in a physician-based outpatient office or a community pharmacy, no specific documentation is required, although it is recommended. The primary purpose of this document is for internal and external auditors to ensure that your medical record documentation supports the CPT levels that you are billing. For all providers, visit documentation is the only consideration for billing. It is for this reason you are advised to involve your practice site billing and/or compliance specialist to sign off on this document.

Key Point Depending on your practice setting and payer mix, you may have the option to bill based on patient complexity or based on time.

Complexity billing is typically how most recognized providers bill, though in certain situations time-based billing is permissible. In the first section of the CPT manual published by the American Medical Association, the criteria for billing for various CPTs for outpatient visits is noted, for example, 99211-99215.[19] The more complex the decision-making process, the higher is the CPT for which a provider may bill. Each organization typically develops a standard by which they code and often have coding specialists who routinely perform internal random audits on provider progress notes to ensure they are in compliance. Noncompliance is considered fraud. The reimbursement for most CPT codes is fixed per payer, and thus one can easily calculate financial projections if the payer mix of the clinic is known. The payer mix simply refers to the percentage of each insurance type of the clinic patients, including Medicare, Medicaid, third-party payers (also known as commercial payers, such as Anthem, United Health Care, Cigna, etc.), self-insured employers, self-pay (uninsured), and health plan patients, as appropriate. You may not have any patients represented by some of these payers and thus would only include payers specific to your patient population when performing financial projections.

If you are billing as a provider, you will likely bill using complexity-based billing and will need to delineate in the billing procedure document what specific criteria you plan to use to bill at the various CPT levels. This will follow the same criteria that other providers are billing under, thus they are likely to have already been established by the coding department or staff at your organization. If you will be billing incident-to a physician in a hospital-based outpatient clinic, you have the option to bill based on time or complexity. The 2010 HOPPS does not specify by which method you may bill. If billing incident-to a physician in a physician-based outpatient clinic, then typically you bill based on complexity. If billing Medicare Prescription Drug Plans as a provider using MTM CPTs, then time-based billing is the default and should be clearly delineated in the billing procedure document. For additional discussion, see Chapter 8 and corresponding web material. (Complexity-based and Time-based Documents)⧉

Chapter Summary

This chapter discussed two of the four tracks that should be traveled simultaneously, namely, clinic operations and policy and procedures. The critical billing and legal tracks are discussed in later chapters and should be reviewed closely. The umbrella term, practice operations, includes defining processes that impact activities on a day-to-day basis. Such activities include office space considerations, scheduling, work flow, and training and credentialing tasks. The first order of business is to ensure that suitable exam room or office space is allocated for your new service. The other tasks may be pursued based on preference and practice site practicality. Which P&P documents are required depends on your practice site and the payers. This may include development of clinic P&Ps, laboratory P&Ps, and a billing procedure document. In some instances, challenges may arise in securing your billing and compliance staff support regarding specific language. However, in the scope of tasks that need to be accomplished in order to set up a new practice site, developing P&Ps is perhaps the easiest.

References

1. Harris I, Baker E, et al. Developing a business-practice model for pharmacy services in ambulatory settings-ACCP white paper. *Pharmacotherapy.* 2008;28(2):7e-34e.
2. Linn W, Carter B, et al. Establishing and evaluating clinical pharmacy services in primary care-ACCP white paper. *Pharmacotherapy.* 1994;14(6):743-758.

3. Unerti K, Weinger M, et al. Describing and modeling workflow and information flow in chronic care disease. *J Am Med Inform Assoc.* 2009;16(6):826-836.

4. Vazquez S, Campbell J, et al. Anticoagulation clinic workflow analysis. *J Am Pharm Assoc.* 2003;49(1):78-85.

5. Xakellis G, Bennett A, et al. Improving clinic efficiency of a family medicine teaching clinic. *Fam Med.* 2001;33(7):533-538.

6. Snella K, Sachdev G. A primer for developing outpatient clinics in the outpatient setting. *Pharmacotherapy.* 2003;23(9):1153-1166.

7. Snella K, Trewyn R, Hansen L, et al. Pharmacist compensation for cognitive services: focus on the physician office and community pharmacy. *Pharmacotherapy.* 2004;24(3):372-388.

8. Hospital Outpatient Regulations and Notices. Centers for Medicare and Medicare Services. Hospital Outpatient Prospective Payment System web site. http://www.cms.gov/HospitalOutpatientPPS/HORD/list.asp#TopOfPage. Accessed July 11, 2011.

9. Incident to Regulations. *Fed Regist.* 2010; 42:410.26. http://edocket.access.gpo.gov/cfr_2010/octqtr/pdf/42cfr410.26.pdf. Accessed July 12, 2011.

10. Point of Care Testing Topic Center. College of American Pathologists web site. http://www.cap.org/apps/cap.portal?_nfpb=true&cntvwrPtlt_actionOverride=%2Fportlets%2FcontentViewer%2Fshow&_windowLabel=cntvwrPtlt&cntvwrPtlt%7BactionForm.contentReference%7D=committees%2Fpointofcare%2Fpoct_topic_center.html&_state=maximized&_pageLabel=cntvwr. Accessed July 11, 2011.

11. Cayirli, T, Veral E, et al. Designing appointment scheduling systems for ambulatory care services. *Health Care Manag Sci.* 2006;9(1):47-58.

12. Blum B. Definition of medication therapy management: Development of profession-wide consensus. *J Am Pharm Assoc.* 2005;45:566-572.

13. Anonymous. Summary of the executive sessions on medication therapy management. *Am J Health-Syst Pharm.* 2005;62:585-592.

14. American Pharmacists Association web site. www.pharmacist.com. Accessed July 11, 2011.

15. National Plan and Provider Enumeration System (NPPES) web site. https://nppes.cms.hhs.gov/NPPES/Welcome.do. Accessed July 11, 2011.

16. Summary of the HIPAA Security Rule. HIPAA PHI Regulations web site. http://www.hhs.gov/ocr/privacy/hipaa/understanding/srsummary.html. Accessed July 11, 2011.

17. Current CLIA Regulations. Centers for Disease Control and Prevention web site. http://wwwn.cdc.gov/clia/regs/toc.aspx. Accessed July 11, 2011.

18. Clinical Laboratory Improvement Amendments. U.S. Food and Drug Administration web site. http://www.fda.gov/MedicalDevices/DeviceRegulationandGuidance/IVDRegulatoryAssistance/ucm124105.htm. Accessed July 11, 2011.

19. Coding Billing Insurance. AMA web site. http://www.ama-assn.org/ama/pub/physician-resources/solutions-managing-your-practice/coding-billing-insurance/cpt.shtml. Accessed July 11, 2011.

Web Resources

Example Referral/Order/HIPPA Consult Form

Physician Fax Form

Example of an Anticoagulation Management Face Sheet

Example Warfarin Monitoring Sheet

Work Flow Diagram

Examples of Clinic Policy and Procedure Documents

    Billing Policy Example

    Medication Management Clinic Policy and Procedure

Examples of Billing Procedure Documents

    Proposed Point-based Billing Procedure for Clinical Pharmacy Services Billing Incident

    -   to Physician

    Proposed Time-based Billing Procedure for Clinical Pharmacy Services Billing Incident

    -   to Physician

New Patient Intake Form

DM Patient Assessment

MTM Patient Note Template

Revised Initial Patient Note

Patient Education Web Resources

Web Toolkit available at
www.ashp.org/ambulatorypractice

Appendix 5-1: Web Resources for Patient Education Material🖥

GENERAL

http://healthfinder.gov

http://medlineplus.gov

http://www.noah-health.org

http://caphis.mlanet.org/
consumer/index.html

www.kidshealth.org

http://girlshealth.gov

http://nihseniorhealth.gov

http://womenshealth.gov

http://www.ashp.org/menu/
InformationFor/Patients.aspx

http://www.ahrq.gov/consumer/
healthy.html

http://jama.ama-assn.org/cgi/
collection/patient_page

FamilyDoctor.org Smart Patient Guide

http://familydoctor.org/online/
famdocen/home/pat-
advocacy.html

Medline Plus Easy-To-Read Health Materials

http://www.nlm.nih.gov/
medlineplus/all_easy
toread.html

American Academy of Pediatrics: Patient Education

http://patiented.aap.org/
categoryBrowse.aspx?
catID=5003

Center for Multicultural Health: Health in Many Languages

http://health.utah.gov/cmh/
multilinguallibrary.htm

Safe Medication: Medication Tips Tools

http://www.safemedication.com/
safemed/MedicationTips
Tools.aspx

DISEASE SPECIFIC

Cancer

http://cancer.gov

Heart Failure

http://www.heartfailure.org/>
http://www.nhlbi.nih.gov/health/dci/Diseases/
Hf/HF_WhatIs.html

http://www.nlm.nih.gov/medlineplus/
heartfailure.html#cat69

http://www.heart.org/HEARTORG/Conditions/
HeartFailure/AboutHeartFailure/About-Heart-
Failure_UCM_002044_Article.jsp

American Heart Association: Tools and Resources

http://www.heart.org/HEARTORG/Conditions/
HeartFailure/HeartFailureToolsResources/Heart-
Failure-Tools-Resources_UCM_002049_Article.jsp

Thyroid

http://www.nlm.nih.gov/medlineplus/
thyroiddiseases.html

COPD

http://www.nhlbi.nih.gov/health/dci/Diseases/
Copd/Copd_WhatIs.html

http://www.nlm.nih.gov/medlineplus/
copdchronicobstructivepulmonarydisease.html

http://www.cdc.gov/copd/#learn_more

http://www.cdc.gov/copd/resources.htm

http://www.lungusa.org/lung-disease/copd/

http://www.lungusa.org/lung-disease/copd/living-
with-copd/copd-management-tools.html

Asthma

http://www.nhlbi.nih.gov/health/dci/Diseases/
Asthma/Asthma_WhatIs.html

http://www.nlm.nih.gov/medlineplus/asthma.html

http://www.cdc.gov/asthma/

http://www.cdc.gov/asthma/publications.html

http://www.lungusa.org/lung-disease/asthma/

Hyperlipidemia and Heart Disease

http://www.nhlbi.nih.gov/chd/index.htm
http://www.nhlbi.nih.gov/health/public/heart/
index.htm#hbp

Appendix 5-1: Web Resources for Patient Education Material🖳 (cont'd)

GENERAL

Safe Medication: How to Administer

http://www.safemedication.com/safemed/MedicationTipsTools/HowtoAdminister.aspx

Medline Plus

http://www.nlm.nih.gov/medlineplus/druginformation.html

Medication Misuse Brochure

http://www.ismp.org/tools/ISMP-Med-Cabinet-10.pdf

Medication Safety in Community/Ambulatory Practice

http://www.ismp.org/tools/communitySafetyProgram.asp

Information for Consumers

http://www.fda.gov/Drugs/ResourcesForYou/Consumers/default.htm

Healthy Living

http://www.cdc.gov/HealthyLiving

Medications Made Easy

http://assets.aarp.org/www.aarp.org_/articles/health/images/meds/meds_made_easy.pdf

Guide for Older Adults

http://www.fda.gov/Drugs/ResourcesForYou/ucm163959.htm

Center for Medicines and Healthy Aging

http://www.medsandaging.org/

Be Med Wise

http://www.bemedwise.org/

DISEASE SPECIFIC

Diabetes

http://www.hearthub.org/hc-diabetes.htm

http://cdc.gov/diabetes/consumer/index.htm

http://www.nlm.nih.gov/medlineplus/diabetes.html

http://www.ndep.nih.gov/

http://diabetes.niddk.nih.gov/dm/ez.asp

http://www.dshs.state.tx.us/diabetes/patient.shtm

http://www.nlm.nih.gov/medlineplus/diabetes.html

http://www.diabetes.org/living-with-diabetes/?utm_source=WWW&utm_medium=GlobalNavLWD&utm_campaign=CON

http://www.diabetes.org/food-and-fitness/?utm_source=WWW&utm_medium=GlobalNavFF&utm_campaign=CON

http://www.ndei.org/v2/website/content/PatientEducation.cfm

Smoking Cessation

http://www.aafp.org/online/en/home/clinical/publichealth/tobacco/resources.html

http://www.acpfoundation.org/files/ht/smo_en.pdf

http://www.cancer.org/Healthy/StayAwayfromTobacco/GuidetoQuittingSmoking/index?sitearea=ped

http://www.cancer.gov/cancertopics/factsheet/Tobacco

http://www.heart.org/HEARTORG/GettingHealthy/GettingHealthy_UCM_001078_SubHomePage.jsp

Arrhythmia

http://www.hearthub.org/hc-arrhythmia.htm

Atrial Fibrillation

http://www.cdc.gov/dhdsp/data_statistics/fact_sheets/fs_atrial_fibrillation.htm

http://www.hrsonline.org/PatientInfo/HeartRhythmDisorders/AFib/index.cfm

Heart and Stroke Facts

http://www.americanheart.org/downloadable/heart/1056719919740HSFacts2003text.pdf

Appendix 5-1: Web Resources for Patient Education Material🖳 (cont'd)

GENERAL	DISEASE SPECIFIC
Senior Series Fact Sheets	**Cholesterol**
http://ohioline.osu.edu/ss-fact/ index.html	http://www.hearthub.org/hc-cholesterol.htm
	http://www.nlm.nih.gov/medlineplus/cholesterol.html
Primary Care Clinic Patient Handouts	http://www.mayoclinic.com/health/high-blood-cholesterol/DS00178
http://www.eric.vcu.edu/home/ resources/pcc_handouts.html	http://www.nhlbi.nih.gov/health/public/heart/chol/ wyntk.pdf
	http://www.patientedu.org/aspx/HealthELibrary/ HealthETopic.aspx?cid=HC0806
	Hypertension
	http://www.hearthub.org/hc-high-blood-pressure.htm
	http://www.cdc.gov/bloodpressure/
	http://www.nlm.nih.gov/medlineplus/ highbloodpressure.html
	http://www.controlhypertension.org/patient/
	http://www.hypertensionfoundation.org/booklets.cfm

Communication & Documentation for an Ambulatory Practice

Seena L. Haines, Tim R. Brown

CHAPTER 6

Chapter Outline

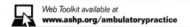
Web Toolkit available at
www.ashp.org/ambulatorypractice

Chapter Objectives

1. Identify the relevance for pharmacists' documentation of clinical services.

2. Compare and contrast manual and electronic documentation systems.

3. Review the common documentation styles and communication techniques used in clinical practice.

4. Recognize the appropriate levels for billing based on an example of documentation.

5. Discuss continuous quality assurance and other safety measures when implementing and maintaining documentation.

Introduction

Regardless of your practice environment, you will need to use electronic and manual methods of documentation to communicate, exchange information, and educate patients, caregivers, and other health care professionals. Like other health care providers, you will primarily use the patient medical record (PMR) for documentation of patient care. Through efficient and comprehensive documentation you can (1) meet professional standards and legal requirements, (2) communicate with other health care professionals, (3) establish accountability for medication-related aspects of direct patient care, (4) strengthen transition and continuity of care, (5) create your record of critical thinking and judgment, (6) provide evidence of your value and workload allocation, (7) justify reimbursement for cognitive services, and (8) provide needed data for tracking of patient health outcomes.[1]

Currently, industry-driven advances in technology are having a profound effect on how pharmacists document and are also creating new challenges. With the passage by Congress of the stimulus package (the American Recovery and Reinvestment Act, or ARRA), expansion of health information technology (HITCH) is now mandated by the U.S. government. ARRA budgeted approximately $150 billion for health care reform and close to $34 billion for health care provider adoption of HITCH and a nationwide health record system by 2014.[2] The most critical element to the e-health system is the electronic medical record (EMR) and the electronic health record (EHR). An EMR is a portal that shares relevant patient information among health care professionals. Likewise, it can perform as a patient scheduler and an intraoffice messaging system as well as assist with laboratory communications, e-prescribing, and billing processing. An EHR is an individual patient medical record digitized from many locations or sources, including the patient and family members. It can interface with evidenced-based treatment algorithms and protocols, outcomes reporting, and quality assurance and is synonymous with what is also called the patient medical record (PMR). An electronic personal health record (ePHR) can be created by patients, physicians, pharmacies, health systems, and other sources, but originates from a patient.[2]

An EMR and EHR can enhance provider communication in all health care settings. EMRs are primarily focused on physician and hospital-based practice, but there is potential for benefit in pharmacy practice with wider implementation. EMR adoption is predicted to bring the following patient and health care provider benefits: lower costs, quality care, improved reimbursement, enhanced productivity, efficiency, effectiveness, and communication.[2]

While the EMR has promise of advancing patient care and can be a resource to capture patient encounters, it is not without its challenges. This is especially true in the primary care setting due to the sheer number and small size of ambulatory organizations. Pharmacists practicing in the ambulatory patient care arena have historically used a modified SOAP (subjective, objective, assessment, plan) note format to document patient encounters, with sections expanded or omitted based on relevance to the practice and scope or service. It has been physician, and not pharmacist, work flow that has driven creation, adoption, and integration of most outpatient EMR and PMR applications. Consequently, it has been difficult to alter or adapt a physician-driven EMR to fit the work-flow dynamics of a pharmacist-provided visit in the ambulatory setting. For example, most templates that fit individual disease states have predetermined signs and symptoms that are consistent with a pharmacist's visit, such as documentation of hypo- or hyperglycemic symptoms for diabetes; however, pharmacists do not perform eye exams routinely, thus documenting a normal eye exam would be inappropriate in the template. This is where the EMR can be tricky for the pharmacist because both are normally included in a diabetes visit template. This is important since it relates to payment for clinical services. Although pharmacists do not perform detailed physical exams, we do address complexity, such as multiple disease states, some aspects of review of systems (ROSs) and physical exams (PEs), monitoring, follow-up, and capturing of outcomes. Documentation on templates is designed to emphasize and ensure that the appropriate information is in place for billing using the correct evaluation and management service codes. Using a template that has incomplete sections or that can be billed inappropriately (physician services versus a midlevel provider services) could result in devastating financial and legal consequences for your organization. Depending on your EMR, investigate whether it has the ability to code and recognize language used in your template to populate other fields in the PMR to ensure correct billing for your services, to collect data related to your services, and to generate a list of patients for whom you have provided care. If not, you should consider a separate clinical pharmacy documentation system to capture your needed documentation. Optimally it should integrate in some form or manner with your organization's EMR.

CASE

In Dr. Busybee's office they have already converted from a paper PMR to an EMR. Now that all the logistics of seeing patients in the office are resolved, you must determine how you want to document your interaction with each patient. After a review of the current EMR you noticed that none of the disease state templates address anticoagulation management; however, the good news is the diabetes management template used by the physicians could be used for your visits as well. Knowing that you have no built-in system to document care given for patients using an anticoagulant, you approach the office manager about changing the EMR. The office manager promptly tells you this is outside their expertise and that they want nothing to do with changing the EMR setup. Dr. Busybee really does not understand why you cannot just type your encounter note into the EMR. You attempt to explain the volume of patients and the time commitment for that type of documentation. His response is "We use the EMR in this office — make it work so I can start referring patients to you as soon as possible."

Because EMRs generally are not created with clinical pharmacy practice in mind, you may have already concluded it will be important for you to collaborate with your institutional information technology (IT) personnel as well as pharmacy management system (PMS) vendors as needed to develop the necessary technical integration solutions that incorporate your work flow and corresponding documentation requirements.[2] This seems like a straightforward solution; however, many IT personnel have no experience with pharmacists seeing patients in an ambulatory setting or with the details of how we document, so they may be unwilling or lack sufficient knowledge to build a special area for a pharmacy visit within the adopted EMR. This can be further complicated by the fact that not all EMRs are created equally, and the adopted EMR may require a major system overhaul or significant financial outlay to accommodate your clinical services. You should be prepared to educate IT personnel on how you document your patient encounters, such as the need for a universal template for all pharmacotherapy-based visits and specific disease-state templates (e.g., diabetes or anticoagulation). An existing physician template may be used with minor or no alterations.

How do you know which type of templates work for you within an EMR? Just like other challenges in the pharmacy world you will need to research and investigate the functionality of the proposed or current EMR at your site. Visit the EMR vendor web page and familiarize yourself with the advantages and disadvantages of the application and whether the system can address the needs of midlevel providers such as the clinical pharmacist. Reviewing articles and attending lecture series as well as professional meetings may help, but usually it requires your review of your particular system to solidify its application to your services. One resource is the American Medical Association's online bookstore.[3] Currently, there are several books available that discuss types of EMRs, as well as incorporation and maintenance of the systems. (AMA web site) Granted, pharmacists rarely have a vote in the decision regarding which system is purchased for outpatient services, but such EMR resources can educate you on which systems allow specialization and customization and which are more restrictive in adapting to midlevel provider patient care services.

Once you understand your EMR's flexibility and how your services will integrate into the EMR system, you can begin to create or adapt your current manual patient care notes to an electronic template format. The majority of EMRs do use a SOAP-based format, but it may appear unrecognizable because many systems follow a point-and-click process rather than use free text for documenting. No matter which format, you will have to integrate your documentation within the systematic approach designed by the EMR's manufacturer. It is imperative that your documentation work flow be developed with your input and feedback to ensure the documentation process is efficient, easy to use, synergistic with the flow of the patient visit, and captures all the needed information. If the process is not scrutinized thoroughly, you may find yourself inefficiently jumping around the screen or having to type a large amount within your template; this leads to less time spent seeing patients and ultimately decreasing productivity and reducing reimbursement, which affects the viability of your practice.

One solution is to critically assess work flow with IT assistance to create an electronic template that is geared toward practice functions (pre-visit information gathering, visit documentation, orders you are able to execute, and billing) as well as the type of patient care visits you encountered. One example is an anticoagulation visit in which the international normalized ratio (INR) is obtained by the nursing staff while they are doing vitals and preparing the patient room for the office visit. You may then enter the room to complete your visit with information already entered into the electronic note. Alternatively, you, a resident, or your advanced practice clerkship student could be responsible for performing vitals, point-of-care testing, and the interview. The work flow and thus the note would be different. The key is to create your template around the structure and flow of your patient visit. No matter which work flow and template is incorporated, your note should always contain the following elements:

- time of arrival and departure
- chief complaint
- history of present illness
- past medical history
- allergies
- social history
- family history
- appropriate referrals
- labs
- medication reconciliation
- assessment and plan

(Example Documentation Elements for EMR/PMR)

CASE

Over the past 3 months you have slowly integrated into Dr. Busybee's practice, and your office hours have gained momentum to where you are seeing approximately 20 patients per week. Dr. Busybee calls you into his office to discuss how the first quarter has gone and wants to know if you are "keeping track" of your impact. After some thought, you admit the last 3 months have been busy and just keeping up with the clinical aspect of your job has taken a great deal of time. Dr. Busybee reminds you of your business plan proposal and would like you to create metrics and outcome measures to ensure you are meeting your goals. In the meantime he has been approached by a local pharmacy school and asked if his office would allow pharmacy students to complete an Ambulatory Care rotation. They are offering compensation for each student, and he believes this is a perfect fit since they have you in their practice. This allows for additional revenue to the office and helps pay your salary. You agree to act as a preceptor with the first student starting in 2 months. The first thought you have is: How will I integrate these students into my clinical practice site, how best can I utilize students to help me accomplish my work, and what hurdles do I face with documentation if I allow students to see my patients?

Once you have your work flow outlined and templates designed, the next step is to ensure the security of your system. The overall security will be created and implemented by the IT department; however if the setting is an experiential training site, you will need to create security measures that limit the access of your pharmacy students. For a thorough experience, students will need access to the EMR with their own log-on information; however, their integration must be limited so they cannot "complete" an encounter note without your preceptor's electronic signature.

Another consideration is integrating pharmacy residents that are completing training at your institution into your documentation process. As pharmacy residents are licensed pharmacists and generally should receive greater autonomy, you may wish to create an electronic preceptor section within the encounter note that allows the preceptor to add addenda and cosign the resident's completed note. This allows supervision by the preceptor, a level of autonomy for residents, and billing for the visit, since technically the precepting pharmacist is the collaborating midlevel provider, not the pharmacy resident.

Despite the many challenges, transitioning to an EMR and computerized provider order entry (CPOE) is the future and a requirement under new Medicare Part D regulations that were effective in 2009. Technological advancement certainly facilitates generation and transfer of documentation and holds much promise to improve patient safety, although many concerns still exist, such as access to data (storage) and patient confidentiality. The American Society of Health-System Pharmacists (ASHP) has an investment to "increase the extent to which health systems apply technology effectively to improve the safety of medication use." ASHP has identified several targets to aid in goal achievement, including enhanced use of CPOE and EMRs, along with enhancement of information access and communication across the health care continuum. Since 2005, pharmacists in 19% of health systems transfer information to promote seamless care of patients with complex medication regimens. ASHP strives to increase integration of technology as the new pharmacy practice model is defined and adopted by practice sites.[2,4]

Documentation Styles

Whether the information is typed or written into a PMR, the documentation of a clinical interview should provide (1) what happened, (2) to whom, (3) who made it happen or the cause of the event, (4) occurrence, (5) rationale for why it occurred, and (6) outcome of action.[1,5-9] A survey among community-based pharmacists identified the following primary characteristics of ideal documentation practices: comprehensiveness, affordable cost, time efficiency, ease of use, and ability to generate patient reports.[5] Additionally, with our improved understanding of the perils associated with patient transitions of care, communication and coordination of care documentation should be added to this list. Several documentation styles can and have been adapted to record pharmacist encounters, including unstructured notes, semistructured notes, and systematic records, all possible in written documentation and growing in popularity within EMR formats. No matter the format and media, documentation should be

- clear,
- concise,
- legible,
- nonjudgmental,
- patient focused,
- standardized, and
- confidential.[1,6-8]

The most common format used in the medical system is systematic documentation, which includes SOAP, TITRS (title, introduction, text, recommendation, signature), and FARM (findings, assessment, recommendations or resolutions, and management). Other examples of structured formats include drug-related problem, rationale, plan (DRP); data, assessment, and plan (DAP); and drug-related problem, data, assessment, and plan (DDAP). TITRS is an assessment approach, and FARM places importance on monitoring, but these formats are not common among pharmacists' documentation and therefore are not discussed in greater detail. The SOAP note is an interventionist approach and considered the standard for most if not all health care providers, including pharmacists.[1,6-8]

Each style of structured or unstructured noting has advantages and disadvantages but should be consistently used in the most effective and efficient manner. Unstructured notes are seen more commonly with traditional manual documentation, and as the name implies, they are free in form, with appropriate language and chronology. Advantages of this style are that the notes can be written expeditiously while still providing a solid, high-quality, general overview. One disadvantage is the note may be incomplete and inconsistent, which limits communication to other health care professionals, leaving practitioners vulnerable to liability. This type of documentation, whether it be manual or electronic, is usually reserved for phone messages and informal communication between practitioners regarding ongoing patient care issues secondary to the limitations.[1,6,7]

To be more complete the majority of manual and electronic documentation follows the systematic approach, allowing for completeness, consistency, and organization. Without a systematic structure, the documentation of the encounter may be time consuming and confusing, especially in regards to the placement of information from different sources. An example of this can be seen when documenting height, weight, and allergies. One clinician may document this information in the subjective findings, and another may place the information within the objective data collection section. The primary determinant for where this information should appear is how the information was collected. Was the information patient reported (subjective) or clinician measured (objective)? This problem may not be as apparent with an electronic documentation since many of the templates allow data to be entered only in certain fields of the encounter note, creating semistructured documentation. This blends different styles for which some fields are more standardized and others are free text. Like unstructured documenting, semistructured documentation may also lack the quality and consistency of the standardized SOAP note. Semistructured noting may be best used when triaging or forming a general impression for referral with no specific action needed by the pharmacist, much like a phone message or reporting of a lab result to the collaborating practitioner.

The more structured SOAP note format is appropriate when follow-up and monitoring are required as well as showing continuity of care provided by the health care practitioner. Both of these documentation styles have been used routinely with written communication and now are slowly being integrated as standards for the majority of EMRs.[1,6,7,10] This is especially true of the SOAP format since it is the primary form for which payers traditionally reimburse.

No matter the format or style, documentation should always be used to demonstrate the impact of your interventions to improve patient care and the overall management of the chronic disease state(s). In addition, the documentation needs to support and allow for reimbursement. All documentation should be complete, complementary, compelling due to supportive evidence, and standardized and systematic to complement the oral communication among providers. Furthermore, documentation should reflect patient agreement with the care plan among multiple providers in terms of medication reconciliation, data collection, continuity of care, and the transitioning of care along the continuum.[1,6-8,11,12]

Knowing this makes it much more apparent that documentation is more than completing forms or capturing data during a patient encounter. No single ideal format can encompass all patient interviews, yet documentation can still provide evidence of the pharmacist's interventions in advocacy and patient management. An example SOAP note (**Figure 6-1**) illustrates a standardized, structured approach to documentation and medication reconciliation, which will be discussed shortly. (Example SOAP Note)

The four distinctive sections of a SOAP note are outlined as follows:[1,6-8]

1. **Subjective**: symptoms, information, and answers to provider questions that the patient verbally expresses or that are provided by a caregiver. These descriptions provide a clinician with insight into the severity of a patient's condition, the level of dysfunction, illness progression, and degree of pain.

2. **Objective**: measurements that are observed (seen, heard, touched, smelled) by clinician or that can be tested. Examples include vital signs, pulse, temperature, skin color, edema, and diagnostic testing.

3. **Assessment**: a prioritized list of assessed conditions. Simply stated, it is what you think are the patient's issues or problems from your perspective as a pharmacist provider. This may consist of a level of control, differentials, potential confounders to control, pertinent positives or negative signs and symptoms related to the condition, reference to evidence-based medicine (EBM), considerations for pharmacotherapy, and adjunctive lifestyle measures.

4. **Plan**: care plan action steps for the patient and health care practitioners. The plan consists of the actions that you initiate or suggest to improve or resolve the issues or problems identified in the assessment. This may in-

clude requests for additional laboratory or diagnostic assessments, alterations in pharmacotherapy, lifestyle recommendations, standards of care, special directions, referrals, self-monitoring, emergency contacts, and time for follow-up appointments.

Date: XX/XX/XX   Time In: 10AM

Pharmacotherapy Note:

S: MM is a 51 YO WM who presents for follow-up regarding his diabetes self-management education (DSME) and follow-up A1C. MM will begin group support classes (part 1 and 2) at the DERC in January. MM does not have a PCP provider at this time since he does not have insurance. He began a new job this month and hopes to have insurance within the next 90 days. Patient does not report any complaints today.

PmHx: Type 2 DM (since June 2009)

Melanoma on forehead

ALL: NKDA

CVD risk factors (–) tobacco (+) HTN (+) DM (+) Low HDL (–) FamHx Ht Dz (+) age (M>45, W>55) = 4 risk factors (1 CVD equivalent)

DM (–) polydipsia, (–) polyphagia but has some increased polyuria last week when starting his new job. Nocturia x 0-2. (–) episode(s) of hypoglycemia since last visit.

(+) tingling in wrist and calves, (–) burning, and numbness of extremities or cramping. Pt reports (–) edema

HTN: (+) HA 2 days ago resolved with ibuprofen and rarely occurs (–) dizziness, (–) chest pain. Trying to keep sodium intake <2g/d.

Trying to follow dietary recommendations (low in sat fat, trans fats, more complex carbs and higher fiber): eating three meals a day. Will review food labels and carb counting in DSME classes.

Soc Hx: (–) Tob, never smoked (–) EToH, (–) illicit drugs, (+) caffeine (1 cup tea in AM with skim milk and sugar subst), not exercising right now due to left toe amputation in June. Works at a hotel and recently changed location, as an auditor on 11-7P M shift.

SurgHx: Left toe amputation (due to DM or other factor)

SMBG: per patient log (10/10-10/13): (FBG only) (133–144). No readings above 140 mg/dL.

Standards of care:

Podiatry appt: to be scheduled   Optometry appt: to be scheduled

Immunizations: flu shot and pneumo needed, refer to health department

O: Sex: M HT: 68 in. WT: 193 (Previous 197, 202)   Race: Caucasian

BMI: 30 (category I)

BP: 148/56 (no HTN medications taken today, caffeine within 30 min of appt)

(Prev) 114/76, 112/72 mmHg

100

PPBG: 122 mg/dL (ate cereal at 8:30 AM)   Prev FBG: 8/17 (184, 1 hr PPBG)

Previous labs: 7-09 (fasting or nonfasting)

K: 4.3

LFT: WNL

Figure 6-1. Example SOAP Note (written by SL Haines).

Scr: 0.73

Lipids: WNL, except low HDL 21 mg/dL

Date: XXX (**fasting**)

TC: 145 TG: 135 LDL: 97 HDL: 21

EsGFR: (7/09) 148 (CG), 120 mL/min (MDRD)

Microalbuminuria (UACR): not assessed

A1C: 5.7%   (12.2% [7/10/09] when hospitalized/diagnosed)

Outpt medications: (medication reconciliation documented and verified)

Metformin 500 mg PO BID (taking)

Glipizide 5 mg PO daily (taking)

Clonidine 0.1 mg PO TID (not taking)

Lisinopril 20 mg PO BID (not taking)

Omeprazole 20 mg PO daily (not taking)

OTC

Recommend ASA 81 mg PO daily (has not been taking)

Herbals

None

A: 1. DM: Controlled based on SMBG log, hyperglycemia symptom improvement and A1C today. Needs education reinforcement for meter instruction technique and importance of checking BG twice a day before breakfast and 2 hr after meals. Needs comprehensive annual foot exam and assessment for microalbuminuria, retinopathy assessment, annual influenza, and low dose ASA. (Goal FBG 70-130 mg/dL, PPBG<180 mg/dL, HbA1C<6%-7% without causing hypoglycemia)

2. HTN: Uncontrolled based BP today in clinic. Patient with adverse effects associated with clonidine: sleepiness, lethargy, dizziness. Inappropriately stopped his lisinopril due to poor knowledge regarding medications. (Goal<130/80 DM)

3. Lipids: Controlled based on recent lipid panel with the exception of his HDL. (Goal TC<200 mg/dL, TG<150 mg/dL, HDL>40 mg/dL, LDL<100, optional goal <70 mg/dL)

4. ADHERENCE: Expected level of patient adherence is: good

P: 1. Discussed the importance of checking blood glucose at least BID and provided log to report values. Provided pt education videos on foot hygiene, meter use, and exercise at home.

2. Discussed the s/sx of hypo/hyperglycemia and what to do should they occur. Confirmed technique for meter instruction and will reassess in 3 months.

3. Reviewed all medications (provided med list) with patient and discussed reinitiation of lisinopril. Will reinitiate lisinopril at low dose 20 mg 1/2T PO daily (10mg) and reevaluate for titration when RTC in 2 weeks.

4. Continue current dose of metformin 500 mg PO BID with meals, ASA 81 mg PO daily, glipizide 5 mg PO daily before breakfast. Discussed side effects to look for regarding his medications.

5. Encouraged to continue low-fat, low-cholesterol, moderate CHO diet (130-150 g/d). Reinforced importance of physical activity as tolerated with his amputation and contingent on provider approval. Alternatives are swimming, stationary bike, as well as reinforcing principles of the DASH diet and TLC to help improve HDL.

6. Refer to NP today for comprehensive foot exam and health department for flu shot.

Figure 6-1. Example SOAP Note (written by SL Haines). (cont'd)

7. Will notify Dr. X (physician) of the pending blood work and assessment today.
8. Will need f/u lipid assessment in November, microalbuminuria assessment, A1C in 3 months and should be screened for colorectal cancer.
9. Call with any problems

Follow-up standards of care

1. Podiatry q 6 months
2. Dentistry q 6 months
3. Optometry q 6 months
4. Nutrition prn

Signature

Seena Haines, PharmD, BC-ADM, CDE
Pharmacotherapy Specialist
Diabetes Education and Research Center

Time Out: 60 minutes spent counseling/coordinating care
Total Time Spent: 1 HR

Figure 6-1. Example SOAP Note (written by SL Haines). (cont'd)

Additional considerations when documenting patient care can be obtained from the *ASHP Guidelines on Documenting Pharmaceutical Care in Patient Medical Records, Guidelines on a Standardized Method for Pharmaceutical Care,* and **Table 6-1** provides other characteristics for documentation in an EMR/PMR.[6,7]

Table 6-1. Example Items for Documentation in an EMR/PMR[1,7,9]

Chronological Marker	Date and Time
Summary of Medical History	CC (chief complaint)
	HPI (history present illness)
	PmHX (past medical history)
	SocHx (social history)
	FamHx (family history)
	SurgHx (surgical history)
	ALL (allergies/reaction)
	Medications/OTC/herbals
	PE/ROS (physical exam/review of systems)
	Laboratory indices/diagnostic procedures
Oral/Written Consultations	From other health care professionals (HCP)
Oral/Written Orders	From physician or other HCP
	- start and stop dates
	- precautions
	- drug interactions
	- protocols
Medication Changes	Adjustment of dose, route, frequency or form
	Intended use

Table 6-1. Example Items for Documentation in an EMR/PMR[1,7,9] (cont'd)

Chronological Marker	Date and Time
Drug-related Problems	Actual and potential - drug-drug - drug-food - drug-lab - drug-disease
Assessment and Plan	Interventions and professional judgment
Therapeutic Monitoring	Rule out duplication Expected adherence Pharmacokinetics Adverse events/toxicity Clinical resolution/symptomatology
Patient Education	Therapy related Adjunctive measures Self-monitoring Etiology and progression of disease
Identifiers	Person(s) involved Documenting pharmacist
Aesthetics	Indelible ink Nonalterable (electronic)
Policies	Code of ethics HIPAA
Reimbursement	CPT codes: 0115T, 0116T, 0117T ICD-9 and Evaluation and Management (E/M) Time in and out, total time spent/rate of service E/M Medicare standards

The SOAP note is an example from a patient-pharmacist diabetes self-management educational encounter in a specialized outpatient ambulatory multidisciplinary diabetes practice. The structured note lists the assessment and plan separately; alternatively, they may also be combined. Both are suitable forms of documentation for reimbursement, and the choice is left to clinician preference or documentation procedure unique to your individual practice site.

SOAP notes can be kept in a PMR for ease of documentation for follow-up visits or in a patient registry to expedite data collection and report clinical indicators. Alternative styles of structured notating can also be integrated with the use of an EMR through a variety of manufacturers as discussed. These alternative styles are contingent on the care setting, funding support, your preferences and access, as well as the structure of your practice site. Some may have the ability to adopt pharmacy-based software for documentation, and others will use the software chosen by their practice site administrators and purchased by their health system. (Community-Based Clinical Pharmacy Documentation Software–Table)

Even as electronic information resources (EMR/EHR) gain momentum, it is apparent many practices will still rely on paper and pen for manual documentation. No matter the form, the same documentation principles apply, and the information contained in a PMR serves as justification for reimbursement, a legal permanent health record, and a quality-assurance tool for practice standards.[1,7,8]

Documentation Elements

Medication Therapy Management Community-Based Core Components

The ability to bill for pharmacist services took effect under medication therapy management (MTM) provision of Medicare Part D.[13] A community-based MTM model was developed in July 2004 under the partnership of several pharmacy organizations and published through the American Pharmacists Association and National Association of Chain Drug Stores. Managed care health systems and payers have acknowledged that pharmacists provide consistent, cost-effective, clinical services that improve patient outcomes and reduce health care expenditures.[14-16] Effective in January 2006, pharmacists were recognized providers of MTM as defined under the Medicare Prescription Drug, Improvement, and Modernization Act of 2003 (MMA) Part D Prescription Drug Benefit.[17] It has been clearly recognized that collaborative MTM can maximize patients' health-related quality of life (HRQOL) and reduce the frequency of preventable drug-related problems. In this team approach, drug therapy decision making and management are coordinated through the collaboration of pharmacists, physicians, nurses, and other health care professionals. This framework identifies five core components: medication therapy review, a personal medical record or list, action plan, intervention and referral, and documentation with follow-up. These are the components you should use when seeing patients, and you should discuss them with IT personnel when they are creating or defining the EMR templates for your patient encounters. MTM is a prime example of why the manual chart and/or the EMR need to be altered to accommodate the pharmacists' role in the patient's care.[16]

CASE

By adopting the office templates for diabetic management and creating a template specifically for anticoagulation visits, you were able to select sections of the SOAP note that worked for your type of visits. You also were able to prompt Dr. Busybee in your note when a patient was due for preventive care visits and even immunizations. Adapting to the existing documentation system also assisted the other practitioners in your office to read and understand your plan of care for patients, which allowed for a team approach to the care of the patient.

When you participate in collaborative MTM, you will document your activities in a PMR that you make available to other health care professionals in a timely fashion through established channels of communication.[1,6,7,17] Since documentation

standards vary state to state, you should develop and implement collaborative practice agreements, patient referral processes, and the practice settings in accordance
with the laws in your state. Please refer back to Chapter 1 for more detail on collaborative practice agreements.

HIPPAA Safety Measures

The issue of patient confidentiality and security of documented medical information continues to be debated and discussed. This has been especially relevant in the
transition to electronic media for the majority of the patient's medical information.
Details on what an organization or provider must do to meet HIPAA requirements
are lacking, but the law does state that health care organizations must "implement
physical safeguards for all workstations that access electronic protected health information, to restrict access to authorized users." As a provider, you are expected to
log out when leaving a workstation, use a privacy screen to prevent viewing by
unauthorized people, and remove workstations from high traffic areas.[18] In response
to these measures, it is important that you have your own access code, whether it is
a password or biometric fingerprint, so that electronic media is secure. Also, you
should not electronically document "under" a physician or nurse practitioner who
may see the patient at the same appointment since this does not reflect your encounter and could lead to confusion over your assessment and plan for the patient.
In addition, students should be blocked from entering any data into the system
without your approval and signature. Maintaining patient privacy is critical. If
needed, you may wish to provide some basic training to students and others on the
inappropriateness of discussing patient information in hallways, elevators, at lunch,
or even with others not working at the site. It is a good idea to have all health care
providers visiting the practice, including students, residents, technicians, etc., sign
a confidentiality statement regarding patient information.

All medical records must be maintained in a safe and secure area with safeguards
to prevent loss, destruction, and tampering. Your documentation within the medical record may physically exist in separate and multiple locations in both paper-
based and electronic formats, depending on the practice site(s). However, chronology is essential, so pay close attention to ensure that documents are filed properly
or the information is entered in the correct encounter record for the correct patient, including appropriate scanning and indexing of imaged documents at all practice site(s). All PMRs are retained for at least as long as required by state and federal
law and regulations and must be maintained in their entirety regardless of form or
format. Note that federal law supersedes state law unless the state is stricter than the
federal government. Written or electronic, no documentation entries may be de-
leted from the record except in accordance with the destruction policy. If your
written PMR is microfilmed or kept on a computer database, there should be a
written policy at your site concerning PMRs, outlining who is custodian and where
the original PMRs are stored. This type of record keeping is crucial as offices implement EMRs yet must maintain the outdated written chart as required by state law.[19]

HIPAA waivers have language requesting patient consent regarding the collection
of information, use in research, and disclosure of patient's personal information as required. This also includes who will be sharing in the information, patients' right to

access their own information (medication list, lab results, and list of diagnoses), and the patients' right to submit a complaint. In addition, print or electronic documentation must be stored appropriately to ensure confidentiality. Patients also need to consent when clinical documentation and other health information is transferred to other providers. No matter what system is used for storage of information, access should be monitored and limited to only those clinicians directly involved with the patient's care.[20]

Documenting Medication Reconciliation

Medication reconciliation and verification of a current and accurate medication list is arguably one of the more important documentation activities performed to maintain patient safety and improve patient outcomes for any transition of care. Medication reconciliation reduces errors in transcription, omission, duplication of therapy, indication for use, and drug-drug and drug-disease interactions.[21] The simple act of comparing the drugs that the patient reports taking at home against a recently documented medication administration record (MAR) in either an office or institutional setting allows a cross-check and can help alleviate the approximately 4.7% of hospital admissions linked to adverse drug reactions. In addition, the impact made possible by pharmacists performing this role will help to create opportunities to build collaborative relationships with other health care professionals and patients.[22]

We are focusing on medication reconciliation because its importance extends beyond the setting of patients entering and leaving the hospital. As we know, the transition of patient care to the outpatient setting and among the various ambulatory providers allows gaps in information, especially since most outpatient sites are not linked with each other or with extended-care facilities, health systems, and their hospitals. Additionally, significant errors occur secondary to the many modifications to medication dosages, over-the-counter (OTC) use, and adherence issues patients experience that are often seen by ambulatory pharmacists in their daily practice. Taking responsibility to resolve or prevent these types of errors is what makes medication reconciliation the backbone of pharmacy clinical services. Your expertise lends itself to a thorough and detailed medication history that is then documented in the PMR. Documentation is essential for medication reconciliation to be effective. It should not stop at the medication list, as records regarding side effects, allergies, drug interactions, and cost issues are often as important as medication history for optimal care of the ambulatory patient.[1,6,7,22,23]

The EMR creates a new dimension in medication reconciliation and medication list collection and storage. However, the record is only as strong as the accuracy of what is being documented. In most cases, the ability to transfer the list electronically to another system does not exist. Gaps remain in documenting medication use in the majority of EMRs. Ernest and colleagues illustrate as many as one of every four medications was associated with discrepant information in the patient medical record.[28] Emphasis has been placed on transition to and from inpatient care, but as previously mentioned, this needs to be taken further by those of us practicing in the outpatient setting. Methods to ensure accuracy and transferability of the medication lists in both the electronic and paper format need to be developed, implemented, and maintained and measured for accuracy.[24] Content standards need to be developed and agreed upon to enable interoperability.

No matter if the documentation system is electronic or manual, medication reconciliation should occur at each office visit and include all medications, not just those associated with a particular visit. Pharmacists play a key role in preventing medication errors and enhancing care by simply documenting and updating medication records on a continual basis.[24]

Communication Techniques

Documentation using a clinical encounter note is an effective way to communicate what has occurred at an office visit. Documentation is only as strong as the data gathered, thus it is very important for you to also effectively communicate with your patients during the visit. Employing communication techniques, such as motivational interviewing or assessing the patient's health care literacy level, will aid you in gathering the most useful information from your patient. Good communication will enable you to synthesize and analyze (assessment) the information gathered to create a specific plan for care that meets the patient's needs.

CASE

Over the last 6 months, your practice continues to grow as other patients and providers of the practice hear about your service. You approach Dr. Busybee about expanding the services you provide by offering to include a formal medication reconciliation services and assessment of each patient's health care literacy level. Since this does not conflict with the office process or the original business model, Dr. Busybee sees this as a win-win for his office and his patients and approves you adding these services to your office hours. You are pleased with his vote of confidence, but realize while medication reconciliation seems easy, some questions remain: what do I need to be effective at performing these new services and how will I document my impact?

Communication Tips

Establish rapport early in the encounter with your patient through a welcoming introduction to you and your clinic. Patients can easily sense authenticity in their providers, so most importantly you should be relaxed, confident, and attentive to the patient and the encounter. After ensuring that you and your patient are comfortable and ready to start the visit, conduct the interview with open-ended questions. Doing so enables patients to tell you their health care story in their own words. It is important to frequently pause and summarize or reflect back to the patient so that you may verify accuracy and your correct understanding of the patient's story. Listening is an important communication tool. Documentation of the encounter can include subjective and objective findings that employ the "basic seven" line of questioning. Other question series commonly used are the Indian

Health Service Counseling Model, the PQRST method, and QuEST Scholar method.[25,26] (See web toolkit.)🖳

Motivational Interviewing

Motivational interviewing (MI) is an effective technique that can be incorporated into the patient interview process. Developed in 1991 by Miller and Rollnick, MI uses a patient empowerment approach throughout the encounter.[27] Although MI and another interview style called the *transtheoretical model* (Prochaska and colleagues, developed in 2004) were developed independently; there is some similarity between them.[28] Both assume that people approach change with varying levels of readiness. Historically, MI has been used for patients with drug and alcohol addiction and works from the assumption that many patients who seek therapy are ambivalent about change, but their motivation changes during treatment. The four basic principles of MI are as follows: (1) express empathy, (2) develop discrepancy, (3) roll with resistance, and (4) support self-efficacy. As a pharmacist, you can assume the role of patient mentor or coach to aid patients in making behavior changes by creating "self-selected" patient goals. Documentation should include these goals, which use the SMART acronym: specific, measurable, attainable, realistic, and time-bound relative to behavioral and lifestyle modification.[29] A great clinical example of how to use MI is in smoking cessation. By helping the patient create goals and then working with him or her on the appropriate pharmacologic management choices, you can play a large role in assisting your patient to kick the habit.

Health Care Literacy

As discussed, there are a number of best practices that apply when conducting a patient encounter, but no matter which communication technique is employed, you must have an understanding of the patient's level of health literacy. Health care literacy is defined as "the degree to which individuals have the capacity to obtain, process, and understand basic health information and services needed to make appropriate health decisions."[30]

The National Assessment of Adult Literacy (NAAL) provided the first measure of U.S. health literacy. Survey findings showed 14% of U.S. adults function at below the basic level, 22% function at the basic level, 53% have an intermediate level of health literacy, and 12% have proficient health literacy. Note that interpreting medication labels requires intermediate skill. This means that 36% of adult Americans have levels of health literacy below what is required to understand typical medication information.[31] Low health literacy is a problem that touches all groups and segments of our society (elderly, minorities, homeless, poor, poorly educated, etc). Several studies have assessed patients' understanding of their medications. Individuals with limited health literacy demonstrated 12–18 times the odds of being unable to identify their own medications and distinguish one from the other. Patients who have difficulty understanding simple instructions such as taking a medication every 6 hours or on an empty stomach have insufficient understanding of common drug mechanisms and side effects and greater misinterpretation of drug warning labels.[32-37]

Several tools are available to analyze the readability of patient education materials. Examples include the Flesch-Kincaid Grade Level and Reading Ease and the Simple Measure of Gobbledygook (SMOG) index. There are also resources to test the health literacy of those who need it, such as the rapid estimate of adult literacy in medicine (REALM) and the test of functional health literacy in adults (TOFHLA), which are validated instruments. Additional assessments available are the tools for real-time assessment of health information literacy skills (TRAILS) and the newest vital sign (NVS) by Pfizer's clear health communication, as well as those from Medline-Plus, National Institute for Literacy (NIFL), Plain English Network, the American Medication Association (AMA), and Harvard School of Public Health. The Agency for Healthcare Research and Quality (AHRQ) has a *Pharmacy Health Literacy Assessment Tool User's Guide* on their web site to assess health literacy for pharmacies and has a survey accessible through the public domain.[38]

Key Point

All patients can benefit from five recommended strategies for patient-centered visits:[32,38,39]

1. Use plain language and avoid medical jargon and vague instructions.
2. KISS (keep it short and simple). Tell patients what they need to know.
3. Ask patients to "teach back" what they have learned.
4. Recognize variation in learning styles and preferences, thus verbal messages should be reinforced with written information and images.
5. Everyone learns better if information is reinforced in multiple ways.

Once literacy level is established, it is essential to document the information within the PMR to assist everyone who is caring for the patient. This is true for both health care literacy and literacy skills in general, including English as a second language (ESOL) and learning disabilities.[38,39] Many times pharmacists are the only ones assessing literacy because we are asked to consult on the nonadherent patient or the patient who cannot seem to use medications correctly. Before you accept that the patient is voluntarily nonadherent, assess literacy level, language skills, and any apparent learning disabilities to determine if they play a role in problems the patient is experiencing. That simple act will make you a hero in the patient's eyes, but it will also affect how they are cared for by others as well as the communication style when educating the patient at future encounters. (Literacy Links)

Medical Liability and Auditing

Performance Evaluation

The scope of professional liability has increased parallel to the increase in pharmacists' scope of practice. Historically, pharmacists have functioned and intervened as learned intermediaries under the direct supervision of a physician's verbal or written orders. This paradigm shift of pharmacists practicing as independent providers places more responsibility on pharmacists as medication therapy experts, thus documentation of care is essential to protect pharmacists from liability.[1]

CASE

It has been 1 year since you submitted your business plan to Dr. Busybee. At three months he reminded you that he expected evidence of the impact you have had on his patient population. At that time you began using the EMR to track HgbA1c levels and INR trends for your patients. When you added medication reconciliation and health literacy screening to your service, you expanded your metrics to include compliance checks as well as number of admissions to the local hospital due to a diabetes and/or anticoagulation complications. Using the EMR you were able to show percentage of your patients that achieved treatment goals including compliance with medications, appointments, and lab work. Dr. Busybee was impressed and shared your impact with his partners, who in turn used the local trends to gauge your impact versus patients who did not have access to a pharmacist.

Awareness of this trend shows that it is vastly important that every pharmacist who participates in direct patient care and documents in the PMR have a mechanism in place that tracks performance, continuous quality improvement, and adherence to practice standards. For those using an EMR for documentation, they may have potential for greater ease of measuring ambulatory care-based quality outcomes and errors; however, all clinical documentation can be used to track impact of care.[40] Outcome tracking mechanisms need to be developed using proper documentation that allows for a standardized approach to find and apply patient data to determine if quality standards have been achieved. Integrating pharmacy service benchmarks into a PMR will require a close look at how it can be used to document the effectiveness of pharmacy services and possibly justify expansion of resources and personnel. You should be planning ahead to determine the capabilities of the PMR format used by the practice so it can be designed to find and track your documentation easily, by using certain parameters. This was alluded to in the first part of the chapter regarding how to create your templates for each of your patient encounters. That upfront research and implementation will pay off as you set up your continuous quality improvement and performance measures for your practice. Chapter 7 will provide greater detail on quality and performance measurement.

An EMR note could be applied to assessing quality by looking at how point-of-care testing is documented within your electronic encounter note. With the EMR, only certain fields of the note may be included in parameter searches, but by creating the right template and choosing the correct field, you should be able to track and graph INRs to illustrate your success in keeping patients with the therapeutic range. Another example of using the EMR is to highlight potential problems before they occur, such as searching a database for patients with diabetes who take metformin and cross reference that information with serum creatinine levels. This type of quality assurance initiative will aid in identifying at-risk patients with a potential for an adverse drug event before it happens.[40]

As we have discussed, some EMRs are more robust than others, so it is imperative to discuss with IT personnel how such information can be gathered and formatted in a searchable field.

Chart Audits

One question that is frequently asked is who will be setting up and evaluating pharmacists' performance. Audits are a tool used by ambulatory professionals to assess if an office is meeting designated thresholds for quality. Audits help deviations from standards in patient care and documentation in the patient care process. Many pharmacists have never heard of chart audits. However, with the greater emphasis on quality in health care reform and as we assume the role of independent practitioners, all pharmacists need to develop a protocol and have procedures in place to monitor the quality of services. Thorough documentation of patient care encounters and compliance with CMS standards are key in meeting standards set forth by you and your practice site. You may wish to perform quarterly chart audits and report on what you and your organization consider to be important performance evaluation parameters.

> **CASE**
>
> Since you were able to show an impact for Dr. Busybee's patients, many of his partners have started referring patients to you for care. Realizing you are taking on more responsibility, you approach Dr. Busybee and ask how he keeps track of his impact. You inquire if there is a way to assure you are providing the appropriate care, not just metrics or outcomes. Dr. Busybee suggests that you become integrated into the chart audit protocol the physicians and nurse practitioner use in the office to assess quality of care.

Audits are commonly conducted through peer evaluation where each member of the outpatient clinical team reviews the PMRs of colleagues using a predetermined set of criteria and threshold quality markers. Areas of emphasis may include appropriate labs ordered, medication reconciliation, monitoring parameters, level of patient adherence, preventative measures, screenings, or clinical outcome measures and goals. This applies to all midlevel providers and all remote sites where you practice, thus your audit does not have to be done by another pharmacist; it can be done by other clinicians in the office. Audit procedures are often handled by a continuous quality (CQI) committee. They create the parameters from established standards and billing requirements that are used in auditing the various providers. The purpose of a chart audit is to provide feedback to the clinician to improve patient care, improve accuracy of information recorded, and to ensure thorough documentation practices.[1] (Auditing Tool)

The key points you should consider in the peer review process are as follows:[41]

- Placement of blame, finger-pointing, and conflicts with other caregivers should be resolved through the quality improvement process and does not belong in medical record.

- Subjective terms should be avoided. Subjective opinions by physicians and nonphysician clinicians (NPC) open up liability issues. Documentation should be as factual as possible.

- Hospital staff, facility, or equipment concerns should be addressed in an incident report completed by the hospital administration.

- Do not document conversations with the attorney, insurance carrier, or risk manager in the medical record. If necessary, document separately.

- Incident reports can be protected from discovery if they are part of a peer-review process, although they can be discovered through a review of the medical record when attorneys become aware of their existence. Likewise, chart audits can ensure adequate coding and complexity to protect against fraud and liability with CMS.

The key points you should consider in the chart audit process are as follows:

- Look for under- or overdocumentation in your charts that can raise flags for improper coding selection.

- Ensure that appropriate levels of service are identified and billed.

- Learn the proper steps for choosing appropriate levels of history, exam, and medical decision making (evaluation and management codes are discussed in Chapter 8).

- Get the chart audit forms to implement your internal audit program.

- Learn how to audit based on coding facts and potentially uncover missed revenue.

- Make the chart audit an essential component of the compliance plan.

Professional Liability

Liability, as it relates to clinical documentation, can be an issue when (1) payment challenge is ensuing for service rendered or not rendered or (2) legal action is ensuing as a result of an action or nonaction taken by the provider. In both situations, your documentation will provide the necessary information to manage the process discovery and review of professional conduct.[1]

The importance of good documentation cannot be any more important than when you are defending your decisions and actions regarding patient care.

This means that documentation must be accurate and organized. By any means, you want to avoid any activity that can be misconstrued as fraud. By CMS definition, fraud is "the intentional deception or misrepresentation that an individual knows to be false or does not believe to be true and makes, knowing that the deception could result in some unauthorized benefit to him/herself or some other person" or "to purposely bill for services that were never given or to bill for a service that has a higher reimbursement than the service produced."[42]

 This definition drives home the point that what we document needs to be accurate, factual, and thorough, since we are all aware that if the chart does not reflect the care given, then the actions never happened according to our legal system.

Historically, we have acted as record keepers for medication use as well as drug interactions and adverse drug events. Now our documentation standards have been adjusted and expanded to show the care we provide as health care practitioners.

A key element that all documentation should include is the assessment of the situation within the realm of care given. If you cannot address the problem, or it is out of your scope of practice, there must be documentation of how other health care team members (referring provider or interdisciplinary colleagues) were involved to address the needs of the patient. In addition, your plan of action must be concise yet complete. The ideal documentation includes how you affected care, planned for upcoming visits, and intervened to provide preventive care. For an example, refer back to the SOAP note and notice how part of the plan was to have the patient follow up with certain specialists (standards of care) as outlined by the ADA guidelines. Many pharmacists forget that as a patient advocate you have the power to ensure appropriate care is given to your patient. By communicating thoughts, actions, and plans for the patient, you can assist the next member of your team to provide high-quality care and protect yourself and others from liability.[1,6,7]

Chapter Summary

As you can see, documentation plays a vital role in your everyday professional life. It allows communication between you and other health care practitioners while also providing evidence of what occurred during the patient encounters. Don't forget that multiple providers impact a patient's care, thus you must continue to develop your communication skills not only with other health care providers and patients but also with each other.

Health information technology is being implemented faster than most realize and, while this advancement has its disadvantages, the one area of improvement will eventually be communication between and within health systems. Electronic documentation is the future; by allowing practitioners to collect patient history, reports, prescription information, and reimbursement data, this format will continue to push for proper and thorough documentation so all health care providers can make the most informed clinical decisions possible for patients. In the end, documentation is an essential component to a successful partnership between providers regardless of their degree, location, or specialty.

References

1. Zierler-Brown (Haines) SL, Brown TR, Chen D, et al. Clinical documentation for patient care: Models, concepts and liability considerations for pharmacists. *Am J Health-Syst Pharm.* 2007;64:1851-1858.

2. Webster L, Spiro RF. Health information technology: A new world for pharmacy. *JAPhA.* 2010;50:e20-e34.

3. American Medical Association. Electronic medical record implementation and technical guides. https://catalog.ama-assn.org/Catalog/product/product_list?_requested=797127. Accessed August 7, 2010.

4. American Society of Health-System Pharmacists. 2015 Initiative. Goal 5: Increase the extent to which health systems apply technology effectively to improve the safety of medications use. Published 2007. www.ashp.org/s_ashp/doc1c.asp?CID=421&DID=4024. Accessed August 7, 2010.

5. Brock KA, Casper KA, Green TR, et al. Documentation of patient care services in a community pharmacy setting. *J Am Pharm Assoc.* 2006;46:378-384.

6. ASHP. *Guidelines on a Standardized Method for Pharmaceutical Care; Best Practices for Hospital and Health-System Pharmacy: Position and Guidance Documents of ASHP, 2005-2006 ed.* Bethesda, MD: American Society of Health-System Pharmacists; 2005:183-191.

7. ASHP. ASHP guidelines on documenting pharmaceutical care in patient medical records. *Best Practices for Hospital and Health-System Pharmacy. Position and Guidance Documents of ASHP, 2005-2006 ed.* Bethesda, MD: American Society of Health-System Pharmacists; 2005:192-194.

8. Rovers JP, Currie JD, Hagel HP, et al. *A Practical Guide to Pharmaceutical Care.* Washington, DC: American Pharmacists Association; 1998.

9. Hepler CD, Strand LM. Opportunities and responsibilities in pharmaceutical care. *Am J Hosp Pharm.* 1990;47:533-543.

10. McDonald CJ, Tierney WM. Computer-based medical records: Their future role in medical practice. *JAMA.* 1998;259:3433-3440.

11. Pronovost P, Weast B, Schwarz M, et al. Medication reconciliation: A practical tool to reduce the risk of medication errors. *J Crit Care.* 2003;18:201-205.

12. ASHP Continuity of Care Task Force. Continuity of care in medication management: Review of issues and considerations for pharmacy. *Am J Health-Syst Pharm.* 2005;62:1714-1720.

13. U.S. Department of Health and Human Services. Centers for Medicare and Medicaid Services. Glossary. www.cms.hhs.gov/apps/glossary/default.asp?Letter=ALL&Language=English. Accessed August 7, 2010.

14. Lee JK, Grace KA, Taylor AJ. Effect of a pharmacy care program on medication adherence and persistence, blood pressure, and low density lipoprotein cholesterol, a randomized controlled trial. *JAMA.* 2006;296:2563-2571.

15. Cranor C, Bunting B, Christenson D. The Asheville Project: long-term clinical and economic outcomes of a community pharmacy diabetes care program. *J Am Pharm Assoc.* 2003;43:173-184.

16. American Pharmacists Association and National Association of Chain Drug Stores. Medication therapy in community pharmacy practice: core elements of an MTM service (version 2.0). *J Am Pharm Assoc.* 2008;1-24.

17. Centers for Disease Control and Prevention. Rules and regulations. *Fed Regist.* 2005;70:4541.

18. HIPAA Requires Organizations to Secure Their Electronic Devices. http://www.ashp.org/menu/News/Pharmacy/News/NewsArticle.aspx?id=884. *Health System Pharmacy News.* Accessed March 25, 2010.

19. American Health Information Management Association (AHIMA). Legal medical record standards. http://www.ahima.org/infocenter/guidelines/ltcs/5.1.asp. Accessed August 7, 2010.

20. U.S. Department of Health and Human Services. The Health Insurance Portability and Accountability Act of 1996. http://www.hhs.gov/ocr/privacy/. Accessed on August 7, 2010.

21. Lee JK, Grace KA, Taylor AJ. Effect of a pharmacy care program on medication adherence and persistence, blood pressure, and low density lipoprotein cholesterol, a randomized controlled trial. *JAMA.* 2006;296:2563-2571.

22. Manasse H Jr, Thompson K. *Medication Safety: A Guide for Health Care Facilities.* Bethesda, MD: American Society of Health-System Pharmacists; 2005:4-5.

23. Shojania KG, Duncan BW, McDonald KM, et al., eds. *Making Healthcare Safer: A Critical Analysis of Patient Safety Practices.* Evidence Report No. 43 from the Agency for Healthcare Research and Quality. Rockville, MD: AHRQ Publication No. 01-E058; 2001.

24. Ernest ME, Brown GL, Klepser TB, et al. Medication discrepancies in an outpatient electronic medical record. *Am J Health-Syst Pharm.* 2001;58:2072-2075.

25. McDonough RP, Bennett MS. Improving communication skills of pharmacy students through effective precepting. *AJPE.* 2006;70(3):Article 58, 1-12.

26. Buring SM, Kirby J, Conrad WF. A structured approach for teaching students to council self-care patients *AJPE.* 2007;72(1):Article 20, 1-7.

27. DiClemente CC, Velasquez MW. Motivational interviewing and the stages of change. In: Miller WR, Rollnick S, eds. *Motivational Interviewing: Preparing People for Change.* 2nd edition. New York, NY: Guilford Press; 2002:217-250.

28. Prochaska JO, DiClemente CC. *The Transtheoretical Approach: Crossing Traditional Boundaries of Therapy.* Homewood, IL: Dow Jones-Irwin; 1984.

29. Miller WR, Rose GS. Toward a theory of motivational interviewing. *Am J Psychol.* 2009;64(6):527-537.

30. U.S. Department of Health and Human Services. Healthy People 2010. 2nd ed. *With Understanding and Improving Health and Objectives for Improving Health.* 2 vols. Washington, DC: U.S. Government Printing Office; 2010.

31. Kutner M, Greenberg E, Jin Y, et al. *The Health Literacy of America's Adults: Results from the 2003 National Assessment of Adult Literacy (NCES 2006-483).* Washington, DC: U.S. Department of Education, National Center for Education Statistics; 2006.

32. Kripalani S, Henderson LE, Chiu EY, et al. Predictors of medication self-management skill in a low-literacy population. *J Gen Int Med.* 2006;21(8):803-900.

33. Kripalani S, Weiss BD. Teaching about health literacy and clear communication. *J Gen Int Med.* 2006;21(8):888-890.

34. Gazmararian JA, Baker DW, Williams MV, et al. Health literacy among Medicare enrollees in a managed care organization. *JAMA.* 1999;281:545-551.

35. Gazmararian JA, Kripalani S, Miller MJ, et al. Factors associated with medication refill adherence in cardiovascular-related diseases: A focus on health literacy. *J Gen Int Med.* 2006;21(12):1215-1221.

36. Fang MC, Machtinger EL, Wang F, et al. health literacy and anticoagulation-related outcomes among patients taking warfarin. *J Gen Int Med.* 2006;21(8):841-846.

37. Davis TC, Wolf MS, Bass PF III, et al. Low literacy impairs comprehension of prescription drug warning labels. *J Gen Int Med.* 2006;21(8):847-851.

38. Weiss BD. *Health Literacy: A Manual for Clinicians.* AMA and AMA Foundation; 2003.

39. Weiss BD. Epidemiology of low health literacy. In: Schwartzberg JG, VanGeest JB, Wang CC, eds. *Understanding Health Literacy: Implications for Medicine and Public Health.* AMA Press; 2005:19.

40. Dunham DP, Baker D. Use of electronic medical record to detect patients at high risk for metformin-induced lactic acidosis. *Am J Health-Syst Pharm.* 2006;63:657-660.

41. Bradshaw RW. Using peer review for self-audits of medical record documentation. AAFP; 2000. http://www.aafp.org/fpm/20000400/28usin.html. Accessed August 7, 2010.

42. U.S. Department of Health and Human Services. Center for Medicare and Medicaid Services. Most common medical rip off and fraud schemes. www.cms.hhs.gov/fraudAbuseforConsumers/04_Rip_Offs_Schemes.asp. Accessed August 7, 2010.

Additional Selected References

Freidland RB. *Understanding Health Literacy: New Estimates of the Costs of Inadequate Health Literacy.* Washington, DC: National Academy on an Aging Society; 1998.

Howard DH, Gazmararian J, Parker RM. The impact of low health literacy on the medical costs of Medicare managed care enrollees. *Am J Med.* 2005;118(4):371-377.

Katz MG, Jacobson TA, Veledar E, et al. Patient literacy and question-asking behavior during the medical encounter: A mixed-methods analysis. *J Gen Int Med.* 2007;22(6):782-786.

Kirsch I, Jungeblut A, Jenkins L, et al. *Adult Literacy in America: A First Look at the Results of the National Adult Literacy Survey.* Washington, DC: National Center for Education Statistics, US Department of Education; 1993.

Community MTM.www.communitymtm.com. Accessed March 25, 2010.

ConXus MTM. www.pdhi.com. Accessed March 25, 2010.
Outcomes MTM System. www.getoutcomes.com. Accessed March 25, 2010.
PIDS-Pocket PC Based MTM System. www.rxinterventions.com. Accessed March 25, 2010.
PillHelps Works. www.pillhelp.com. Accessed March 25, 2010.
Medication Management Systems. www.medsmanagement.com. Accessed March 25, 2010.
Mirixa Pro & Mirixa Edge. http://www.mirixa.com. Accessed March 25, 2010.
EPIC Integrated Software. http://www.epic.com. Accessed March 25, 2010.
MCKesson Practice Partner. http://www.practicepartner.com. Accessed March 25, 2010.

Web Resources

Chart Audit Tool

Example Documentation Elements for EMR/PMR

Examples of Community-based/Clinical Pharmacy Documentation Software Web Sources

Example of Electronic Documentation of a Pharmacy Office Visit

Example SOAP Note and 7 Lines of Questioning

Link to AMA Web Site for Bookstore (three books on EMRs)

 Web Toolkit available at
www.ashp.org/ambulatorypractice

Quality Assurance for Ambulatory Patient Care

Mary Ann Kliethermes

CHAPTER

7

Chapter Outline

1. Introduction
2. What Is Quality?
3. Understanding Your System of Care and Opportunities for Quality Improvement and Measurement
4. Establishing a Quality Improvement Program
5. Quality Related to Staff Competency
6. Credentialing and Privileging
7. Chapter Summary
8. References
9. Web Resources

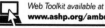
Web Toolkit available at
www.ashp.org/ambulatorypractice

Chapter Objectives

1. Describe the rationale for developing a robust ambulatory clinical patient services quality improvement program.
2. Apply key quality principles to the structure of your clinic or service in order to provide quality services.
3. Implement the PDSA method for quality improvement in your practice.
4. List the skills desired for an ambulatory clinical patient-care pharmacist.

Introduction

Over the past 20 years, attention to quality in health care services has escalated due to limited and shrinking resources, fueling a demand for quality at the best value/cost ratio tied to improved patient outcomes. Incorporating measurements of quality into health care work flow and relating them to patient outcomes has proven to be a daunting challenge. As an industry, health care is just beginning to understand how to measure quality, evaluate which measures provide meaningful information, and determine how well the measures reflect optimal patient outcomes. We as ambulatory clinical pharmacists are not immune from the process and will need to understand how to assess the quality of services we provide and embed quality measurement into our daily practices. As ambulatory pharmacists, we are under greater pressure to show quality and value because clinical ambulatory pharmacy services are relatively new and do not currently enjoy stable or established revenue sources. Whether you are starting your ambulatory program, or currently have a program, the time to think about building quality measurement into your processes is now. Being proactive in this process not only will save you time and resources down the line, but it will allow you to have timely data when the demand inevitably arrives. This chapter will help you establish a framework for your ambulatory clinical care pharmacy quality improvement program, recommend a process for improvement for you to incorporate in your practice, and discuss how to ensure your staff is adequately skilled to provide quality patient care.

If you need to be convinced or need to convince someone regarding the importance of quality measurement, start with the report *To Err Is Human: Building a Safer Health System* released by the Institute of Medicine (IOM) Committee on Quality in America in 1999. This defining event elevated quality to priority status in health care because it brought to everyone's attention the extent of harm being done to patients in our current health care system by reporting approximately 100,000 patient deaths in hospitals yearly due to medical error.[1,2] The importance for pharmacy clinicians is the fact that medications were found to be the source of a significant portion of medical errors. Although data from the ambulatory setting was not included in the report, there is little doubt similar if not greater numbers of medication-related problems exist in this setting.[3,4] The United Sates spends the most money to provide health care yet rates poorly in quality of care when compared to other industrialized countries.[5,6] Compared with other industries concerned with public safety and quality, health care lags far behind.[7] We enjoy the benefit of a safe airline industry, where the *quality gap* for safety between the highest performing airline and an airline performing in the middle of the industry's quality range is less than 1%. Contrast that with data on the U.S. health care system reported by the National Committee on Quality Assurance (NCQA), where the quality gap is 20% or greater for a number of health care measures.[8]

Consequently, quality improvement and measurement programs are moving forward at a feverish pace. Multiple organizations, including accreditation organizations, are developing a whole host of quality measures for health care performance. Health care reform, and in particular The Patient Protection and Affordable Care Act enacted into law in 2010, has as major themes improved health care quality and affordable health care.[9] Payers are increasing their reliance on attainment of quality measures for health care provider reimbursement in pay-for-performance models.[10,11]

Key Point In order to effectively participate and survive in the current health care environment, the ambulatory care pharmacy clinicians will need to understand the basics of quality improvement in health care and their roles and responsibilities in the process. Because medication problems compose a significant portion of the quality chasm, ambulatory clinical pharmacists need to be leaders in narrowing the quality gap in medication-related services provided at the individual patient and population level.

What Is Quality?

Exactly what is meant by quality health care services, let alone quality clinical pharmacy services, and who is defining it? Thus far, the definition has been elusive, as a consensus definition does not currently exist.[12-15] The IOM defines quality of care as the degree to which health services for individuals or populations increase the likelihood of desired health outcomes and are consistent with current professional knowledge.[16] This definition connects quality to the experiences of patients and their outcomes, but it also broadens its scope to the general population level, which may provide a more significant impact for the entire health system. This definition implies that sound evidence-based research should direct services and the efforts to measure them. Less clear is exactly what the desired health outcomes are for any individual or population and who should define them: the patient, the provider, the payer, or a governmental agency.[15] Approaching quality from each of these perspectives may result in very different sets of desired health outcomes. The patient-centered care movement and health care quality leaders advocate that quality efforts focus on the needs, desires, and circumstances of the individual patient. When patient-centered quality care is justly provided in this manner, quality will apply to larger populations and the entire health care system.[14,17]

> The ambulatory patient-care pharmacists will experience pressures from a variety of sources when establishing their quality program. Improving the care and experience of patients served should always be the mission of any quality program.

Understanding Your System of Care and Opportunities for Quality Improvement and Measurement

Today, providing care for illness and improving health for any particular patient or population group is exceedingly complex. Numerous points of interaction occur not only between one patient and one provider but also between one patient, multiple providers, health care-related organizations and payers, and subsequent countless interaction points with each additional patient served. An intricate layer of varying interdependence between these points creates a multitude of opportunity for cracks, flaws, and subsequent error, danger, and poor outcomes. Ambulatory care pharmacists must understand how their patient-care services interact with each patient's unique system of care. Using the guidelines for a practice framework discussed in this book, your own focus on quality in your practice, as well as recommendations to follow in this chapter, will help you overcome this barrier.

Key Point

Failure to recognize the complex connections can result in changes in care made with good intentions but that result in unexpected or untoward effects in another part of the patient's system of care.

Eighteen months after their initial report, the IOM released a follow-up report, *Crossing the Quality Chasm*, which described a framework of four levels of care where opportunities for quality improvement may occur.[18] The first level is the experience of the patient and the patient's community, or satisfaction with the health care provided. The components of care at this level focus on professionalism, which includes compassion, empathy, judgment, responsibility, fostering relationships, and communication. Patient satisfaction surveys are a useful means of measuring goals within this section. The second level constitutes the microsystems of care, or the small units (i.e., pharmacist-pharmacy technician, pharmacist-physician-nurse-office staff, etc.) that directly provide the care to the patient (**Table 7-1**). The IOM believes focusing on this level will provide the most meaningful and sizeable quality improvement. This is the level at which the majority of ambulatory patient-care pharmacists practice, and it is an ideal area to concentrate your quality improvement program. The third level is the health care organization. This level is responsible for health care resources and the supportive infrastructure that allows the microsystem to efficiently and effectively care for patients. The final level, the health care environment, focuses on financing, regulating, accrediting, and litigating the system; educating the workforce; and social policy.

Table 7-1. Examples of What May Constitute Ambulatory Microsystems with an Ambulatory Patient-Care Pharmacist

- Anticoagulation Clinic: Clinical pharmacist, registered nurse, medical physician, front desk appointment clerk, biller
- Medication Therapy Management Clinic: Clinical pharmacists, pharmacy technician, dispensing pharmacist, pharmacy manager
- Diabetes Clinic: Clinical pharmacist, diabetes nurse educator, dietician, endocrinologist, clinic support personnel, biller
- Patient-centered Medical Home: Primary care physician, nurse practitioner, pharmacist, physical therapist, certain specialists, dietician, office staff

Key Point

In order for your clinic or service to work well and achieve the highest possible levels of quality care, each level must work in tandem and provide an acceptable level of quality.

The first two levels of care are under your control and therefore areas where you can demonstrate quality and improve the care of your patients. For your service or microsystem to be successful, however, health care organizations and policy and rule makers need to provide a framework within which you perform improved care. Elements of quality at the third and fourth level are less within the control of practitioners in the microsystem.

As an ambulatory practitioner, you should understand what elements of quality are needed at the higher levels of care in order for you to accomplish your goals and actively work with your administrators at level three and your policy makers and pharmacy associations at level four so they understand what you need to achieve those goals.

Before embarking on the details of your quality program, there are some principles for quality measurement that you should consider.[17] Establishing principles for your program by which you choose your quality goals and measures will keep you focused and assist you in defining quality for your particular practice. It will help prevent goals and measures "gone wild," where you may succumb to a significant amount of work collection data on measures that result in little meaningful improvement or quality in patient care. The principles are as follows:

- Knowledge-based care: The care you provide in your service is and continues to be based on current evidence and current standards of care. The service you provide and the quality measures you choose to evaluate your service should stem from the best known science and practice.

- Patient-centered care: The patient care you provide honors individuality, values, and ethnicity, and is sensitive to disparities and information needs for each patient. Your improvement plans and measures of quality embrace this principle.

- Systems-minded care: Your service is part of a complex matrix of patient care, and therefore you place a high value on cooperation and coordination of care across organizations, disciplines, and roles. When creating and interpreting your quality measures, you understand and consider this interplay.

- Measure what is important: Measure what will result in direct improvement to your patient population and what is high priority to you, your patients, and your organization. Measure what you can directly impact. For example, medication adherence may be problematic in your organization, so choose adherence as a measure with an associated clinical measure such as blood pressure or CD4 count, which will reflect a patient outcome related to improved adherence.

In addition you should examine the underlying framework of your system or services. If you lack a solid infrastructure, your aims of improvement may be sabotaged by an unexpected weak link. We know lapses in performing care or the system of patient-care process leads to lapses in quality and subsequent medical errors that affect patient safety and create poor outcomes and unnecessary costs.[19] The IOM provides a simple set of 10 rules for a microsystem (i.e., your system or service) to use to evaluate the design of services (**Table 7-2**). Adopting these rules will increase the odds of your progress toward improvement and quality.

Measuring and ensuring an acceptable quality standard and patient centeredness within the structure, process, and direct provision of patient care in your system is critical to improving patient outcomes.

Establishing a Quality Improvement Program

As you get started in your quality improvement program, it is helpful to start with three simple but extremely useful questions that will set in motion your plan. This approach is based on a well-established quality process used by many industries, referred to as the plan-do-study-act (PDSA) cycle.[20] As stated by Glasgow, the PDSA cycle is akin to the scientific method in that it provides an overlying framework for approaching a problem, but does not explicitly proscribe the best methods for solving a problem.[21] This allows you to customize your organization. Consider the first question:

· What are we trying to accomplish?

The answer to this question stems from the mission and vision of your particular clinic or program. You may be an anticoagulation clinic whose purpose is the safe use of anticoagulants, or a medication therapy management clinic (MTM) whose mission is to improve medication adherence and decrease adverse drug events. You may be planning to establish a diabetes service to address a large number of poorly controlled diabetes cases in your patient population or a heart failure clinic to address frequent hospitalizations noted in your health system's population. In the first two examples, your next step will be to collect a sufficient sample of key data to determine if indeed you are meeting the goals that you are trying to accomplish. For example, in the anticoagulation clinic or the MTM clinic you may want to look at hospitalizations due to warfarin complications or medications problems. In the latter two examples, your institution or payer source may have already collected and provided you with the number of HgA1c readings greater than 8 or the number of yearly hospitalizations for patients with a heart failure diagnosis. If not, you may need to collect that baseline information.

This brings you to the next question:

· What change can we make that will result in improvement?

With this question, you critically evaluate and adjust your current services or proposed services, using the best scientific evidence and standards of practice, to create a solution that will accomplish your goal. Review similar pharmacy-run (or other provider-run) clinics that have published what they did to improve outcomes of their patient population. For example, you know your medication adherence program population is elderly, with low health literacy and declining cognition. In a review of the literature, you find a study by Lee et al., who provided comprehensive pharmacy services similar to yours, but they also used a "pill box" concept and had impressive adherence rates with improved clinical markers as their outcome. The

Table 7-2. Rules to Ensure Quality in Your Service or Microsystem

Rules For Health Care Quality in Microsystems of Care	Comments	Ambulatory Pharmacy Patient-Care Example
1. Care is based on continuous healing relationship.	Care by the ambulatory pharmacist should be available whenever the patient needs it and may occur in many forms (face-to-face, Internet, telephone, etc.). The focus is on access to care.	A patient instructed on subcutaneous administration of a medication (e.g., insulin or low-molecular-weight heparin) is confused after hours. The patient has a method to contact you or a colleague after hours.
2. Care is customized according to patients' needs and values.	Care systems are designed to meet most patient needs but have the capacity to provide care for variations in patients' choices and preferences such that deviations in the system do not impede that patient's care experience.	In your clinic, you recognize that certain patients due to cognitive or psychological issues may need added visit time. You identify those patients and provide flexible visit times instead of limiting them to any set or standard times.
3. Patients are in control of their care.	Patients should be given necessary information to exercise the degree of control and decision making they choose, and the service should be able to accommodate patient differences in this area.	You run an anticoagulation clinic; your policy for high vitamin K foods is to educate and work with patients to develop a habit of consistency in their diet versus completely avoiding these foods when that is not what they desire.
4. Information and knowledge is shared.	Patients should have unfettered access to their own medical information, communication should be open, and knowledge should be shared.	Any tests results you perform are part of the information you provide to patients with each visit (i.e., blood pressure, pulse, blood sugar results, INR test results, etc.).
5. Decision making is based on evidence.	The system needs to ensure that practitioners are up-to-date and their practice incorporates current evidence and guidelines.	In your clinic, you have a process of continuing education and policy and procedure updating that incorporates current changes in evidence or guidelines in a timely manner. For example, a diabetes clinic may have a yearly evaluation of the ADA guidelines published every January.
6. Safety is the responsibility of the entire system.	Shifts blame for errors from the individual involved with the error to the system that allowed the error to occur with that practitioner. Encompasses a culture change from punitive, hidden error to discussion to open disclosure, with all efforts to correct the flaws that led to the error.	You have a system to identify, discuss, disclose, tabulate, and evaluate errors as they occur, and you use that data as a basis for your quality improvement plan.

Table 7-2. Rules to Ensure Quality in Your Service or Microsystem (cont'd)

Rules For Health Care Quality in Microsystems of Care	Comments	Ambulatory Pharmacy Patient-Care Example
7. Transparency is necessary.	Information on any aspect of the practice (i.e., safety performance, satisfaction, qualifications, quality measurement, etc.) is available.	You share information on your practice and your quality improvement results with others, from the patients you service to other providers.
8. Needs are anticipated.	Reacting to patient needs prolongs access to care. Anticipation or having a proactive mind-set regarding needs allows for a patient's plan of care to quickly identify and addresses needs.	You identify patients who are high risk and you devise a system of follow up. This is an ideal strategy for detecting and acting on adverse drug events.
9. Waste is continuously decreased.	Neither resources nor patient time should be wasted; however, cost-reduction approaches that hinder application of evidence-based care need to be avoided.	You have a hypertension clinic; instead of using your favorite medications, you individualize them to patients with both therapeutic and cost in mind so that tiered copay policies don't prevent a patient from affording an evidenced-based therapy.
10. Cooperation among clinicians is a priority.	Care is collaborative with a team focus. The hierarchy of professionals does not impede or block appropriate patient care. This is analogous to a pilot and the crew preparing a plane for flight.	Within your clinic team, all members including students and technicians are versed in appropriate patient care and empowered and instructed to act when that care is compromised.

ADA = American Diabetes Association;

change you decide to propose is to add the use of pill boxes to your services. The best way to approach this is through the microsystem team. Including the entire team will provide the unique perspective from each member when devising the plan for change and therefore strengthen the plan by reducing unanticipated barriers. Being inclusive will also gain you "buy in" from the team so that members personally care about the change, improving your chances of successes.

· How will we know that a change is an improvement?

This final question stresses the importance of carefully choosing your quality measures. If available, you may want to use measures already published in the health care quality literature that have been tested, and are known to reflect a level of improvement. Reviewing the literature on similar clinics or services and evaluating what they used as measures may provide you some benchmarks as well as identify barriers. However, a measure important to your particular practice may not have such scientific validation. A good strategy in this situation is to run a small pilot of the measure to assure it is providing you the information that reflects what you have implemented.

The essential steps to the PDSA model are outlined below. We will take a closer look at each step. You may wish to use the PDSA work sheet (**Figure 7-1**) to begin to formulate your particular project as you go through the remainder of the chapter.[22]

The Planning Phase

1. Set aims: Define what you are trying to fix or accomplish.

2. Find promising strategies for change: Use your team, literature review, innovation, and problem-solving skills to reengineer the patient-care system and services.

3. Define measurements: Choose tools that measure the level of achievement of the aims.

The Do Phase

4. Implement the change: As a team, inform all involved (patients, other providers, etc.) of the change and implement it in an organized manner.

The Study Phase

5. Test those ideas: Determine if the new ideas for change result in improvement.

The Act Phase

6. Take results from the study phase and restart the PDSA cycle until you are performing at your goal of quality for that particular aim.

Getting Started: The Planning Phase

Setting Aims

Establish aims for your program by determining the direction of improvement or the desired goals your microsystem wishes to achieve. Setting aims is similar to setting patient therapeutic goals. Aims need to be specific so that they are attainable and measurable. Just as setting a patient's blood pressure goal at 120/80 mm Hg or less is specific and measurable, so should the quality aim be specific so measurement of an improvement and an optimal end point can be determined. Aims should be ambitious so the value of the work required in the PDSA cycle yields significant and sustainable improvement. A collaborative team or process should be involved in aim establishment so that the influence of the various touch points of a patient's unique system of care is optimally considered. The aims chosen should always result in improvement in patients' needs and their experience of care.

Setting aims is similar to setting patient therapeutic goals. They should be specific, designed to be attainable, and measurable.

Plan to Develop or Improve _____ **Services**

- **Aims**: What are the one or two high-level goals you have for your program?

  Aim 1.

  Aim 2.

- **Strategies**: What are the strategies you intend to pursue to achieve your aims?

  Strategy 1.

  Strategy 2.

  Strategy 3.

  Strategy 4.

- **Objectives**: For each goal, what are your desired objectives and outcomes?

  Aim 1.
  - O1:
  - O2:
  - O3:

  Aim 2.
  - O1:
  - O2:
  - O3:

- **Key Performance Measures:** For each objective, how will you measure success?

  Measures

  A1-O1:

  A1-O2:

  A1-O3:

  A2-O1:

  A2-O2:

  A2-O3:

Figure 7-1. PDSA Worksheet

Adapted from Rollinson R, Young E. *Strategic Planning for the 21st Century: A Practical Strategic Management Process.* 1st ed. Chicago, IL: LookingGlass Publishing; 2010.

Adapting a commonly used business strategy termed "a balanced scorecard" to the health care environment ensures that all aspects of the microsystem of care are simultaneously evaluated and improved.[23] When a business focuses on just one aspect at the expense of another, it tends to be less successful, for example focusing on the bottom line at the expense of the service provided. In health care, if the focus is only on patient outcomes without balancing attention to structure, process, and value, the chances of notably improving outcomes is diminished. Within the "balanced scorecard" concept, several major goals are set within each perspective (**Figure 7-2**). Direction in choosing the aims or goals for each section of your balanced scorecard will be driven by your microsystem's mission and vision statements, the values deemed important by your clinic, and the needs and desires of your patients. Once determined and prioritized, objectives and measures can be applied to each aim.

Finding Strategies for Change

Just as you did when setting aims, you should use your microsystem team to brainstorm ways to create a system or process for a new service or to change your current system in order to achieve your aims. Researching the literature and communicating with others to get a sense of what works and what does not is an excellent beginning strategy. Citations that describe in varying detail diverse ambulatory pharmacy patient-care services are on the web. Some models are well established

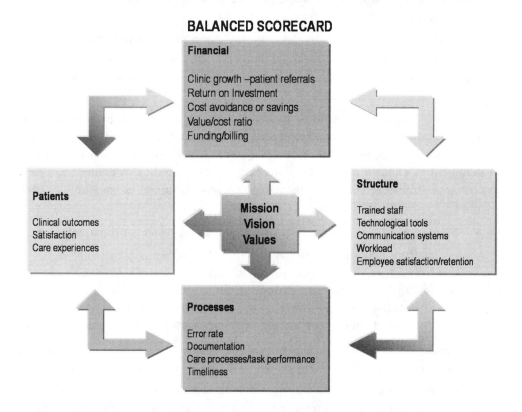

Figure 7-2. Balanced Scorecard for the Ambulatory Patient-Care Pharmacist

Adapted from Kaplan RS, Norton DP. *Balanced Scorecard: Translating Strategy into Action.* Boston, MA: Harvard Business School Press; 1996.

and reproducible, such as anticoagulation, whereas others are still in need of further innovation, such as medication therapy management. A number of pharmacy organizations as well as disease- or therapy-specific specialty organizations have practice sections and Listserves that can facilitate your research for this task. In the present environment of technology, much of your research can be found with a simple question and a click.

Choosing Quality Measures

Once aims and your strategy for change are determined, the next step is setting one or more objectives for each aim. This will provide the specificity that will allow meaningful measurement and produce the outcomes you desire.

> **CASE STUDY**
>
> In Dr. Busybee's clinic process, your current strategy is to have 20 minutes allotted for each patient visit. Your aim is to provide enough time for patient visits yet to be cost effective in staff or resource use. Your objective may be to accommodate 90% of your patients in that visit range in order to keep your providers feeling they have adequate time to provide services to your patients and avoid poor patient experiences with excessive waiting times. Your measure would then be number of patient visits within the 20 minutes as the numerator and total number of patient visits as the denominator over a set time span. You may consider an additional measure of patient or provider satisfaction with this change.

Measures in health care tend to be categorized into what has been termed the three dimensions of health care: structure, process, and outcome.[24] This concept fits nicely into the goals of the balance scorecard, with the addition of financial measurement as a fourth dimension. Thinking of "measure" in this context will help you connect a measure to your aims and objectives. Examples of measures in each category include the following:

- *Structure*: Measures the effect of resources and systems on patient care
    o Staffing hours per clinic day
    o Number of patient visits per clinic day
    o Average wait times per patient in clinic
    o Pharmacist time spent arranging clinic visits for patients
    o Pharmacist time spent arranging transportation for patients

- *Process*: Measures the interaction of the health care provider or ambulatory pharmacist with the patient or the care and services provided
    o Number of reconciled medication services provided per patients seen
    o Number of blood pressure measurements performed compared to number of patient visits
    o Percentage of times adherence to medications is documented per patient visit

- o   Number of visits with sufficient documentation compared to number of visits total
- o   Number of visits with comprehensive patient education

- *Outcomes*: Measures the effect the program has on the patient(s) served (further discussed below)

- *Finance*: Measures related to cost/value (the value of the service measured through other outcomes such as clinical or humanistic), return on investment (ROI), growth, billing
  - o   Amount collected compared to amount billed
  - o   Successful collection compared to billing code used
  - o   Staffing costs compared to cost savings from improved outcomes
  - o   Service growth

Patient outcome measures have been the primary focus of most quality measurement in the clinical arena, including clinical pharmacy. They have their own categorization of measures called the ECHO (economic, clinical, humanistic, outcome) model on patient outcomes. Examples of these types of measures are listed below.

- Clinical outcome measures describe patients' health status with two subcategories.
  - o   Primary outcomes
    - -   Number or percentage of patients who die
    - -   Number or percentage of patients who suffer an adverse drug event
    - -   Secondary outcomes that relate to a disease or treatment
      - ·   Blood pressures at goal
      - ·   Number of patients with 10% reduction in blood pressures
      - ·   Number of patients with at-goal lipid values
      - ·   Number of patients achieving 90% medication adherence for HIV medications
      - ·   Number of patients with HgA1c values less than 7

- Humanistic outcome measures evaluate customers' (usually patients') satisfaction with the program and their quality of life
  - o   Number of patients with improved health
  - o   Number of patients who feel they have improved understanding of how to use their medications
  - o   Number of patients who feel less anxiety regarding their medical care

- Economic outcomes measure the economic value of a program to the patient or population through cost savings
  - o   Percentage reduction in hospitalizations or emergency room visits
  - o   Reduction in testing due to improved clinical disease control

To use ECHO, you select several high-priority aims that represent key aspects (balanced scorecard) of your program that you believe need evaluation for quality or improvement. Under each of those aims, you create or redesign processes or services to achieve certain objectives. For each objective you select or create a measure for which you can collect data to inform you if, indeed, the change you made has achieved your objective and ultimately your aim.

Fortunately, as previously stated, quality measurement development is a booming field with a multitude of resources to assist the practitioner (**Table 7-3**). The majority of these measures have been tested, or validated. Advantages to using these measures are that they have the potential to allow comparisons on a large scope. You now can compare yourself to others who provide the same services nationally or in your city or state. A number of these sites have catalogued large numbers of measures and have search functionality to find those measures related to topics of interest.

The quality measures you choose should possess three important characteristics related to your particular practice; measures should be meaningful, feasible, and actionable.[25] Diligence in selecting program aims and objectives will greatly enhance the meaningfulness of the measures you chose. Meaningfulness that extends outside your organization is enhanced if measures are evidence based and validated. Due to the infancy of the field, many publically available measures vary widely in possession of these traits although in most instances the measures are created based on knowledge gained through scientific evidence. The majority of measure development organizations use comprehensive processes with expert input for both the topic of measurement and measure development, and rigorous evaluation processes are used before measures are endorsed or made available for public use. Using best practice or minimal acceptable care can guide the meaningfulness of a measure.

Key Point Choose quality measures that possess three important characteristics related to your particular practice; measures should be meaningful, feasible, and actionable.[25]

For a quality program to be manageable and effective, the measures chosen must be feasible and actionable. You must be able to collect data on the chosen measure with minimal interruption in patient care and often without the luxury of additional resources. When determining if you will be successful using a particular measure, important questions to answer as you develop your plan are as follows (**Figure 7-3**) (Quality Measure Feasibility Checklist is available on the web):

- Is the data readily available to collect?
    - o Where in the process of care will data be collected?
    - o Will collecting data significantly disrupt the care or efficiency of providing care?
    - o On what population will the data be collected?

Table 7-3. Resources for Information on Quality Improvement and Developed Health Care Measures

Source	Location	Description
The Quality Alliances: Hospital Quality Alliance (HQA), Ambulatory Quality Alliance (AQA), and Pharmacy Quality Alliance PQA	http://www.hospitalquality alliance.org/ http://www.aqaalliance.org/ http://www.pqaalliance.org/	The HQA drives hospital-based quality measures. The AQA drives ambulatory care improvements, primarily geared toward physician providers. PQA develops and validates medication-related and pharmacy-driven quality and efficiency measures. Refer to approved or proposed measure sets.
ASHP (American Society of Health-System Pharmacists) Quality Improvement Initiative (QII)	http://www.ashp.org/qii	Site provides resources to support pharmacist leadership and engagement in health care quality initiatives that improve patient outcomes and reward performance excellence.
Customer Assessment of Health Plans and Systems (CAHPS)	http://www.cahps.ahrq.gov/con-tent/products/PROD_Amb Care-Surveys.asp	Patient satisfaction surveys/metrics for ambulatory care including some measures that could be impacted by pharmacy services. Note: A pharmacy-specific CAHPS survey is undergoing review for approval as of 2010.
CDC (Centers for Disease Control and Prevention) Healthy People 2010	http://www.cdc.gov/nchs/ healthy_people.htm	CDC project that provides science-based, 10-year national objectives for promoting health and preventing disease, including health and wellness metrics.
CMS (Centers for Medicare and Medicaid Services) Physician Reporting Quality Initiative (PRQI)	http://www.cms.hhs. gov/pqri/ see "Measure Codes"	Contains current measure sets for ambulatory care, including measures targeting medication-related and chronic condition outcomes.
Institute for Healthcare Improvement (IHI) Strategic Initiatives	http://www.ihi.org/IHI/Pro-grams/StrategicInitiatives/	IHI does not develop quality measures but does drive quality innovation and support national quality initiatives. Ideas for quality measures or clinical target areas can be found in the Strategic Initiative area of the IHI site.
The National Committee for Quality Assurance (NCQA)	http://www.ncqa.org and select "HEDIS and Quality Measure-ment"	The Healthcare Effectiveness Data and Information Set (HEDIS) is a tool used by more than 90% of U.S. health plans to measure performance on important dimensions of care and service.
National Quality Forum (NFQ)	http://www.qualityforum.org/ Measuring_Performance/ Measuring_Performance.aspx	May view the current list of NQF-endorsed standards.

Table 7-3. Resources for Information on Quality Improvement and Developed Health Care Measures (cont'd)

Source	Location	Description
National Quality Measure Clearinghouse	http://www.qualitymeasures. ahrq.gov/	A searchable public repository, sponsored by AHRQ, for evidence-based quality measures and measure sets that also provides guidance on how to apply measures. Use the "browse" category to find measure types.
Quality improvement organizations (QIOs)	http://medqic.org/dcs/Content Server?pagename=MedqicMQ Page/Homepage http://www.ahqa.org	QIOs are state-based private organizations that contract with the federal government to monitor the appropriateness, effectiveness, and quality of care provided to Medicare beneficiaries.
The Joint Commission (TJC)	http://www.jointcommission.org Do a state search for Accreditation http://www.jointcommission.org Do a state search for National Patient Safety Goals	TJC provides accreditation for institutions providing ambulatory care and has standards that include quality goals. Also, TJC surveys on the National Patient Safety Goals (NPSG) for ambulatory care.
Physician Consortium for Performance Improvement (PCPI)	http://www.ama-assn.org/ama/ pub/category/2946.html	AMA organization to develop, test, and implement evidence-based performance measures for use at the point of care for the goal of enhancing quality and patient safety and fostering accountability.

> o Is the entire population feasible, or a will a subset provide accurate information?
>
> o How are you going to collect the data: manually or electronically?
>
> o Do you have the resources and time to collect the data in the manner chosen?

- Are the data collected accurate and reliable, such that confidence exists in the results obtained?

- Can you afford to collect the data?
  - o How burdensome is collecting the data?
  - o Will you need to process the data by case-mix adjustment or risk stratification (i.e., adjusted for vulnerable populations, disparate populations, or other added complexities)?

When assessing if a measure is actionable, the following attributes are key:
- Are the results interpretable such that areas of improvement can be identified?
- Are the resulting opportunities for change under your control?
- Do norms, benchmarks, or standards exist?

Question	Yes/No	Value Yes = 1 No = 0	Comments
Are the data readily available to collect?			
Are the data being collected during the process of care?			Where in the process?
Will collecting data significantly disrupt the care or efficiency of providing care?			
If yes, is it acceptable disruption?			
Will the data be collected on the entire population?			If not, which group?
Are you able to collect the data electronically?			
Do you have the resources to collect the data?			
Do you have the time to collect the data?			
Will the data provide you timely information?			
Are there problems with accuracy for your data?			
Will the collection of data be costly?			
Do the data need to be case-mix adjusted or risk stratified (i.e., adjusted for vulnerable populations, disparate populations, or other added complexities)?			
Will the information provide you ways to improve?			
Is the ability to change what you are measuring under your control?			
Do norms, benchmarks, or standards exist?			

Optimal measure = 10–12; Acceptable measure = 5–10; Difficult measure < 5

Statistical Resources on the Web

Free statistical software: http://statpages.org/javasta2.html

http://www.freestatistics.info/stat.php

http://www.statsci.org/free.html

http://statistical-package.smartcode.com/

Figure 7-3. Quality Measure Feasibility Checklist

Addressing all of the recommended measure characteristics can be a daunting task. Measures do not need to be perfect; they need to provide information so that you as an ambulatory pharmacist can learn and identify less than optimal areas in your patient-care services in order to improve. Taking a large problem or significant aim and breaking it down into small steps within the PDSA cycle may be the most efficient method for improvement.

Implementing the Quality Improvement Process: The "Do" Phase

When implementing your change and its measurement plan, be transparent to all involved. Inform patients and other providers involved about the changes, why you are changing your service and process, and how you plan to evaluate whether it will work. Making sure you touch all the points of interaction and interdependent processes and services discussed earlier will decrease unforeseen barriers and reduce unexpected events. The quality of the data and tolerance of any disruption in the work process will be best achieved if all participants are engaged and understand the aims and objectives of the measures.

CASE

Using our previous example of changing visit times to 20 minutes, you will need to inform patients why their visit times are changing. You may need to inform other health care providers in your clinic, the information desk, the billing department, etc. about the change as well. You may explain your goal of accommodating 90% of patients in this time frame and that you will be assessing if patients and the providers feel they have enough time to accomplish visit goals in that time frame.

Do plan for deviations or the unexpected complication to occur by anticipating and providing a process to deal with these potential occurrences. Barriers will arise: Planning a process to deal with them will reduce the likelihood of the barriers derailing your program. For example, you may decide to have a weekly (or other reasonable time frame) huddle of key people involved in your project to address any deviations or barriers that pop up. Establish a reasonable and feasible time line to collect and assess the data. Be cautious of extended time lines since current data can be more meaningful. Build routine follow up into your plan, such that review and reporting are not burdensome, but turnaround is frequent enough to keep participants engaged in the quality work process.

Key Point   The more current the data, the greater meaning and impact it will have on your program.

Evaluating Measure Results: The "Study" Phase

Once sufficient measure data are collected, assessing it is the next step. Measure results should always be reviewed for inconsistencies and discrepancies to ensure that data are reliable. Poor or unreliable data can provide erroneous results and ineffective actions for change. The data should make sense and be plausible on review by the providers within the microsystem. Appropriate methods of analysis and display of the data should be determined. Descriptive statistics often are adequate to convey the desired information. The resources and skills of your organization will determine the extent of analysis and presentation you can perform. Graphs and tables are useful tools for which software resources are readily available.

Key Point   The most important outcome of the data analysis is the answer to the query, "Do the data provide sufficient information for you to make a change to improve?"

CASE

Returning to our sample case of evaluating visit time length. The results are as follows:

Case Figure 1. Number of Patient Visits at This Time Range/Total number of Visits over 2 Months (%)

(A)

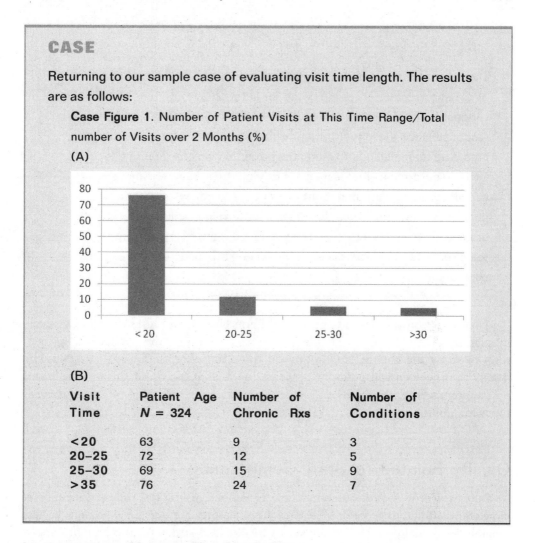

(B)

Visit Time	Patient Age N = 324	Number of Chronic Rxs	Number of Conditions
< 20	63	9	3
20–25	72	12	5
25–30	69	15	9
> 35	76	24	7

Implementing Change: The "Act" Phase

Reacting to measure results, developing promising change concepts, and acting on the change concept are the most important parts of the PDSA process.[17,20] Reacting to measure results requires leadership and participation from key members of the microsystem. Through problem solving, using the skills and knowledge of the microsystem employees, and brainstorming, solutions for improvement can be envisioned for clinic structure, patient-care processes, or services provided based on the measure results. Finding several ideas to test may give the organization options to act quickly if one concept fails. Taking small manageable steps toward improvement to achieve your quality improvement aims is the essence of the entire PSDA process. Resistance to change may be the most formidable challenge to overcome in this step. Empowering the microsystem with time, authority to make change, and a safe harbor (i.e., no idea is a bad one) are important strategies for overcoming resistance.

CASE

The results of our sample show that you are not meeting your goal of 90% of patients adequately being cared for in the 20-minute time slot. The data suggest that older patients and those with more medications appear to be responsible for the longer patient visits. The team meets to review the data. The team decides to study the patients who are requiring longer visits to determine what issues are driving the increased time, such as a specific drug, condition, patient characteristic, knowledge deficit of pharmacy staff, etc. Once the cause is determined, the team will brainstorm how to streamline the specific drivers of longer visits. The team restarts the PDSA cycle, planning what to measure in the outlier population.

Finally, act on the desired and agreed upon change and restart the PSDA cycle by planning the change idea implementation, performing the change, using measures to study the change, and acting on the result. The PDSA cycle sustains the quality improvement program by perpetuating a state of continuous change based on the premise that the status quo is never good enough. In every program there is room for improvement.

Quality Related to Staff Competency

Measures for process and outcomes for the various health and illness domains are large and continue to expand. Where quality measures are lacking is around the less tangible yet equally crucial first level of health care structure: the patient experience. These measures of quality include provider judgment, knowledge, compassion, and communication.[15] The subjective nature of these characteristics renders them difficult to measure. A process to ensure quality in this critical part of an organization's structure is to establish measures or criteria for staff selection and competency in order to provide ambulatory pharmacy patient-care services.

Traditionally, measures of competency have relied on knowledge base, licensure, and certificates of training. To ensure the ambulatory patient-care pharmacists possess the needed judgment, compassion, and communication skills to provide patient-centered care, competency needs to encompass both knowledge base and interpersonal and social skills. A recent proposed taxonomy on professionalism provides an excellent and comprehensive set of aims and objectives for assessing the quality of the skill set necessary for ambulatory pharmacy patient-care providers.[26] In their taxonomy, Brown and Ferrill describe three hierarchal domains that convert well to aims within the structure portion of an organization (**Figure 7-4**). Within each domain are lists of objectives that describe desirable traits for the practitioner (**Table 7-4**).

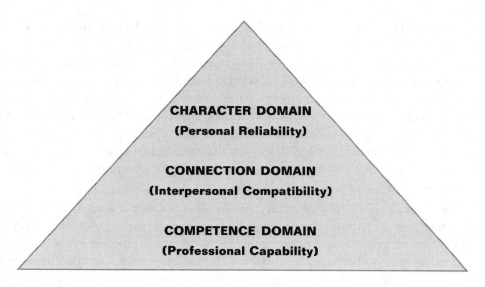

Figure 7-4. Brown and Ferrill's Professional Pyramid

Reprinted with permission from Hermann, RC, Palmer RH. Common ground: A framework for selecting quality measures for mental health and substance abuse. *Psychiatr Serv.* 2002;53:281-287.

Table 7-4. Brown and Ferrill's Taxonomy of Professionalism[25]

Competency Domain	Connection Domain	Character Domain
1. Knowledge	1. Compassion	1. Honesty/Integrity
2. Self-directed learning	2. Empathy	2. Humility
3. Applied skill	3. Self-control	3. Responsibility
4. Proactivity	4. Kindness	4. Service
5. Wisdom	5. Influence	5. Moral courage

Establishing Competency

Knowledge clearly is a primary objective within the competency domain. A number of references are available outlining in detail the suggested knowledge base required for a clinical patient-care pharmacist.[27-29] The type of services provided and the requirements of the patient population to being served will dictate the knowledge and training needed for a particular site. Generally, a sound knowledge base of the medical conditions or disease states of the patient population, including evidence-based literature and guidelines; the appropriate physical assessment skills; laboratory and test management and interpretation; and knowledge of optimal drug therapy, are essential. To attain the prerequisite knowledge, various practice model-specific traineeships, certificates, and other similar venues are available through pharmacy organizations and schools of pharmacy. For many practitioners, however, that option may not be feasible. Using acquired research and self-learning skills may offer a satisfactory option to achieve the necessary knowledge competency.

Health care is not static, as it constantly and quickly changes; therefore, a vital attribute includes being a self-directed learner. Practitioners should seek to answer clinical questions as they arise and have a sense of responsibility for continued learning in order to maintain their knowledge base. Knowledge is wasted, however, if the pharmacist is unable to apply that knowledge to patient care. Patients and their particular circumstances generally do not mimic the perfect textbook disease case. The ambulatory pharmacist needs critical-thinking and problem-solving skills in order to apply knowledge and skills such that wise decisions are made in the care of individual patients. Having sound judgment reflects the wisdom the pharmacist needs to possess and needs to continue to develop.

The ambulatory clinical pharmacy patient-care practice is a relatively new and expanding area. Practitioners may often find themselves carving out their position and developing or growing a new practice. To successfully function in this capacity, pharmacists need to be proactive and have the initiative to define and create their roles in the ambulatory setting, persevering over barriers and obstacles that will inevitably emerge.

Making Connections

The connection domain reflects communication skills and the ability of the pharmacist to develop positive working relationships with people at all levels, including other health care providers, colleagues within the practice, and patients with varying cognition and health literacy skills. Pharmacists should posses confidence in their personal communication style and be able to adapt their knowledge to patients by effectively translating complex information into what patients find understandable and usable. Critical communication skills include listening and observing. The ambulatory patient-care pharmacist must not only listen well to what patients verbally state but also observe and interpret what patients are expressing nonverbally.

Compassion and empathy are particularly important traits when working with chronically ill patients. One-to-one communication is enhanced when patients sense their provider listens well to their concerns, and further, when patients believe the practitioner cares and understands how they feel and think. For patient-centered care, the pharmacist must treat all the patients' concerns and provide care for the whole patient, not just a particular disease or test result.

The health care environment is often unpredictable and can occasionally become chaotic, with heavy workloads, taxing situations, and challenging patients. The ability to maintain self-control in trying circumstances, while still showing understanding and kindness, is an important ability. Being ill, especially chronically, is not pleasant, and often the pharmacist will need to effectively connect with patients when they are not at their best.

The most difficult proficiency will be that of influence. This need may present itself in a variety of ways. It may be changing poor prescribing habits of a provider, or shifting less than optimal patient-care practices within an organization, or altering patient behaviors such as medication adherence or poor health habits. The pharmacist will need to discern an individualized tactic or plan in each situation to effect overall improvement in outcomes of patients and the services provided. The ability to influence may prove to be a crucial skill set in the ambulatory environment.

Evaluating Character

At the top of the professional pyramid are character traits and the moral and ethical base of an individual. The placement at the top of the pyramid conveys its importance, yet it may prove to be the most difficult to measure and quantify. For the highest quality of patient care, the personal behaviors of honesty, integrity, responsibility, etc. are essential. The ambulatory patient-care pharmacist should serve as the patient's advocate regarding all medication issues. No medication need or patient-care task should exist that is viewed by pharmacists as beneath them or not considered their role to solve. This sense of humility and responsibility is necessary for multidisciplinary teamwork to positively affect patient care. Their approach to patient care should be one of striving for excellence. This sense of duty for excellence elicits personal responsibility to ensure all patient needs are addressed, minimizing to the fullest any lapses in care.

As a pharmacist, you should have knowledge of current ethical standards and have a strong sense of what is right and wrong. You should possess the moral courage to do what is right even when it is difficult or unpleasant. Patient service is the major role of the ambulatory care pharmacist; therefore, your work ethic should be guided primarily by the desire to help, and your work satisfaction should stem primarily from having helped.

Credentialing and Privileging

Sometimes it is difficult for a manager or an organization leader to identify a competent staff candidate even with the guidance presented here. Interviewing and selecting candidates that may meet your needs is a skill that often requires practice and experience. You may decide to use more concrete criteria in the selection of your staff. In certain situations, laws, regulations, payers, and other providers may want specific evidence of current and continued competency to perform ambulatory patient-care services. Consequently, there are a number of avenues available to establish competency, from licensure to privileging (**Table 7-5**).

Deciding on whether you require or desire specialized training for the clinician practicing in your organization depends on a number of factors. First is the type of clinic you have. Does your clinic provide basic, complex, or specialty clinical services? Your clinic may focus on a basic pharmacy service such as medication reconciliation and decide that a 6-year PharmD training is sufficient for medication reconciliation activities. However, for a diabetic care clinic service you may want to ensure a different level of training and experience. How advanced is your scope of practice, and how independently will the clinical pharmacist be practicing? For a comprehensive medication therapy management program with a collaborative practice agreement to adjust medication dosages to the therapeutic goal, you may desire a practitioner with residency training and board certification competency. As stated, there may be state laws or payer stipulations on what type of credentials or training a provider of certain services must possess. For pharmacists to provide immunizations, state laws require completion of training and certification from a recognized immunization program. Other health providers, physicians who assume

Table 7-5. Examples for Evidence of Ambulatory Patient-Care Competency

Training	*Post BS PharmD*: Programs that provide in-depth disease state, therapeutics, patient care and assessment training
	6-year PharmD: Current entry pharmacy degree ensures entry level competence for medication distribution and basic patient-care services.
	Postgraduate Residency Training: Provides additional practice experience and clinical and research training. First-year programs provide minimal clinical competence. Second-year programs provide more in-depth knowledge and experience, often in a specialty area (infectious disease, oncology, ambulatory etc).
	Fellowships: Further training after residency, geared toward practice research experience
Experience	*Clinical work history portfolio*: Practitioners who have gained experience in direct patient care through work experience
Peer Review by Credentialing Committees	*Credentialing*: Process of obtaining, verifying, and assessing the qualifications of an applicant to provide patient care, treatment, and services to patients within a health care organization.[30]
	Privileging: Process by which a health care organization grants a specific practice or practitioner the authorization to provide specific patient-care services and defines the scope of service.[31]
Certification	Process by which a nongovernmental agency, such as a professional association, grants recognition after assessment of an individual who has met certain predetermined qualifications specified by that organization.
a. Testing	1. Board of Pharmacy Specialties (pharmacotherapy, ambulatory, oncology, etc; www.bpsweb.org)
	2. Commission for Certification in Geriatric Pharmacy (www.ccgp.org)
	3. National Certification Board for Diabetes Educators (www.ncbde.org)
	4. Certified Anticoagulation Care Provider (www.ncbap.org)
b. Training and testing	Numerous program examples include:
	Immunization, anticoagulation, heart failure, etc. (search colleges and pharmacy associations)
	Anticoagulation (several colleges provide)

responsibility for midlevel providers such as clinical pharmacists, may insist on a skill level afforded only by advanced training, certification, or experience. Examples include specialized services such as treating heart failure or diabetes; these diseases need team-based management, are complex, and often require additional experience and training. Finally, availability of adequately trained candidates in your area may affect your choices. You may need to consider hiring and then using a certificate program for training in such situations.

Generally, the more complex the services, the greater the level of training needed to ensure standards of care and appropriate level of risk and liability. Each step of training provides additional practice and experience to tackle the complexity of clinical problem solving, make optimal patient-care decisions, know how to best communicate those decisions, and measure such decision's effect on patient outcomes. Therefore, you may make the decision that for your practice site, your ambulatory clinical staff (or at a minimum its leadership) must have a certain level of training and certification.

Although residency training provides important supervised and guided practice experience for the novice practitioner, and certification testing ensures a level of knowledge, they are not foolproof in ensuring competency for an individual. Many organizations also use credentialing and privileging for health care professionals providing complex patient care. This process is common for physicians and nurse practitioners in many institutional settings and is gaining popularity for pharmacists involved in complex and specialized patient-care roles. Organizations create a credentialing and privileging committee of experienced peers who establish practice qualification standards and performance markers for practitioners who provide complex or high-risk patient-care services.[31] They also define scope of services, approve collaborative practice agreements, and develop policy and procedures for the application and approval process. Credentialing and privileging not only grant a practitioner the ability to provide services within the organization, but they are also responsible for the maintenance of the practitioner's privileges through review and reappointment on a periodic basis.

As a pharmacist, the application process may include evidence of your training and previous experience through your curriculum vitae, any certifications you have achieved, and professional references. Confirmation of skill in patient care may be supplied through the submission of sample patient notes, both initial visit and SOAP notes.[32] Samples of patient-care documentation should provide examples of your ability to appropriately assess patients, a demonstration of your problem-solving skills, and your thought process in patient care as described in Chapter 6. Ongoing competency and privileging would be based on review over some time frame, such as annual or biannual. This may include an evaluation of any quality measures affiliated with your clinic and patients, evidence that you are maintaining and improving your knowledge base, and continued peer review of your work through submission of sample documentation of patient care.

Ensuring competency of providers is an important component of quality. Although there is no perfect method, every practice site should address the competency and skills of its staff to perform the functions they are assigned. Not only is this an activity required by accreditation organizations such as the Joint Commission, but also it is vital to providing optimal patient care.

Chapter Summary

This chapter provides the elements necessary to create and maintain a quality improvement program for your ambulatory patient-care practice. Quality care, however, is not just about the steps in a program. To have true organizational improvement, a culture and desire to improve the experience of each patient must exist among the leadership and staff. Fixing those identified areas that impede optimal patient care should receive high priority and sufficient resources. The reality of health care reform and the future of the industry are based on how well organizations understand how to cost effectively and efficiently improve the experiences and care of their patients. To ensure an effective quality improvement program you not only will need to use the tools discussed in this chapter but also build your program on key principles outlined by Glasgow in his commentary.[21]

- Make your quality improvement efforts about quality and not about meeting a requirement. Keeping your program centered on the patient will help you accomplish this.

- Aim for real change, not just education. Do not stop at identifying a problem and then trying to fix it by only educating on what is being done wrong. People generally are trying very hard to do things right. The system usually needs to be changed to help the practitioner consistently provide optimal care.

- Empower and excite. Leaders need to identify, communicate, and empower. It is usually the frontline workers who understand best how to improve a process that improves quality.

- Start small, dream big. Taking on smaller achievable goals builds confidence and buy-in to improved quality, which, in the long run, usually results in achieving the larger goal.

References

1. Kohn LT, Corrigan JM, Donaldson MS. *To Err is Human: Building a Safer Health System. Committee on Quality in America.* Washington, DC: Institute of Medicine, National Academy Press; 1999.

2. Chassin MR, Galvin RW, the National Roundtable on Health Care Quality. The urgent need to improve health care quality. *JAMA.* 1998;280:1000-1005.

3. Gurwitz JH, Field TS, Harrold LR, et al. Incidence and preventability of adverse drug events among older persons in the ambulatory setting. *JAMA.* 2003;289:1107-1116.

4. Ghandi TK, Burstin HR, Cook EF, et al. Drug complications in outpatients. *J Gen Intern Med.* 2000;15:149-154.

5. Bureau of Labor Education, University of Maine. The U.S. health care system: Best in the World, or Just the Most Expensive. 2001. http://dll.umaine.edu/ble/U.S.%20HCweb.pdf. Accessed October 2009.

6. Docteur E, Berenson R. How Does the Quality of U.S. Health Care Compare Internationally? Urban Institute, Robert Wood Foundation. August, 2009. http://www.rwjf.org/files/research/qualityquickstrikeaug2009.pdf. Accessed October 2009.

7. McGlynn EA, Asch SM, Adams J, et al. The quality of health care delivered to adults in the United States. *N Engl J Med.* 2003;348:2635-2645.

8. NCQA. *The State of Health Care Quality: 2004.* Washington, DC: National Committee for Quality Assurance; 2004.

9. http://www.opencongress.org/bill/111-h3590/text. 112th United States Congress. HR3590 - Patient Protection and Affordable Care Act.

10. Rosenthal MD, Landon BE, Normard SL, et al. Pay for performance in commercial HMOs. *N Engl J Med.* 2006;3518:1895-1902.

11. Epstein AM, Lee TH, Hamel MB. Paying physicians for high quality care. *N Engl J Med.* 2004;3504:406-410.

12. Blumenthal D. Quality of care—what is it? *N Engl J Med.* Pt. 1. 1996;335:891-894.

13. American Medical Association. Quality of care. *JAMA.* 1986;256:1032-1034.

14. Wharam JF, Sulmasy D. Improving the quality of health care: Who is responsible for what? *JAMA.* 2009;301:215-217.

15. Wharam, JF, Paasche-Orlow MK, Farber NJ, et al. High quality care and ethical pay-for-performance: A society of general internal medicine policy analysis. *J Gen Intern Med.* 2009;24:854-859.

16. Institute of Medicine. *Medicare: A Strategy for Quality Assurance.* Washington, DC: National Academy Press; 1990.

17. Berwick D. A user's manual for the IOM's Quality Chasm Report. *Health Affairs.* 2002;21:80-90.

18. Institute of Medicine. *Crossing the Quality Chasm: A New Health System for the 21st Century.* Washington, DC: National Academy Press; 2001.

19. Wolf SH. Patient safety is not enough: Targeting quality improvements to optimize the health of the population. *Ann Intern Med.* 2004;140:33-36.

20. Berwick DH. Education and debate: A primer on leading the improvement of systems. *Br Med J.* 1996;312:619-622.

21. Glasgow J. Introduction to Lean and Six Sigma Approaches to Quality Improvement. Expert Commentary. National Quality Measures Clearinghouse. May 16, 2011. http://qualitymeasures.ahrq.gov/expert/printView.aspx?id=32943. Accessed May 19, 2011.

22. Rollinson R, Young E. *Strategic Planning for the 21st Century: A Practical Strategic Management Process.* 1st ed. Chicago, IL: LookingGlass Publishing; 2010.

23. Kaplan RS, Norton DP. *Balanced Scorecard: Translating Strategy into Action.* Boston, MA: Harvard Business School Press; 1996.

24. Donabedian A. The quality of care. How can it be assessed? *JAMA.* 1988;260:1743-1748.

25. Hermann, RC, Palmer RH. Common ground: A framework for selecting quality measures for mental health and substance abuse. *Psychiatri Serv.* 2002;53:281-287.

26. Brown D, Ferrill MJ. The taxonomy of professionalism: Refraining the pursuit of academic professional development. *Am J Pharm Ed.* 2009;73:1-10.

27. Burke JM, Miller WA, Spencer AP, et al. ACCP white paper: Clinical pharmacist competencies. *Pharmacotherapy.* 2008;28:806-815.

28. The ACCP Clinical Practice Affairs Committee. Practice Guidelines for Pharmacotherapy Specialists: A position statement of the American College of Clinical Pharmacy. *Pharmacotherapy.* 2000; 20:487-490.

29. American Society of Health-System Pharmacists. *Preceptor's Guide to the RLS.* 3rd ed. Bethesda, MD: American Society of Health-System Pharmacists; 2008.

30. Blair MM, Freitag RT, Keller DL, et al. ACCP white paper: Proposed Revision to the Existing Specialty and Specialist Certification Framework for Pharmacy Practitioners. *Pharmacotherapy.* 2009;29:3e-13e.

31. Galt KA. Credentialing and privileging for pharmacists. *Am J Health Syst Pharm.* 2004;61:661-670.

32. Claxton KL, Woital P. Design and implementation of a credentialing and privileging model for ambulatory care pharmacists. *Am J Health-Syst Pharm.* 2006;63:1627-1632.

Web Resources

PDSA Worksheet

Quality Measure Feasibility Checklist

Example case: Medication Therapy Management Clinic

Additional Selected References

Ambulatory Care Pharmacy Suggested Resource Web Sites

Resources for Information on Quality Improvement and Developed Health Care Measures

Web Toolkit available at
www.ashp.org/ambulatorypractice

Reimbursement for the Pharmacist in an Ambulatory Practice

Sandra Leal, Betsy Bryant Shilliday, Amy L. Stump

CHAPTER

8

Chapter Outline

1. Introduction
2. Billing Models
3. Other Methods and Models
4. Chapter Summary
5. References
6. Additional Selected References
7. Web Resources

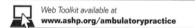
Web Toolkit available at
www.ashp.org/ambulatorypractice

Chapter Objectives

1. Compare and contrast the most common models of billing for ambulatory pharmacist services, including incident-to, facility fee, medication therapy management codes, and employer-sponsored wellness programs.

2. Explain how alternative routes of revenue generation, such as grants, demonstration projects, and relative value units, can be used when creating a pharmacist service.

3. List resources to use when creating a sliding fee scale for self-pay patients.

Introduction

The profession of pharmacy is continuously changing to include delivery of comprehensive clinical, consultative, and educational patient care services. No longer is the profession defined solely by products and dispensing, but instead it is enhanced by collaborative practice that is recognized by 47 states, the Department of Veterans Affairs, and the Indian Health Service.[1] Pharmacists, however, are not recognized under Title XVIII of the Social Security Act, thus resulting in lack of reimbursement eligibility under Medicare B due to lack of provider status.[2]

Historically, pharmacists have lobbied for provider status to create reimbursable services that are self-sustaining in a health system.[3] Although provider status recognition has not occurred for Medicare Part B, some progress has resulted in recognition under Medicare Part D, certain Medicaid plans in some states, and some individual third-party payers. Other strategies you may consider for payment include funding programs through indirect reimbursement methods such as "incident-to" billing.

In many instances, you may not be able to create a sustainable clinical practice based solely on the direct and indirect billing. Because of this, other creative reimbursement opportunities have surfaced that allow for supplementation of revenue to continue successful practice expansion. This chapter will address the reimbursement strategies that currently exist, along with other creative opportunities to provide guidance to initiate billing, expand billing, or generate funding opportunities that will allow your practice to succeed.

Billing Models

The gold standard for medical billing is the U.S. government and the Centers of Medicare and Medicaid Services (CMS). Although other payers such as commercial payers and state Medicaid may develop and use any model they wish, most use the Medicare billing model as their base. Doing so greatly decreases the billing process burden for providers of medical care and their patients. It is a system that has worked for a number of years. This chapter will focus on Medicare billing rules and processes and note how it may differ in the commercial sector or state Medicaid space. If your organization has a large non-Medicare-insured population, the compliance officer in your organization is responsible for understanding the billing process of the payers with which your organization may contract. This is another good reason for you to get to know your compliance officer.

Medicare Structure

To understand Medicare billing, it helps to understand how Medicare is structured. There are four separate arms of Medicare:

1. Medicare Part A is responsible for the rules, regulations, and reimbursement of all institutional services for Medicare beneficiaries, including hospitals, long-term care facilities, hospice, and some home health services. All Medicare beneficiaries have Medicare Part A benefits.

2. Medicare Part B is responsible for the rules, regulations, and reimbursement for all medically necessary outpatient services. This includes physicians, midlevel practitioners that have Part B provider status, some preventative services, and some home care services. Medicare beneficiaries usually have Medicare Part B, but not everyone does. Those without Social Security benefits or those who opted out of this benefit due to coverage with commercial insurance may not have Part B.

3. Medicare Part C, also called the Medicare Advantage Plan, is a managed care program that a beneficiary may opt to use. It is administered by a vari-

ety of commercial payers. Medicare pays a monthly fixed amount for the beneficiary to the private insurer who then manages the care and sets reimbursement for providers. Comparatively, this is a small part of Medicare.

4. Medicare Part D is the prescription benefit plan with which most pharmacists are familiar. This plan is administered by commercial companies that contract with Medicare, referred to as prescription drug plans or PDPs. Medication therapy management (MTM) services are included in the administrative fees that Medicare pays to the PDP.

CMS contracts part of the administrative responsibilities for Medicare Part A and/or Medicare Part B to private insurance companies, called fiscal intermediaries (FIs) or regional carriers. They have two primary functions: reimbursement review and medical coverage review. We will elaborate on the impact they have on ambulatory pharmacy patient care services later on in the chapter.

The majority of patient care pharmacy services that occur in outpatient clinics or independent physicians' offices are for Medicare beneficiaries and fall under Medicare Part B rules, regulations, and processes for billing. Reimbursement in the Medicare Part B space is called fee for service: in other words, you provide a service and you get paid. You may also run into ambulatory organizations that do business in the managed care arena and contract with Medicare Advantage plans. This model uses a capitated reimbursement method in which the organization receives a monthly set fee to manage the health care of a patient. The organization's reimbursement is also based on meeting or exceeding certain quality clinical and service benchmarks. As already stated, MTM services for Medicare are administered under Medicare Part D.

Incident-to Billing in a Noninstitutional Ambulatory Setting

Medicare Part B Billing

Since pharmacists are not recognized as Medicare Part B providers, the only method available to bill for the services provided by the pharmacists to Medicare beneficiaries in the outpatient clinic or ambulatory setting is "incident-to" billing. Incident-to billing is an indirect billing mechanism whereby pharmacists provide patient care services under direct supervision of a physician or other approved Medicare Part B provider (defined by Medicare to be a physician, physician assistant, nurse practitioner, clinical nurse specialist, nurse midwife, or clinical psychologist).[4] We will use "physician" as the term for this provider throughout the remainder of the chapter when speaking about Medicare Part B incident-to billing, with the understanding that Medicare has recently expanded incident-to to include the list of providers mentioned. Incident-to billing is not just for pharmacists, but for any auxiliary personnel that furnish a necessary service that is under and integral to the service provided by the physician or other approved Medicare Part B provider. Currently, incident-to billing is one of the most common means by which you might bill for clinical services.

In order for pharmacists (or other auxiliary personnel) to bill incident-to the physician, Medicare stipulates that certain criteria must be met (**Table 8-1**). The patient must be an established patient of the practice; there must be a prior face-to-face visit with the physician for the same problem; the service must be medically necessary and be an "integral, although incidental, part of the physician's professional services"; it must be a service commonly furnished in the physicians' office and commonly rendered without charge or included in the physician's bill; and it must be furnished by the physician or auxiliary personnel under the physician's direct supervision.[4-6]

> **Key Point**
> An established patient is defined as a patient initially seen by a physician in your practice within the previous 3 years for the same problems you are going to see the patient. The physician establishes a plan of care for the patient that includes or authorizes your service and must continue to be actively involved in that plan of care.[4,5]

Actively involved means the physician continues to see the patient face-to-face and provides evaluation and management (E&M) services for the identified problem(s). Reviewing or signing the notes of your visit does not constitute active involvement. Although CMS rules do not define specifically how often the patient's physician must be involved in the ongoing treatment and management of the patient when using the incident-to model, many fiscal intermediaries for CMS have interpreted a "one of three rule." This interpretation means that for Medicare patients, the physician must see the patient every third visit.

Table 8-1. Medicare Requirements for Incident-To Billing

1. Before the pharmacist can provide an "incident-to" service, the patient must have been seen by the physician or other Medicare Part B–approved practitioner for the same problem. The provider must have provided an evaluation or Medicare-covered service.

2. The physician or Medicare Part B–approved provider must have provided authorization for the service, and the authorization is included in the medical record.

3. The physician or Medicare Part B–approved provider must provide subsequent services at a frequency that reflects his/her active participation in management of the course of treatment. Review of the medical record does not qualify.

4. The service is of the type that is commonly furnished in a physician's or Medicare Part B–approved provider's office or clinic.

5. The service must be medically appropriate to be given in the provider's office or clinic.

6. A physician or Medicare Part B–approved practitioner must be on the premises, but not necessarily in the room, when incident-to services are performed. The supervising practitioner must be part of the organization defined as that which performs Medicare-billable services for patients within the organization.

7. The pharmacist providing the incident-to service must be an employee, leased or contracted to the physician or Medicare Part B–approved provider. The practice must have some legal control over the person and his or her services, and the person must represent an expense to the practice. (The expense is not required to be salary.)

Direct supervision is defined by the CMS as "the physician being present in the office suite and immediately available to provide assistance and direction throughout the time the aide is performing services."[4] There are no Medicare-required qualifications for auxiliary personnel; however, Medicare does state that the auxiliary personnel must be a financial expense to the physician and that reporting of their services should be to the physician.[4,7] Usually in the case of the ambulatory pharmacist, they may be employed, leased, or contracted; in essence, the pharmacists have some type of legal relationship to the physician.

This does not necessarily have to translate into salary expenses. In the contract, the financial expense incurred by the physician's practice may include nonsalary support to the pharmacist, such as providing clerical, nursing, billing, and technical staff support, in addition to providing exam room space, office supplies, and common waiting room space.

Through the incident-to billing model, pharmacists bill for their services incident-to the sanctioned Medicare Part B provider using evaluation and management (E&M) codes (99211-99215) for established patients of the practice.

> **Key Point**
>
> Most if not all FIs or regional carriers of CMS have interpreted the incident-to billing rules, for the noninstitutional arena, to mean pharmacists can only bill at the E&M 99211 level unless a physician physically sees the patient and adequate service documentation supports the higher level. The FI rulings revolve around the fact that pharmacists are not recognized Medicare Part B providers, therefore are not allowed to bill at a level higher than the lowest, 99211, nurse-level visit.

If the Medicare Part B provider sees the patient with you, the provider must provide adequate attestation on your visit note stating that he or she has seen the patient. An example of such attestation may be as simple as "I have seen and assessed this patient. The patient was discussed with the midlevel provider. I agree with the encounter assessment and plan above." To find the specifics of your region, we suggest contacting your regional CMS carrier directly. You can find your regional carrier contact at http://www.cms.gov/ContractingGeneralInformation/Downloads/02_ICdirectory.pdf. Reimbursement for these services also varies by region and institution type but may be accessed at https://www.cms.gov/apps/physician-fee-schedule/search/search-criteria.aspx.

These visits should then be appropriately documented in the patient's medical record. Although there are no CMS requirements for visit documentation of a 99211 visit, your service should be documented in the patient's medical record in the standards outlined in Chapter 6 to show that the interaction occurred and should contain the names of the supervising physician and person providing the service.

Non-Medicare Billing

For non-Medicare incident-to billing, individual state Medicaid rules and commercial payers may allow a pharmacist to bill higher codes as long as services and documentation support the higher billing (99212-99215). Some clinic administrators and compliance officers within institutions may interpret billing rules from these payers conservatively and follow Medicare regulations for non-Medicare payers too. If your institution allows you to bill at a higher level, adequate documentation must be noted to substantiate the higher bill. When documenting to meet the requirements of a higher-level visit, there are three key portions to include: history, physical exam, and medical decision making. In order to bill at these higher levels, you must address and document at least two of these three key portions. The level of billing would depend on the extent of history, physical exam performed or complexity of medical decision making involved. A comprehensive billing card is provided in Appendix 8-1, listing all the required documentation elements required for the various levels of billing. Pharmacists most commonly bill at levels 99211, 99212, and 99213; however, with appropriate documentation, you may bill higher provided all elements are satisfied. Let us now break down the three key areas one by one and discuss the detailed documentation necessary for each component, based on the level billed.

1.   History: The first pertinent area of documentation is the history, which is subcategorized into history of present illness (HPI), including chief complaint for the visit; review of systems (ROS); and past, family, and social history (PFSH). The various elements within the HPI, ROS, and PFSH are included in Appendix 8-1 and **Table 8-2**.[8] The HPI would be considered brief if the documentation includes one to three elements and extended if four or more elements are described or the status of at least three chronic or inactive conditions are noted.

CASE

You are now an established practitioner seeing patients within Dr. Busybee's office, and he has referred Ms. Honeybee to you so that you can assist in the management of her uncontrolled diabetes. An example documentation of a history you may create for this diabetic patient at her first appointment is as follows: "Ms. Honeybee is a 56 yo Caucasian female presenting to the office today with a chief complaint of uncontrolled blood sugars. HPI includes 2-week history of polyuria, polydipsia." If this is a 99214 visit, you may document further to list "elevated glucose readings in the 300s with home monitoring and burning on urination."

The second area under history is the ROS, which can be broken down into three levels: problem pertinent (1 system), extended (2–9 systems), or complete (at least 10 systems). A problem-pertinent review corresponds to a lower-level visit (99211–99213), an extended review correlates to a 99214 visit, and 10 or more systems constitute a detailed 99215 visit (Table 8-2). The findings of this review may be positive or negative, but each must be documented regardless of its positivity or negativity. If you wish to be more succinct in your documentation of negative findings, "all other systems negative" may be used to indicate a complete ROS was done.[8]

CASE

The 99213 visit may include focus on the endocrine system, whereas a 99214 visit may go further into documenting blood pressure, lipid labs, etc., as well as the cardiovascular system.

The third and final element of the history is documentation of PFSH. There are two levels to this area of documentation: pertinent (consisting of one of the three areas of past, family, or social history) and complete (for established patients having two of the three areas documented); see **Table 8-2**.

CASE

A 99213 does not have to contain PFSH, but a 99214 visit would expand to cover at least one element of the PFSH, such as one of the following: a mother with type 2 diabetes mellitus, medication review, or use of tobacco or alcohol.

Table 8-2. Established Outpatient Visits

Document two of the three portions at the level billed.

		99211 (Nurse visit)	99212 (PF)	99213 (EPF)	99214 (Detailed)	99215 (Comprehensive)
History		n/a	PF	EPF	Detailed	Comprehensive
	HPI	n/a	Brief: 1-3 elements	Brief: 1-3 elements	Extended: 4+ elements	Extended: 4+ elements
	ROS	n/a	n/a	Pertinent systems	Extended: 2–9 systems	Complete: 10–14` systems
	PFSH	n/a	n/a	n/a	Pertinent: 1 of 3 areas	2 of 3, 3 of 3 areas
PE		n/a	PF	EPF	Detailed	Comprehensive
	97 Guidelines	n/a	1-5 elements	6–11 elements	12+ elements	2 elements from 9 systems
	95 Guidelines	n/a	Limited exam of affected system/ area	Limited affected system + other symptom/ related systems	Ext exam of affected system + other related system(s)	8 or more systems
MDM		n/a	SF	Low	Moderate	High
Approx Time (min)		5	10	15	25	40

PF = problem focused; EPF = expanded problem focused; Hx = history; PE = physical exam; MDM = medical decision making; SF = straightforward.

In summary, there are four levels of billing based on the history component of the visit: problem-focused visit (99212) must contain a brief HPI; an expanded problem-focused visit (99213) must contain a brief HPI and a pertinent ROS, but does not have to contain a PFSH; a detailed visit (99214) must contain an extended HPI (4 or more elements), ROS (2-9 elements), and one PFSH element. A comprehensive visit (99215) must contain an extended HPI, complete ROS (10 or more systems), and documentation of past, family, and social history components (see Table 8-2).

2.   Physical exam: For each level of billing (99212, 99213, etc.) a physical exam is a required element of the visit. The physical exam of the visit may be a general multisystem exam or any single-organ system exam. There are currently two physical exam guidelines that may be used for documentation: the 1995 guidelines and the 1997 guidelines. Both of these are valid; however, the 1995 guidelines are not as detailed and therefore are easier to meet criteria. **Table 8-3** and **Appendix 8-1** provide the specific elements required for the physical exam for both the 1995 and 1997 guidelines.

Table 8-3. Physical Exam Components for Documenting E&M Codes

	Physical Exam		
Level	**97 Guidelines**	**OR**	**95 Guidelines**
99211	n/a		n/a
99212	1–5 elements		Limited exam of affected system/ area
99213	6–11 elements		Limited affected system + other symptom/related systems
99214	12+ elements		Ext exam of affected system + other related system(s)
99215	2 elements from 9 systems		8 or more systems

CASE

For Ms. Honeybee, the physical exam would likely include an assessment of the endocrine and genitourinary systems based on her presenting symptoms and thus easily meet the 1995 guidelines for a 99212 or 99213 visit. Depending on the extent of your workup, the visit could reach a 99214 with additional lab workup, reviewing CV system, vitals, etc. A 99214 visit could be reached based on billing with elements in the HPI and MDM, discussed in the next section.

---

3.   Medical decision making (MDM): Finally, the medical decision-making component is based on the number of diagnostic and/or management options, amount and complexity of data, and risk (**Table 8-4**). Diagnostic and management options can be scored based on a maximum of 4 points in each of five criteria:

Table 8-4. Medical Decision Making Component Requirement for E&M Documentation and Table of Risk Levels

Medical Decision Making Components

Level of MDM	Diagnosis/Mgmt Options (points)	Amount of Data (points)	Overall Risk
Straightforward	0–1	0–1	Minimal
Low	2	2	Low
Moderate	3	3	Moderate
High	4	4	High

Level of Risk	Presenting Problem(s)	Diagnostic Procedure(s) Ordered	Management Options Selected
Minimal	• One self-limited or minor problem, e.g., cold, insect bite, tinea corporis	• Laboratory tests requiring venipuncture • Chest x-rays • EKG/EEG • Urinalysis • Ultrasound, e.g., echocardiography • KOH prep	• Rest • Gargles • Elastic bandages • Superficial dressings
Low	• Two or more self-limited or minor problems • One stable chronic illness, e.g., well-controlled hypertension, non-insulin dependent diabetes, cataract, BPH • Acute uncomplicated illness or injury, e.g., cystitis, allergic rhinitis, simple sprain	• Physiologic tests not under stress, e.g., pulmonary function tests • Noncardiovascular imaging studies with contrast, e.g., barium enema • Superficial needle biopsies • Clinical laboratory tests requiring arterial puncture • Skin biopsies	• Over-the-counter drugs • Minor surgery with no identified risk factors • Physical therapy • Occupational therapy • IV fluids without additives
Moderate	• One or more chronic illnesses with mild exacerbation, progression, or side effects of treatment • Two or more stable chronic illnesses • Undiagnosed new problem with uncertain prognosis, e.g., lump in breast • Acute illness with systemic symptoms, e.g., pyelonephritis, pneumonitis, colitis • Acute complicated injury, e.g., head injury with brief loss of consciousness	• Physiological tests under stress, e.g., cardiac stress test, fetal contraction stress test • Diagnostic endoscopies with no identified risk factors • Deep needle or incisional biopsy • Cardiovascular imaging studies with contrast and no identified risk factors, e.g., arteriogram, cardiac catheterization • Obtain fluid from body cavity, e.g., lumbar puncture, thoracentesis, culdocentesis	• Minor surgery with identified risk factors • Elective major surgery (open, percutaneous, or endoscopic) with no identified risk factors • Prescription drug management • Therapeutic nuclear medicine • IV fluids with additives • Closed treatment of fracture or dislocation without manipulation
High	• One or more chronic illnesses with severe exacerbation, progression, or side effects of treatment • Acute or chronic illnesses or injuries that pose a threat to life or bodily function, e.g., multiple trauma, acute MI, pulmonary embolus, severe respiratory distress, progressive severe rheumatoid arthritis, psychiatric illness with potential threat to self or others, peritonitis, acute renal failure • An abrupt change in neurologic status, e.g., seizure, TIA, weakness, sensory loss	• Cardiovascular imaging studies with contrast with identified risk factors • Cardiac electrophysiological tests • Diagnostic endoscopies with identified risk factors • Discography	• Elective major surgery (open, percutaneous, or endoscopic) with identified risk factors • Emergency major surgery (open, percutaneous, or endoscopic) • Parenteral controlled substances • Drug therapy requiring intensive monitoring for toxicity • Decision not to resuscitate or to deescalate care because of poor prognosis

From: http://www.med.unc.edu/compliance/education-resources-1/RiskTable2.doc

1. self-limited, minor (1 point)

2. established problem stable, improved (1 point)

3. established problem worsening (2 points)

4. new problem, no additional workup planned (3 points)

5. new problem, additional workup planned (4 points)

The amount and complexity of data can be scored on the following: review of clinical lab, radiologic study, or noninvasive diagnostic study (1 point each); discussion of diagnostic study with interpreting physician (1 point); independent review of diagnostic study (2 points); decision to obtain old records or get data from source other than patient (1 point); and review/summarize old medication records or gather data from a source other than the patient (2 points). Risk includes the presenting problem, diagnostic procedures, and management options listed in **Table 8-4**. Selecting the level of MDM would then be based on cumulative scores in 2 of the 3 above areas (Table 8-2, Appendix 8-1). Other areas that should be documented are amount of time spent providing patient counseling, coordination of care, problem severity, and time spent with the patient.[9] If greater than 50% of the visit is spent counseling the patient, one should document the time spent in the visit and note greater than 50% of the face-to-face visit was spent in direct patient counseling. With this notation, time could then be considered the key factor for qualifying the visit for a Current Procedural Terminology (CPT) code.[10]

CASE

For Ms. Honeybee, you would accrue 4 points based on the fact that she presents with a new problem requiring further workup. You will be reviewing clinical labs. The amount and complexity of data includes the review of those clinical labs and would provide 1 point. The overall risk based on Table 8-4 would be moderate, based on prescription drug management. Therefore, the MDM would be moderate and therefore qualify as a 99214 visit when combined with the other required visit elements discussed above.[9]

Special Billing Situations

Another option for pharmacist revenue generation has been through the use of G codes.

There is a separate set of G codes designated for diabetes education for the purpose of teaching patients diabetes self-management and training if you are a certified diabetes educator (CDE). Medicare Part B recognizes CDEs as providers, therefore pharmacists who are CDEs may bill using these codes. Many commercial payers and state Medicaid programs also recognize the CDE codes. These G codes for diabetes education are G0108 for individual visits and G0109 for diabetes education group visits.

These visits are billed and paid in increments of 30 minutes, with indication of the number of 30-minute increments noted on the billing form. For example, if a diabetes group education class lasts for 240 minutes, you would indicate "G0109 x 8" on the billing form. There must be a signed order from the physician stating the number of initial or follow-up hours needed (maximum of 10 hours per year), topics to be covered in training, and whether the patient should receive individual or group visits. The documentation must be maintained in a file that includes the original order and special instructions. When the order is changed, the new order must also be maintained in the file.[11] G codes may be billed in addition to the usual E&M codes if these services are provided in addition to the E&M visit with all the required documentation or alone if those E&M requirements are not met.

In 2005, Medicare began reimbursing for smoking and tobacco use cessation counseling through the use of G codes as well.[12] In July 2009, CMS replaced these counseling G codes with CPT codes and clarified that the services could be provided incident-to the physician by qualified personnel as long as proper documentation was provided. Effective January 1, 2011, in addition to CPT codes 99406 and 99407, two G codes, 0436 and 0437, were created for billing tobacco cessation counseling services to prevent tobacco use in nonsymptomatic patients.

Key Point — Medicare reworded the language to say these services must be "furnished by a qualified physician or other Medicare-recognized practitioner."[13] Therefore, pharmacists are once again not able to bill for these services until they become Medicare-recognized providers.

Another caveat with incident-to billing exists when two providers within the same clinic see a patient on the same day. In this case, two separate bills may not be generated.

CASE

For example, if Ms. Honeybee sees Dr. Busybee today for hypertension and she sees you for diabetes, two bills may not be generated on the same day of service. If two bills are submitted, CMS will default to and reimburse the lesser charge, which could create a significant financial impact on your clinic. However, Dr. Busybee could combine the two services, and instead of billing a problem-focused visit, rather bill for an expanded-problem visit or higher, if between the two sets of notes the two services meet the above criteria for documentation and billing. If a patient was seen in the ophthalmology clinic and the general medicine clinic on the same day, then two bills may be generated because these are two separate clinics.

Currently, only a physician or nurse practitioner can bill by time for Medicare Part B billing. Time cannot be used because the definition of time is "face-to-face time with the *physician*."[14,15] A key point to remember is in the past manual documentation could have gaps in information pertaining to the patient encounter leading to a decrease in reimbursement, many EMRs code and bill the visit based on inputted information and could make the billing process more efficient and thorough.

Charges for pharmacist services using the incident-to model should be billed using the clinic's usual billing mechanism for physician visits, usually performed by designated billing staff. All Medicare outpatient provider visits are documented and filed using a CMS 1500 form, which is the standard claim form used by a noninstitutional or ambulatory care provider or supplier to bill Medicare carriers and durable medical equipment regional carriers (DMERCs). It is typically filed electronically but may also be filed using the paper form found on the CMS web site (www.cms.hhs.gov/cmsforms/downloads/CMS1500805.pdf).[16] The 1500 form is also used by many commercial payers. If filed electronically, there is quicker turnaround for reimbursement, and typically it is the preferred method for clinics to date. (Review a case study and example SOAP note written by a pharmacist after a patient encounter to test your ability to determine the appropriate incident-to code [99211–99215] for the patient encounter based on the documentation provided.) (Anticoagulation E/M Documentation Standards)

Medicare Incident-to Billing or Facility Fee Billing in an Institutional Outpatient Setting

Facility fee billing is another method of billing frequently used by pharmacists for Medicare patients in institutional-based clinics (i.e., hospitals and health systems). This method of billing was created by CMS under the Outpatient Prospective Payment System (OPPS) in August 2000 to standardize the facility fee with an Ambulatory Payment Classification system (APC) based on corresponding CPT codes in cases where the hospital operates the clinic.[17] It was updated in 2010 and is referred to as Hospital Outpatient Prospective Payment System (HOPPS). The major changes in 2010 were supervision requirements (reported in this chapter), quality measurement requirements, and payment for medications and biologicals.[18] CMS states that hospital employees may bill for services, but they do not delineate who the employee is or in what manner the services should be billed.[19] In other words CMS does not state the employee must be a Medicare Part B provider or limit the employee to one level of billing. Facility fee billing is not billing for a professional fee but rather for the use of the facility or technical resources. This type of billing is generally not used by commercial payers. You will need to check the rules for your contracted private payers.

Incident-to billing and E&M codes are used in this setting, and many of the incident-to billing rules need to be followed; that is, the patient must be an established patient (seen within the past 3 years) of the facility in order to obtain care by the pharmacist in this model. The hospital must ensure the services rendered are medically necessary, sufficiently documented, and reflect the level of resources used. The billing is then converted from the incident-to codes to the Ambulatory Payment Codes (APCs), as mentioned above. **Table 8-5** shows how the CPT E&M codes are mapped to the appropriate APC codes.[17]

Table 8-5. Corresponding E&M Codes to Ambulatory Payment Codes

E&M Code	APC Code
99211	604
99212	605
99213	605
99214	606
99215	607

CMS does not provide guidance with tools or instructions on how to calculate charges for the E&M/APC code but rather leaves it up to the individual hospitals. However, CMS does require facilities be compliant with reporting, documenting, and billing for these services. There are existing companies that hospitals can hire to assist them with the creation of "point tools" to determine the level of billing. The point tool is typically a one-sheet document with various assessments, tasks, and education listed in columns, rows, or sections in increasing intensity (**Figure 8-1**). For instance, all the simple tasks, limited number of medications, assessments, and simple education of 1–5 minutes may be listed in the same column that is worth 10 points each (see Figure 8-1). More intermediate tasks, assessments, larger number of medications, and higher involvement of education may be listed in another column, each worth 20 points, etc. Typical point tools will include sections for tasks, assessment, education, and plan. The task section allows nurses to document their contribution to the visit, such as obtaining vitals, assessing pain, or other operations, such as wound care or specimen collection, with more points assigned as the complexity of the task increases. If a task, such as blood pressure check, needs to be repeated, then more points are accrued for each repeated measurement. If medication lists are reviewed, there are typically more points assigned to patients with a large number of medications versus those with few medications, and the point tool may determine that cutoff for assignment of points. Some institutions have procedures such as blood draws charged as a procedure separate from the point tool and therefore it should not count toward the points in the point tool. The assessment section is also based on the complexity of the visit, with a more complicated visit being assigned a higher point value. Also, the more disease states assessed, the more points received. The education component of the visit is based on time spent; time spent in more in-depth counseling receives higher points. Finally, the points associated with the plan of the visit are based on the coordination of care and procedures or education involved. In addition, if physicians are consulted because of the complexity of the visit, then higher points are often assigned to those tasks due to the increased staff and resource time. Once all points have been accounted for in the various areas, a total tabulation of points is performed and assigned to the corresponding level to be billed to the patient. (Facility Fee Point Tool)

THIS HOSPITAL CHARGE FORM FOLLOWS PATIENT UNTIL THE END OF HIS/HER VISIT. 1 FACILTY FEE PER PT/PER CLINIC/PER DAY. CHECK ALL SERVICES PERFORMED BELOW.

Ind #	#	10 POINT VALUE	Ind #	20 POINT VALUE	Ind #	30 POINT VALUE	Ind #	40 POINT VALUE
		Initial Vital Signs (including BP)		ASSESSMENT - SIMPLE		ASSESSMENT - COMPLEX		Adverse Reaction Management: Call MD to discuss and obtains additional orders
		Pain Assessment-Simple- Grade ≤5		Ambulation Assistance		Pain Assessment-Complex-Grade >5 F/U w/ MD		Altered Mental Status
		Repeat Vitals (10 pts for each repeat)		Orthostatic BP (count each REPEAT set)		Additional Nursing Assistance Required		Multidisciplinary Support: Coordinate care with multiple providers during same visit
		Additional BP (10 pts for each repeat)		Specimen Collection: Urine, sputum, etc.		Symptom Management: Simple (does not require call to MD)		Symptom Management: For extreme system(s) not anticipated/ prompts call to MD.
				Evaluate Labs for Tx (labs w/in range)		Evaluate Labs for Tx (lab outside of range-Call MD, document f/u)		
				Medication Order & Administration - PO/PR/Topical (count each 'drug' given, not		Meter/Pump-Download and Coordinate Info		Meter/Pump/Logs-Data Assessment
				Coordinate/Arrange Social Worker/Patient Counselor/ Beacon Counselor				Arrange Interpretation Services (sign language, foreign language)
				Schedule/Coordinate/Counsel Future Tests/Procedures				
				Treatment Plan Simple-1 Disease State		Treatment Plan Complex >1 Disease State		
		Patient Education 1-5 mins		Patient Education 6-10 mins		Patient Education 11-24 mins		Patient Education 25 mins to 1 hour (first hour)
								Patient Education Each ADDITIONAL 30 mins up to 1 hour
		<== Total Column 1		<== Total Column 2		<== Total Column 3		<== Total Column 4
		LEVEL 1 = 0 - 30 POINTS		LEVEL 2 = 40 - 60 POINTS		LEVEL 3 = 70 - 90 POINTS		LEVEL 4 = 100-120 POINTS
		LEVEL 5 = ≥ 130						
Pharmacist Signature:		Date:						

NOTE: For electronic use of this form patient name and identifiers, provider identifiers such as the NPI number, diagnosis codes and supervising physician identification are connected to this charge electronically through a separate screen and/or process. For paper versions of this charge tool, this information is captured on the reverse side.

Figure 8-1. Hospital Facility Fee: Pharmacist Charge Form

CASE

Using the point sheet (Figure 8-1) and the previous case of Ms. Honeybee from earlier, let's work through what a point tool may give us in terms of billing. Let's assume you checked Ms. Honeybee's blood pressure and found it to be 150/90. You then repeated it and found it to be 140/80. You asked her to rate her pain, as this is standard practice in your clinic. You then collect a urine specimen for urinalysis (which ends up being abnormal) and download her home glucose monitor to evaluate her glucose control. The total visit was 30 minutes, and you spent half that time performing patient education regarding elevated blood glucose, glucose control, and infection, and you increase her diabetes medications and hypertension medications. What level would you bill in this facility fee model?

The downside of facility fee billing is the extra financial burden on the patient. A hospital-based clinic typically bills a facility fee for Medicare Part B non-recognized providers who are employed, contracted, or leased by the hospital and a professional plus facility fee for the Medicare Part B recognized providers (physicians, nurse practitioners, or physician assistants) who may be employed, contracted, or leased by the institution. Thus, if the patient is seen by a pharmacist the same day as a physician, the physician would bill a professional fee using E&M codes and a facility fee. A separate facility fee would be billed for the pharmacist or any other non-recognized provider such as a nurse who may have provided patient services during that same visit. In this scenario, the patient would get two bills: a bill for the professional fee for the physician, which is an E&M code (99211-99215) and their facility bill; and a separate facility fee bill that combines the services provided by the nursing staff and the pharmacist in the clinic. This is a common practice and is no different from a patient receiving X-ray services. That patient would have his or her X-ray read by a radiologist and an X-ray technician obtaining the X-ray. The patient receives a provider bill from the radiologist and a hospital bill for services performed by the X-ray technician.

Facility fees may be lumped into the deductibles or the coinsurance with commercial payers and not as part of a flat primary care provider copay, so until the patient meets the deductible, he or she will have to pay 100% of the cost (adjusted per contracts between the payer and the hospital) and then a percentage after the deductible is met. Due to the complexity of this billing process, clinics will often have patients sign a waiver stating they understand part of the visit may not be covered by their insurance and they are responsible for the payment out of pocket. This billing method also makes it difficult to track pharmacist-specific revenue since the nurse and pharmacist are using the same billing form. Some institutions create an identifiable tag or number they can use to track and separate the charges, but they may not have an easy way of identifying reimbursed dollars specific to the pharmacist versus the nurse.

Billing in the facility fee model can follow the usual billing mechanisms of the facility but would be included on a "superbill," which is typically transmitted electronically. However, paper transmission using a CMS-1450 (also known as UB-04 and previously noted as UB-92) form, specific to facility fee billing, may be used. (Go to the web toolkit, and use the same the SOAP note of a patient's visit to determine the appropriate code for the encounter using the facility fee billing.)🖳

Other Items Required for Billing

We have spent a good portion of this chapter describing procedure codes and proper documentation of those procedures for billing. Although they are the most complex and difficult to understand for pharmacists, procedure codes are not the only requirements for successful billing. The following are also needed in the billing process:

1. Patient Identification - This is the patient's insurer ID number (Medicare Part B number, Medicaid number, etc.).

2. Medical Necessity - Services that you provide must be deemed medically necessary. CMS defines medically necessary as: Services or supplies that are proper and needed for the diagnosis or treatment of a medical condition, are provided for the diagnosis, direct care, and treatment of the medical condition, meet the standards of good medical practice in the local area, and are not mainly for the convenience of the patient or the provider (http://www.cms.gov/apps/glossary/default.asp?Letter=M&Language=English<http://www.cms.gov/apps/glossary/default.asp?Letter=M&Language=English>).

3. ICD-9/ICD-10 code - Medicare and most insurers require a diagnosis code using the International Classification of Diseases 9th Revision (ICD-9) for coding diagnoses. As noted in Chapter 5, starting in 2012 with final conversion in October 2013, diagnosis codes will be using the updated and revised ICD-10 classification.

4. Provider Number - Medicare providers (physicians, nurse practitioners, physician assistants, etc.) under Part B have two numbers that are used for billing: the Provider Identification Number (PIN) and the National Provider Identifier (NPI). (Referred to as BPNs in Chapter 5.) The NPI is a nationally assigned alphanumeric identifier unique to each individual provider and is to be used on all administrative and financial transactions. The PIN number identifies the provider and site of service. An individual Medicare provider will have only one unique NPI number but may have several PIN numbers depending on the site of service where they are billing.

   Although pharmacists presently cannot bill directly to Medicare, it is recommended that all health care providers obtain an NPI number. Your organization may require you to obtain this number for internal tracking purposes. Non-Medicare payers may require this number for you to submit a bill. An NPI number can be obtained at https://nppes.cms.hhs.gov/NPPES/StaticForward.do?forward=static.npistart.

Summarizing Billing

Now that we have presented to you all the nuances of incident-to billing, let's see if we can summarize the process for better understanding, using the perspective of your practice site (**Figure 8-2**). If you practice in an independent physician's office

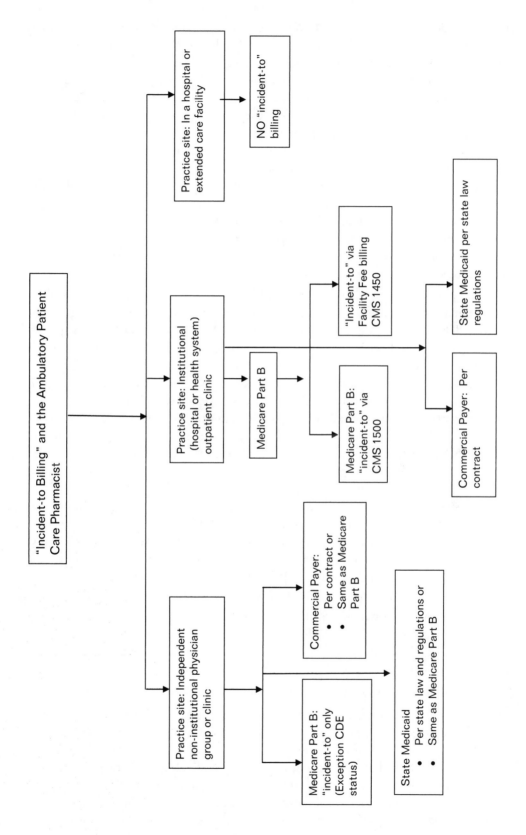

Figure 8-2. "Incident-to Billing" Pharmacist Flow Chart

or clinic, which means you are not connected to an institution in any legal manner, your only avenue for reimbursement under Medicare Part B is incident-to the physician(s) who practice in that office or clinic. For Medicare, you are restricted to billing at the 99211 level, and you must use the electronic or paper 1500 claim form. The one exception is if you also are a CDE, then you may bill Medicare Part B for diabetes education and training using the codes described because CDEs are a recognized Medicare Part B provider. In this setting, if you have contracts with commercial payers or you have a state Medicaid program that recognizes you, the clinical pharmacist, as a provider, then you may bill in whatever manner (some use the MTM codes, which is discussed later) and at whatever level is negotiated in the particular contract or stated in the state regulations. If you do not have a commercial contract or state regulation allowing you to bill differently, most organizations follow the more prudent path of billing commercial payer and state Medicaid as you would Medicare Part B. Most non-Medicare payers use and recognize the Medicare methodology of incident-to E&M codes and the 1500 claim forms.

If you practice in a hospital or health system-based clinic that falls under HOPPS CMS regulations, then you may bill incident-to services in one of two different methods. The first method is exactly like the independent noninstitutional physician office or clinic described in the previous paragraph. The other option is facility billing. As stated under the facility billing section, technically you are not billing your cognitive services but rather the use of the institution's facilities. However, incident-to billing processes are still used because of the requirement for documentation, reporting, assuring medical necessity, supervision, treating an established patient, etc. The incident-to codes are then converted to an APC code and placed on a CMS-1450 claim form for submission to Medicare for reimbursement. Each institution needs to review HOPPS and the two billing options to determine the optimal method for the midlevel providers, such as the clinical pharmacist, practicing in the institution. Like the noninstitutional setting, a hospital or institution may contract with a commercial payer or state Medicaid that recognizes the pharmacist as a provider and bill and reimburse as dictated by the contract or regulations. Again, when no separate contract or state law exists, most organizations will follow the policies and procedures used for Medicare.

As a final note of clarification, incident-to billing methods cannot be used within an institution or the in-patient setting. So if you are providing clinical services in a hospital or in an extended care facility, even if you are under an independent physicians' group not affiliated with the hospital except for admitting privileges, you cannot bill incident-to for any work you perform in that space.

Barriers to Billing for Pharmacist Services

The first barrier to billing for your services is learning all the language as it relates to billing. For example, what is a CPT code, an E&M code, which model of billing do you fall under, and what are all the logistics required for billing in that model? Pharmacists have very limited training in this area and often must learn this on the job. Resources you should use to learn more include talking with your accounting department and having your employer send you and other pharmacists to the billing and coding training all providers go to. Other resources are the Medicare web site (www.cms.gov), the American Medical Association web site (www.ama-assn.org/), or your clinic's ICD-9/ICD-10 CM International Classification of Diseases book.

In addition, billing is an ever-changing topic. Just when you think you have a system of billing for your services, new codes or interpretations by FIs are released. An example of this is for smoking cessation, mentioned earlier, or that patients with stable INRs should not be billed for the visit. Many times you must discuss and negotiate with your institution's compliance and billing departments regarding the need to change. Compliance departments or officers within your practice are helpful resources. These departments are usually present in large institutions and help with internal audits to ensure that health care providers are documenting and billing appropriately. All organizations are subject to external audits from Medicare and other payers to verify billing comliance. A major role of the compliance officer and the compliance or billing department is to ensure the organization or clinic will satisfactorily pass these external audits.

The billing department within your institution can help you find these compliance officers. If you are working in a private physician's office, then the person in your billing office or the clinic manager may be your best contact for ensuring that the required documentation is present for your visits. If they are not knowledgeable, then consider contacting the physician director or performing a literature search on billing documentation. The billing department within your practice should be informed of changes in billing rules and regulations. With anticoagulation, many pharmacists have been able to demonstrate to their compliance departments that monitoring of anticoagulation is a medical necessity and therefore qualifies for reimbursement when appropriate evaluation and documentation supports the billing. Sometimes the assistance and support of physicians in discussion with the compliance personnel can aid your efforts. You may also see that rulings may be written in a manner that can be interpreted in multiple ways. Many times the compliance department will not want to call FIs or Medicare to clarify the ruling as they do not want to raise "red flags" that may lead to audits, investigations, etc. In these circumstances, the compliance department assumes responsibility for the institution and therefore assumes the risk if there were an audit that could unveil problems and therefore incur reimbursement costs. If a compliance department is willing to accept risks, then document according to its recommendations. In addition, written directions from the compliance department regarding its recommendations would be advisable to protect you in the future, if necessary.

The best means of dealing with these billing issues is to establish close relationships with someone in your compliance and billing departments so they serve as a resource to you. If they are aware of your services, they can alert you when changes in your practice area occur. Or when you hear of issues arising with other colleagues across the country, you can call and get their input on the topic and how it may affect you.

Medication Therapy Management

Although the management of medications has been a foundation of the pharmacy profession for years, the term *medication therapy management services (MTMS)* is relatively new. In 2003 the U.S. Congress approved the Medicare Prescription Drug, Improvement and Modernization Act (MMA), which created Medicare Part D.[20] In addition to creating a prescription drug benefit, the MMA also requires insurers to provide MTMS to certain beneficiaries.[20] The MMA identifies three elements of MTMS: education to improve enrollees' understanding of their medications, programs to increase medication adherence, and detection of prescription medication misuse and adverse drug reactions.[21] The legislation specifically states that payment should be provided for MTMS, but does not suggest fee schedules or create a coding mechanism to be used.[21] Interestingly, the MMA does not require that MTMS services be provided by a pharmacist, but rather services must be developed in cooperation with licensed pharmacists and physicians and provided by pharmacists or other qualified providers. Of note, Medicare Part D plans must submit a MTMS program description each spring to CMS for approval. "Positive changes" are allowed to be submitted midcycle if they are in the best interest of the Medicare beneficiary or reflect MTMS best practices. More information on MTMS can be found at the CMS website, http://www.cms.gov/PrescriptionDrugCovContra/082_MTM.asp#TopOfPage.

As the MMA definition of MTMS is relatively vague, multiple pharmacist organizations developed their own definitions of the term. In an attempt to unify the profession, the Pharmacy Stakeholders Conference on MTMS was held in 2004 to develop a consensus on the definition of MTMS.[22,23] A total of 11 pharmacy organizations were involved in the process. The development of a more detailed consensus definition of MTMS was an important step in the creation of Current Procedural Terminology (CPT) codes to be used in billing for MTMS provided by a pharmacist. See **Tables 8-6** and **8-7**.

Overview of Codes

The MTMS CPT codes first appeared in 2005 as Category III (emerging technologies). The codes were changed to Category I (permanent) in CPT 2008.

Key Point

Important items to note when using the MTMS codes include the following: services must be provided by a pharmacist, visits with patients must be face-to-face, and documentation of visits should specifically include the length of the visit in addition to other clinically relevant information to justify the codes utilized.[24]

One important clarification regarding the codes is the medical billing definition of an established patient. An established patient is a patient that has received professional services (face-to-face) within the last 3 years from a provider or by another provider of the same specialty within the same clinical group.[24] For example, if two clinical pharmacists work in a diabetes management clinic, and a patient who routinely sees pharmacist A makes an appointment with pharmacist B, pharmacist B would consider the patient to be established even if they have never met. Thus the pharmacist would code the encounter using the established patient codes.

Although the creation of the MTMS CPT codes was a step forward for pharmacists, their existence does not guarantee payment for services. Currently, the CMS

Table 8-6. Summary of MTMS Consensus Definition and Practice Recommendations[17,18]

MTMS Component	Key Recommendations
Patient care	1. Performing or obtaining necessary assessments of the patient's health status
	2. Formulating a medication treatment plan
	3. Selecting, initiating, modifying, or administering medication therapy
	4. Monitoring and evaluating the patient's response to therapy, including safety and effectiveness
	5. Performing a comprehensive medication review to identify, resolve, and prevent medication-related problems, including adverse drug events
	6. Documenting the care delivered and communicating essential information to the patient's primary care providers
	7. Providing verbal education and training designed to enhance patient understanding and appropriate use of his or her medications
	8. Providing information, support services, and resources designed to enhance patient adherence with his or her therapeutic regimens
	9. Coordinating and integrating medication therapy management services within the broader health care management services being provided to the patient
Practice management	1. High-risk patient identification: multiple chronic diseases, multiple drugs, high costs
	2. Patient recruitment: outreach to patients, caregivers, and physicians
	3. Qualifications of the MTMS provider: pharmacist as primary provider, eligibility of all pharmacists, need for exploration of credentialing
	4. Quality assurance: need to develop MTMS outcome measures and document outcome improvements
	5. Preference for face-to-face patient interactions

Table 8-7. CPT codes for Medication Therapy Management by Pharmacist[19]

Code	Definition
99605	Medication therapy management service(s) provided by a pharmacist, individual, face-to-face with patient, with assessment and intervention if provided; initial 15 minutes, new patient
99606	Initial 15 minutes, established patient
99607	Each additional 15 minutes (List separately in addition to code for primary service) (Code first 99605, 99606)

has not assigned a monetary value to these codes, and most private insurances will not reimburse for the codes either.[24] Thus, contractual agreements between the MTMS provider and the patients' insurance or the patients themselves must be negotiated in order to obtain reimbursement.

Barriers to Successful Use of the MTMS CPT Codes

The largest barrier to using the MTMS CPT codes is lack of universal reimbursement for the codes. This has led many pharmacists who are currently charging for services using the incident-to or facility fee models to avoid these codes as a viable alternative. Tremendous effort must be put into negotiating contracts with payers in order to obtain reimbursement with the MTMS codes. Often, pharmacists have little experience and/or training in how to approach potential payers. Frequently, payers are not interested in contractual agreements for payment because Medicare does not currently reimburse the MTMS CPT codes. Additionally, many payers do not care to negotiate with pharmacists because they are not eligible to be credentialed as providers in the payers' health plans. One possible way to get around this barrier is to credential the physical pharmacy as the provider of health services. If a pharmacy processes insurance for prescription drug claims, then it is credentialed with those prescription plans. When considering providing MTMS for Medicare patients under Medicare Part D, this may be a very viable billing option, although contractual payment schedules may still need to be negotiated. Unfortunately, not all pharmacists work in a pharmacy, and therefore this option is not a good fit for everyone. Finally, it is important to remember that the MTMS codes cannot be used in addition to the incident-to or facility fee models. Therefore, if you have used the incident-to or facility fee models in the past and switch to the MTMS codes without successful payment negotiation, your revenue generation may decrease to zero.

Community-based Nature of Codes

Even though reimbursement with the MTMS CPT codes is not universal or easily obtained, there are many examples of successful MTMS practices available. Many of these are state Medicaid demonstration projects, community pharmacies that have successfully negotiated with Medicare Part D plans, or employer-based disease state management programs.[25] You can find links to more information regarding successful practice models using the MTMS CPT codes in the web resource section of this chapter. Once again, you can review the SOAP note of the pharmacist visit on the web to determine the appropriate way to code the encounter using the MTMS codes.

Employer-based Reimbursement

In an effort to cap rising health care costs, some businesses have collaborated with pharmacists in creative ways to improve patient outcomes. A pharmacist participating in this type of employer-based reimbursement model, typically an employer-sponsored wellness program, contracts with an employer to provide specific services for payment. Services can vary widely from immunization clinics to chronic disease management. Sometimes you provide the service on-site at the business involved. Other times, the business employees come to you. All aspects of the service are negotiated between the pharmacist and employer, such as number of employee visits allowed and length of visit, type of pharmacist service provided and where the visit will occur, payment schedule, what information will be reported back to the employer for outcomes measurement, and which employees will be eligible for the service.

Most commonly, businesses that participate in these types of programs are self-insured employers. You will find that these types of businesses are the most approachable when you are trying to create an employer-based reimbursement situation because they have more control over what services their health plan allows and are more acutely aware of the rising health care costs for the members covered in their health plan. Additionally, the people who make the decisions regarding the health plan are usually local. This gives you greater access to key decision makers for the health plan and a greater chance at successfully negotiating a contract.

Approaching Potential Employers

When approaching a potential employer group, you should be well versed in recent medical literature that shows the benefit of the employer-based wellness program model. The Asheville Project, one of the most widely recognized and replicated models of this kind, has published outcomes data on diabetes, asthma, hypertension, and dyslipidemia management, all demonstrating the ability of the pharmacist to decrease health care costs.[26-28] Additionally, it is beneficial for you to obtain certain health plan information, such as number of covered lives in the plan, number of members with high-cost chronic diseases (e.g., diabetes, dyslipidemia, COPD, heart failure), average health care costs per member per year, and average health care costs per member per year for patients with certain high-cost chronic diseases. Discussion of these costs with the employer allows the estimation (based on outcomes from current medical literature) of how much money the employer could save by partnering with you. For example, diabetes outcomes from the Asheville Project showed a mean direct medical cost decrease of $1,200–$1,872 per member per year.[26] If a given employer had 100 members with diabetes and each member had an average of $5,000 in mean direct medical costs per year (total cost = $500,000), then implementation of the pharmacist-provided wellness program could decrease employer mean direct medical costs to $3,128–$3,800 per member per year for patients with diabetes (total cost = $312,800–$380,000). This would demonstrate a potential cost savings on average of $120,000–$187,200 in direct medical costs per year for patients with diabetes if all members participated in the program. The cost savings information should be shared within the context that as health care costs continue to rise, the pharmacist-provided wellness program will cause health care costs to decrease in this subset of patients. This may be one of your most powerful talking points to share when beginning negotiations with an employer, especially if the subset of patients identified is the most costly on the health plan.

Wellness Incentives

One of the hallmark features of employer-based reimbursement programs is the use of wellness incentives to encourage employees to participate in the program. In the Asheville Project diabetes model, for example, patients who enroll in the disease management program are able to receive all of their diabetes-related medications and testing supplies at no cost.[26] In contrast, patients in the Asheville Project hypertension and dyslipidemia model receive reduced copays on blood pressure and cholesterol medications in exchange for program participation.[28] Another program, the Hickory Project, used both copay reduction and waivers as incentive for patient participation.[29] Although this may appear to be an unnecessary cost, and at times a hard sell to a potential employer group, incentives have proven to be quite powerful in patient recruitment and retention.

CASE

Ms. Honeybee has been amazed at the attention she has received from you and how well her sugars are doing with your help. She is so pleased that at her quarterly appointment with Dr. Busybee she raves about you and says she wishes she could share you with some of her co-workers who are struggling with diabetes. Dr. Busybee sees money signs and approaches you after she leaves to suggest you approach Ms. Honeybee's employer, Big Town Exterminators, to investigate if they would be interested in contracting with the practice to manage their employees' diabetes. As he walks away you wonder, "How am I going to make this happen?"

Barriers to Successful Implementation of the Employer-Based Reimbursement Model

One barrier to implementing an employer-based reimbursement model is identification of employers interested in partnering with you. Again, self-insured employers are generally the businesses that are most receptive to this model. Small business coalitions, city or county governments, and local health systems are often great places for you to start identifying potential partners. Unfortunately, getting human resources representatives from these organizations to return your calls is sometimes difficult. It is important to clearly explain what you would like to discuss with the employer and, if possible, meet with owners and leaders within the company to find a champion. At the first meeting, be sure to present data from nationally recognized programs such as the Asheville Project to demonstrate the value and cost savings that you are offering the employer. Also highlight data regarding decreased employee sick days and increased productivity in addition to cost savings for the health plan. If your first meeting is successful, next steps may include obtaining employer-specific health plan data to determine the best services to provide and cost savings that may be expected. These data are best obtained by meeting with the employer's third-party administrator in addition to human resource representatives familiar with the health plan. A second barrier is the contract negotiation itself. Employers often have a difficult time spending money up-front to pay for pharmacist time and employee incentives in order to save money 3–5 years down the road. Placing emphasis on the cost savings to come and being reasonable in what is expected for pharmacist reimbursement and employee incentives can help your negotiation be successful.

Self-Pay Patients

When considering the various models of charging for pharmacist services, most of the emphasis is typically placed on how to obtain reimbursement from insurance or other payers. Many times the uninsured or self-pay patients are simply forgotten. Depending on the demographics of the community where your service is located, it may be important to consider self-pay patients. The reason for this is twofold. First, many self-pay patients would benefit greatly from pharmacist services, but due to inability to pay, may chose to not participate. Second, self-pay patients may choose to participate, but due to inability to pay end up having bills sent to collections. The collections process can be a major contributor to lost time and money for a pharmacy. An easy solution to this problem is the creation of a sliding fee scale for uninsured patients.

CASE

Unfortunately, Big Town Exterminators was not interested in partnering with your practice. After a few months, it became apparent why . . . they filed for bankruptcy, leaving Ms. Honeybee without a job and health care benefits. She presents today crying, saying she can no longer afford two "docs" all the time so she has made the decision to see Dr. Busybee only in extreme emergencies. You realize all the success you and she have achieved could be compromised if she does not seek care on a routine basis. After some discussion with your office manager, you start researching some options for Ms. Honeybee.

Sliding Fee Scales

To create a sliding fee scale, you will need the following items: current federal poverty income guidelines (available at http://aspe.hhs.gov/poverty/09extension.shtml) and the pharmacist service's fee schedule for codes that would otherwise be submitted to insurance. The federal poverty income guidelines are a useful resource to ensure the sliding fee scale is applied fairly to all patients, and there are clear definitions as to why an individual patient is receiving a particular discounted charge. In addition to adjusting charges based on the poverty level, you should consider a graduated system for discounting charges for patients who are near (e.g., 150% or 200%) but not at the poverty level. Thus, a tiered charge system can be created based on the pharmacist service's fee schedule and the federal poverty guideline income requirements. (UWFM SFS as an Example)

Finally, it may be useful for you to create an intake form to use with all uninsured patients to document patient income and qualification for the sliding fee scale. Note that it is not necessary to have proof of income when using a sliding fee scale. Therefore, institutional policy will dictate whether patient report is sufficient to qualify for discounted charges. (UWFM Intake Form) Institutional policy will also dictate how often a patient should reapply for sliding fee scale eligibility as well as any payment plan arrangements.

Barriers to Reimbursement with Self-Pay Patients

The balance between providing needed patient care services and obtaining adequate reimbursement is the largest issue regarding self-pay patients. If your service has a high number of uninsured or underinsured patients, it may be prudent to seek out government or grant monies that can be used to offset expenses when caring for this population.

Other Methods and Models

Financial sustainability and growth is possible despite full provider status recognition. Pharmacists have used various vehicles to create funding for their practices, allowing them to expand services. Some of these reimbursement opportunities include the use of relative value units (RVU), participating in studies, demonstration projects, and pay-for-performance projects that can help to create partnership with local, state, and national organizations.[30,31]

Relative Value Units

In order to fully understand reimbursement for health care services, you should also examine the Medicare Resource-Based Relative Value Scale (RBRVS). The RBRVS is a physician reimbursement model created as a standardized method of analyzing resources involved in the provision of health care services or procedures.[32] In this model, three factors are considered: physician work, which encompasses the complexity and difficulty of the patient seen or procedure performed; practice expense; and liability insurance.[33] These factors are considered, and then a RVU is created and assigned to each CPT code. A RVU is a nonmonetary, relative unit of measure that indicates the value of health care services and resources consumed when providing different procedures and services.[33] RVUs vary across the United States as they are adjusted based on geographic location using the geographic practice cost indexes or GPCI (referred to as "gypsies" in billing and coding circles). Once the RVU for a certain service is determined, it is multiplied by the Medicare current year conversion factor to be converted into a dollar payment amount.[34] Although CMS developed the RBRVS, the American Medical Association makes recommendations to CMS for RVU value assignment.

Pharmacists who charge for their services using CPT codes already see the effects of the RBRVS in their practices. For example, the Medicare payment associated with the use of the code 99211 in a physician's office-based clinic would be determined by multiplying the geographically adjusted RVU for this code by the Medicare current year conversion factor. This explains why a pharmacist practicing in North Carolina would receive a different reimbursement from a pharmacist practicing in Wyoming, even though they may perform a similar service and use the same billing code. The CMS web site is a useful tool for looking up RVUs for specific codes as well as finding out the Medicare payment for particular codes

based on geographic location and type of institution (see http://www.cms.hhs.gov/
PFSLookup/). Additionally, the American Medical Association web site is an excellent resource for learning more about the RBRVS (http://www.ama-assn.org/ama/
home/index.shtml).

It is important to note that the medication therapy management codes (99605–
99607) previously discussed in this chapter do not have RVUs assigned to them.
RVU assignment would be a beneficial step in obtaining reimbursement for these
codes because the value of health care services and resources used when providing the service described by the codes would be more apparent to payers. This
may allow for more successful negotiations for payment or standard payment because payers are already familiar with the RBRVS. Finally, the RBRVS system is an
imperfect one because pharmacists must bill the 99211 code for all Medicare
patients. This decreases reimbursement as well as RVU credit that pharmacists
may receive for a potentially complex patient visit. You are curious about the
RVU and Medicare reimbursement in your area. Using the CMS web site listed
above, determine the Medicare rate and RVU for your geographic area associated
with the incident-to code that you felt was most appropriate for the patient encounter found on the web. Compare this to the Medicare rate and RVU associated with the code 99211.

Patient-Centered Medical Home

An emerging concept in the delivery of primary care is the patient-centered medical home (PCMH). Increasingly, you may find yourself providing services as one
part of the PCMH team. In 2007, the Patient Centered Primary Care Collaborative
(PCPCC) issued a statement of principles describing the characteristics of the PCMH.
One of these principles is payment for services (see http://www.pcpcc.net/content/
joint-principles-patient-centered-medical-home). Currently, there is no standard
way for providers (including both physicians and pharmacists) to charge for services as part of a PCMH. Models range from continued use of fee-for-service and
incident-to methods to a medical practice receiving a lump sum based on the number of patients with certain disease states (capitated payment system). You should
be aware of the PCMH concept and look for ways to be reimbursed for the value
you add to this interdisciplinary team care concept.

Developing Partnerships with Schools of Pharmacy

Partnerships with academic organizations may serve as a key ingredient to help
organizations maintain sustainable practices. With more than 100 schools of pharmacy in the United States, there are opportunities to collaborate with schools of
pharmacy by providing faculty practice sites and experiential sites for the increasing numbers of students enrolling in these programs. Relationships such as these
can be mutually beneficial because funding for the faculty position could be negotiated so that the academic institution pays for a portion of your salary. Various
examples of successful practices have integrated faculty in clinical care opportunities, resulting in exciting opportunities for both the practitioners and students to
gain invaluable experience by using community partners.[35] One such example of

this is occurring with the University of Arizona College of Pharmacy and El Rio Health Center partnership.

In the University of Arizona College of Pharmacy strategic plan for 2009 to 2013, they note one of their goals is to develop the health care system of the future through interprofessional collaboration on research, education, and patient care. Because El Rio Health Center has similar goals, a partnership was developed to create a faculty position to expand direct patient care services at the center using matching funds, all while creating research and rotation opportunities for students in collaborative care ambulatory practice.

Grants for Research

Linking academia and local knowledge can also lead to opportunities for funding. By tapping into academia, such as by contacting local school of pharmacy professors or by creating practice sites that offer potential research populations, you can and should explore opportunities to pursue. For example, current funding opportunities at the National Institutes of Health (NIH) include community-based participatory research on health promotion, disease prevention, and health disparities jointly conducted by communities and researchers to target medically underserved areas and medically underserved populations. Because of the nature of the request for proposals, it is imperative that you be involved in research partnerships with academic institutions, health agencies, and communities to create relationships that can enhance research, population outcomes, and funding opportunities to show the value you can have on a multidisciplinary team.[36]

Grants from Donors

Seeking funding from foundations, corporations, local businesses, government, individuals, families, and estates can offer another source of revenue for successful practices. One of the key strategies for you to access these resources is to document outcomes and market your services and successes with these groups to engage them into the practice. These opportunities can be sought only if you work to partner and build relationships.

Grant donors give money for a number of reasons:

1. They care enough about a particular issue or issues that they want to get involved.
2. They have the financial capacity and ability to donate.
3. They want to contribute to the community.
4. There may be a financial benefit to corporations or other for-profit entities that donate grants, expertise, or items in kind.
5. They have personal experience or interest in the areas being addressed.
6. Governments, including federal, state, counties, and tribes, that offer grants may be directing federal grant dollars into their jurisdiction to the benefit of their community. Government may also be aware of a specific problem uniquely plaguing their community and may allocate some of their own local budget to fight this problem (such as diabetes, asthma, etc.).

7. Health care reform and the Accountable Care Act have allocated grant money to study a number of initiatives where pharmacists and MTM services fit well into the specifications of the grants available. Much of this funding is through the Agency for Healthcare Quality and Research (AHRQ) (see http://www.ahrq.gov/).

Ultimately, those who donate grant money do so because they appreciate the work and may want to get involved. Donors want to see their donation and efforts affect outcomes in the community. Donors may want to establish successful partners in the community for future projects. If you keep in mind why your grant donor is involved, the partnership will help you both benefit your community.[37]

Grant money can often be the seed money needed to create or expand pharmacy services. By maximizing these funding opportunities and documenting the value of the services being delivered, it will allow for longitudinal reporting of outcomes. This strategy can be used to seek funding for an employer-based reimbursement program, a demonstration project such as a pay-for-performance plan with a payer, or direct contracts from third-party payers. Additionally, donors would appreciate knowing their initial contribution was used to create a sustainable service that will continue to impact the community in a positive way. This kind of reputation in itself creates capital for other potential donors.

Demonstration Projects

Pharmacy demonstration projects can be an excellent opportunity to show the impact and value of your interventions, all while generating revenue. Several examples have been documented in the literature, including the Pharmacy Quality Alliance (PQA), the Diabetes Ten City Challenge, and Health Resources and Services Administration's (HRSA's) Clinical Pharmacy Demonstration Projects.

In the PQA project, the mission was to improve the quality of medication use across health care settings through a collaborative process in which key stakeholders agree on a strategy for measuring and reporting performance information related to medications.[38] Several of these demonstration projects have become available in recent years in which pharmacists can participate. By becoming involved in these types of efforts, a source of revenue can be established, but more importantly, involvement can lead to improved patient care and data that can be used to negotiate with payers.

In the Diabetes Ten City Challenge, the American Pharmacists Association Foundation, along with support from GlaxoSmithKline, collaborated to establish a pharmacist intervention to improve care in patients with diabetes, a program modeled after the Asheville Project of North Carolina. The benefit to pharmacists, aside from improving patient care, was that reimbursement was negotiated with the employers to cover these services for their employees.[39]

Finally, in the Department of Health and Human Services HRSA, $1 million became available for clinical pharmacy demonstration projects during fiscal year 2000. The goal of this project was to demonstrate how access to needed pharmaceuticals, when delivered as a part of comprehensive pharmacy services, makes a substantial and affordable contribution to improving the health status of the patient population, and that such a service should become a standard component of health delivery systems.[40]

These unique opportunities are just a small sampling of previous and current opportunities pharmacists have participated in, and continue to participate in, every day. They highlight various models of reimbursement, including employer-based reimbursement, grants, and research.

Barriers to Other Reimbursement Models

The most common barrier in identifying alternate models for reimbursement is the time factor. Partnerships with schools or pharmacies, research, grants, and demonstration projects require constant cultivations of relationships and dialogue, and it might sometimes feel like a full-time position along with the requirements of the actual practice. Furthermore, these models might lead to initial funding but not to sustainable methods of maintaining a practice by themselves. However, it may be what you need to get started. Measuring your outcomes and your value, as described in Chapter 7, will be critical to achieving sustainability.

Chapter Summary

Pharmacists have made significant inroads in creating opportunities to generate revenue to fund their practices. Despite these inroads, continued efforts need to be made for the profession to be recognized as a vital partner in health care delivery. Pharmacists must document their outcomes, market their results, and create partnerships with patients, other health professionals, and the communities they serve.

References

1. Rochester CD, Leon N, Dombrowski R, et al. Collaborative drug therapy management for initiating and adjusting insulin therapy in patients with type 2 diabetes mellitus. *J Am Health-Syst Pharm.* 2010;57:42-48.

2. O'Brien DM. How nurse practitioners obtained provider status: Lessons for pharmacists. *J Am Health-Syst Pharm.* 2003;60:2301-2307.

3. Cantwell HM, Kwong MM. Achieving provider recognition. *J Am Health-Syst Pharm.* 2001;58:973.

4. Medicare Benefit Policy Manual. Chapter 15—Covered Medical and Other Health Services. http://www.cms.hhs.gov/manuals/Downloads/bp102c15.pdf. Accessed January 21, 2010.

5. HCFA clarifies "incident-to" billing by pharmacists. *Am J Health-Syst Pharm.* 2000;57:1557-1558.

6. Snella KA, Trewyn RR, Hansen LB, et al. Pharmacist compensation for cognitive services: focus on the physician office and community pharmacy. *Pharmacotherapy.* 2004;24(3):372-388.

7. Gosfield AG. The ins and outs of "incident to" reimbursement. *Fam Pract Manag.* 2001;(Nov/Dec):23-27.

8. University of North Carolina School of Medicine Compliance Office. Powerpoint presentation for Detailed E&M Coding Course. http://www.med.unc.edu/compliance/education-resources-1/refresher%20course%20detailed.ppt#273,14, Review of Systems (ROS). Accessed January 19, 2010.

9. University of North Carolina School of Medicine Compliance Office. Table of Risk. http://www.med.unc.edu/compliance/education-resources-1/RiskTable2.doc. Accessed January 19, 2010.

10. Kuo GM, Buckley TE, Fitzsimmons DS, et al. Collaborative drug therapy management services and reimbursement in a family medicine clinic. *Am J Health-Syst Pharm.* 2004;61:343-354.

11. CMS Medicare Preventative Services, Medical Learning Network. *Training Medicare Patients on Use of Home Glucose Monitors and Related Billing Information.* http://www.cms.gov/MLNMattersArticles/downloads/SE0905.pdf. Accessed May 20, 2010.

12. CMS Medicare Preventative Services, Medicare Learning Network. Information for Medicare Providers. Smoking and tobacco-use cessation counseling. *MLN Matters.* http://www.cms.hhs.gov/MLNMattersArticles/downloads/MM3834.pdf. Accessed October 28, 2005 and January 25, 2010.

13. CMS Medicare Preventative Services, Medical Learning Network. Counseling to prevent tobacco use. *MLN Matters.* http://www.cms.gov/MLNMattersArticles/downloads/MM7133.pdf. Accessed March 5, 2011.

14. Centers for Disease Control and Prevention. Rules and regulations. *Fed Regist.* 2005;70:4541.

15. U.S. Department of Health and Human Services. Centers for Medicare and Medicaid. http://www.cms.hhs.gov/home/medicare.asp. Accessed August 7, 2010.

16. Centers for Medicare and Medicaid. 1500 Health Insurance Claim Form. www.cms.hhs.gov/cmsforms/downloads/CMS1500805.pdf. Accessed January 19, 2010.

17. Nutescu E. Controversies for Billing for Clinical Services. http://www.ashp.org/DocLibrary/MemberCenter/SHACCP/Anticoag_Controversies_Billing.pdf. Accessed January 25, 2010.

18. Centers for Medicare and Medicaid Services. 42 CFR Parts 410, 416, 419. Medicare Program: Changes to the Hospital Outpatient Prospective Payment System and CY 2010 Payment Rates; Changes to the Ambulatory Surgical Center Payment System and CY 2010 Payment Rates; Final Rule. *Fed Reg.* Friday, November 20, 2009; 60315–61012.

19. Centers for Medicare and Medicaid Services. Is it appropriate for a hospital to bill a visit code under the Outpatient Prospective Payment System (OPPS) for care provided to a registered outpatient if the patient was not seen by a physician? http://questions.cms.hhs.gov/app/answers/detail/a_id/8810. Accessed October 16, 2008; January 29, 2010; October 22, 2010.

20. Summary of HR 1 Medicare Prescription Drug Improvement, and Modernization Act of 2003, Public Law 108-173. http://www.cms.hhs.gov/MMAUpdate/downloads/PL108-173summary.pdf. Accessed January 24, 2009.

21. HR 1 Medicare Prescription Drug Improvement, and Modernization Act of 2003, Public Law 108-173.http://frwebgate.access.gpo.gov/cgibin/getdoc.cgi?dbname=108_cong_public_laws&docid=f:publ173.108.pdf. Accessed January 24, 2009.

22. Bluml BM. Definition of medication therapy management: Development of professionwide consensus. *J Am Pharm Assoc.* 2005;45:566-572.

23. Anonymous. Summary of the executive sessions on medication therapy management. *Am J Health-Syst Pharm.* 2005;62:585-592.

24. Gabbert W, Kachur K, Tameka L, et al., eds. *Current Procedural Coding Expert* 2009. Minnetonka, MN: Ingenix; 2008.

25. Pellegrino AN, Martin MT, Tilton JJ, et al. Medication therapy management services definitions and outcomes. *Drugs.* 2009;69(4):393-406.

26. Cranor CW, Bunting BA, Christensen DB. The Asheville Project: Long-term clinical and economic outcomes of a community pharmacy diabetes care program. *J Am Pharm Assoc.* 2003;43:173-184.

27. Bunting BA, Cranor CW. The Asheville Project: Long-term clinical and economic outcomes of a community-based medication therapy management program for asthma. *J Am Pharm Assoc.* 2006;46:133-147.

28. Bunting BA, Smith BH, Sutherland SE. The Asheville Project: Clinical and economic outcomes of a community-based long-term medication therapy management program for hypertension and dyslipidemia. *J Am Pharm Assoc.* 2008;48:23-31.

29. Lee GC, Mick T, Lam T. The Hickory Project builds on the Asheville Project—An example of community-based diabetes care management. *J Managed Care Pharm.* 2007;13(6):531-533.

30. Felt-Lisk S, Sorenson T, Glenn Z, et al. Report to HRSA: *Opportunities to Advance Clinical Pharmacy Services in Safety-Net Settings.* Washington, DC: Mathematica Policy Research, Inc.; January 2008.

31. Felt-Lisk S, Harris L, Lee M, et al. *Evaluation of HRSA's Clinical Pharmacy Demonstration Projects: Final Report.* Washington, DC: Mathematica Policy Research, Inc.; 2004.

32. American Medical Association. The Resource-Based Relative Value Scale. http://www.ama-assn.org/ama/no-index/physician-resources/16391.shtml. Accessed January 25, 2010.

33. American Medical Association. Overview of the RBRVS. http://www.ama-assn.org/ama/pub/physician-resources/solutions-managing-your-practice/coding-billing-insurance/medicare/the-resource-based-relative-value-scale/overview-of-rbrvs.shtml. Accessed January 23, 2010.

34. American Medical Association. The Medicare Physician Payment Schedule. http://www.ama-assn.org/ama/pub/physician-resources/solutions-managing-your-practice/coding-billing-insurance/medicare/the-medicare-physician-payment-schedule.shtml. Accessed January 23, 2010.

35. Connor SE, Snyder ME, Snyder ZJ, et al. Provision of clinical pharmacy services in two safety net provider settings. *Pharm. Prac.* (Internet) 2009; Apr-Jun 7(2):94-99.

36. Viswanathan M, Ammerman A, Eng E, et al. *Community-Based Participatory Research: Assessing the Evidence.* Evidence Report/Technology Assessment No. 99 (Prepared by RTI—University of North Carolina Evidence-Based Practice Center under Contract No. 290-02-0016). AHRQ Publication 04-E022-2. Rockville, MD: Agency for Healthcare Research and Quality; July 2004.

37. Specter A. Why Do Donors Give Grants At All? *Seeking Grant Money Today.* October 2006. http://thegrantplant.blogspot.com/2006/10/why-do-donors-give-grants-at-all.html. Accessed January 22, 2010.

38. The Pharmacist's Role in Quality: A PQA Demonstration Project. Slide presentation from the AHRQ 2009 Annual Conference (text version). December 2009. Agency for Healthcare Research and Quality, Rockville, MD. http://www.ahrq.gov/about/annualconf09/conklin.htm. Accessed January 23, 2010.

39. Wokchik J. Diabetes pilot program yields big cost savings. *Business Insurance.* Available at: http://www.businessinsurance.com/article/20090412/ISSUE01/100027458. Accessed January 29, 2010.

40. $1M Approved by HRSA for clinical pharmacy demonstration grants. *Medscape Medical News.* http://www.medscape.com/viewarticle/411857. Accessed January 29, 2010.

Additional Selected References

Barr MS. The patient centered medical home: Aligning payment to accelerate construction. *Med Care Res Rev.* 2010;67(4):492-499.

Centers for Medicare and Medicaid Services. Form CMS-1500 At a Glance. www.cms.hhs.gov/MLNProducts/downloads/form_CMS-1500_fact_sheet.pdf. Accessed January 19, 2010.

Gosfield AG. The ins and outs of "incident-to" reimbursement: If you work with nonphysician providers, you can't afford to ignore these rules. *Fam Pract Mgmt.* 2001;8(10).

Heidelbaugh JJ, Riley M, Habetler JM. 10 Billing & coding tips to boost your reimbursement: Keep more of what you earn by avoiding these costly coding missteps. *J Fam Pract.* 2008;57(11):724-730. www.jfponline.com.

Hill E. Understanding when to use 99211. *Fam Pract Manag.* 2004; Jun11(6):32-34. www.aafp.org/fpm.

International Classification of Diseases, 9th Rev., Clinical Modification (ICD 9 CM). Washington, DC: CMS; 2010.

Kuo GM, Buckley TE, Fitzsimmons DS, et al. Collaborative drug therapeutic management services and reimbursement in a family medicine clinic. *Am J Health-Syst Pharm.* 2004; 61:343-354.

Snella KA, Trewyn RR, Hansen LB, et al. Pharmacist compensation for cognitive services: Focus on the physician office and community pharmacy. *Pharmacotherapy.* 2004;24(3):372-388.

Web Resources

Coding Reference Card Outpatient

Pharmacists' Specific Facility Fee Point Sheet

Sliding Fee Scale

Patient Intake Form

SOAP Note/Patient Case

Trinity Anticoagulation E/M Documentation Standards

Web Toolkit available at
www.ashp.org/ambulatorypractice

Appendix 8-1: Coding Reference Card Outpatient

Documentation of Outpatient/Office Visit Evaluation & Management Codes

Est. Pt.	New / Consult	HPI	ROS	PFSH	= History Level	Physical Exam 97 Gdelnes	Physical Exam OR 95 Guidelines	Phys Exam	Medical Decision (MDM)	Approx Time Est / New / Con
The Chief Complaint is										
99211 (Nurse Visit)		NA	NA	NA		NA	NA		NA	5 supv.
99212	99201	Brief (1-3)	NA	NA	Problem Focused	1-5 elements	limited exam of affected system or area	PF	I	10 / 10 / 15
99213	99202	Brief (1-3)	Pertinent	NA	Expanded PF	6-11 elements	limit. affected sys. + other symptom/related systems	EPF	Low/Straightfrwd	15 / 20 / 30
99214	99203	Extended (4+)	Extended (2-9)	Pertinent (1 of 3)	Detailed	12+ elements	ext. exam of affected system+other related sys	D	Moderate/Low	25 / 30 / 40
99215	99204	Extended (4+)	Complete (10-14)	2 of 3 / 3 of 3	Comprehensive	2 elements from 9 systems	8 or more systems	C	High/Moderate	40 / 45 / 60
X	99205	Extended (4+)	Complete (10-14)	Complete (3 of 3)	Comprehensive	2 elements from 9 systems	8 or more systems	C	High	X / 60 / 80

2 of 3 areas: History, Exam, MDM

3 of 3 areas

HPI: Review of 3 or more chronic diseases satisfies for Extended

ROS: May use "all others negative" once pertinent pos & neg documented

PFSH: 1) Past 2) Family 3) Social

Physical Exam Types: Problem Focused (PF) Expanded Problem Focused (EPF) Detailed (D) Comprehensive (C)

If >50% of encounter is counseling, record entire amount of time for encounter, document substance of discussion, bill corresponding level

Appendix 8-1: Coding Reference Card Outpatient (cont'd)

HPI elements:
- location
- quality
- severity
- duration
- timing
- context
- modifying factors
- assoc signs & symptoms

ROS systems:
Constitutional symptoms (e.g., fever, weight loss)
Eyes
Ears, Nose, Mouth, Throat
Cardiovascular
Respiratory
Gastrointestinal
Genitourinary
Musculoskeletal
Integumentary (skin and/or breast)
Neurological
Psychiatric
Endocrine
Hematologic/Lymphatic
Allergic/Immunologic

Past History
Current medications
Prior illnesses/injuries
Dietary status
Operations/hospitalizations
Allergies and/or immunizations

Family History
Health status/cause of death of parent, sibling, children
Diseases related to complaint
Hereditary or high risk diseases

Social History
Living arrangements
Marital status
Sexual history
Occupation, history or current
Use of drugs, tobacco, alcohol
Education
Other

95 Physical Exam Systems / Body areas

Organ Systems:
Constitutional
Eyes
Ears nose mouth throat
Cardiovascular
Respiratory
Gastrointestinal
Genitourinary
Musculoskeletal
Skin
Neurologic
Psychiatric
Hema./lymphatic/immun

Body Areas:
Head (incl. face)
Chest
Abdomen
Genitalia, groin, buttocks
Back, incl. Spine
Each extremity

'97 Physical Exam:

General Multi-system Exam
or

Single organ system exam:
Cardiovascular
Ears, Nose, Mouth and Throat
Eyes
Genitourinary
Hematologic/Lymph/Immun.
Musculoskeletal
Neurological
Psychiatric
Respiratory
Skin

Amount and complexity of data (max=4):
Review/order of 1)clinical lab 2)radiologic study 3)non-invasive diag study (1 for ea type max)
Discuss diag study w/interpreting phys. (1)
Independent review of diagnostic study (2)
Decision to get old records/dta from other source (1)
Summarize old med records or gather data fr source other than pt (2)

Diagnostic and/or management options (max=4):
Self-limited, minor (1 ea)
Est problem stable, improved (1 ea)
Est. prob. worsening (2 ea)
New problem, no add'l workup planned (3 ea)
New problem, add'l workup planned (4 ea)

Risk: (See Table of Risk)
Presenting problem
Diagnostic procedure
Management options

Selecting the level of MDM:

Diag./Mgmnt. options	0-1	2	3	4
Amt./complexity of data	0-1	2	3	4
Overall risk	Minimal	Low	Mod.	High
Type of MDM	Strghtfwd	Low	Mod.	High

(Choose level met in 2 of 3 areas)

Inpatient E&M code documentation guidelines

Level	History	Exam	Decision	Time
Initial hospital / Observation				
1	Detailed	Detailed	Straightfrwd/Low	30 / X
2	Comprehensive	Comprehensive	Moderate	50 / X
3	Comprehensive	Comprehensive	High	70 / X
Subsequent hospital visits / Follow up inpatient consults				
1	Problem focused	Problem focused	Straightfrwd/Low	15 / 10
2	Expanded PF	Expanded PF	Moderate	25 / 20
3	Detailed	Detailed	High	35 / 30

Maximizing Your Ambulatory Practice: Planning for the Future

Stuart T. Haines, Jill S. Borchert

CHAPTER
9

Chapter Outline

1. Introduction
2. Planning for Growth
3. Contributing to Our Knowledge
4. Training Future Ambulatory Care Pharmacy Practitioners
5. Anticipating Changes in Health Care Delivery and Financing
6. Keeping Up with Changes
7. Chapter Summary
8. References
9. Additional Selected Resources
10. Web Resources

 Web Toolkit available at
www.ashp.org/ambulatorypractice

Chapter Objectives

1. Develop a plan for growth for your clinical services by analyzing the demand and need for services.

2. Contribute to practice-based research to expand knowledge regarding ambulatory care pharmacy practice.

3. Create an environment conducive to training future ambulatory care pharmacy practitioners, including postgraduate year 1 and postgraduate year 2 residents.

4. Anticipate changes in health care delivery and financing that may impact ambulatory care pharmacy practice.

Introduction

Building a successful ambulatory care practice requires more than a personal commitment to helping patients achieve optimal health outcomes. It requires a long-term vision and a strategic plan. You'll soon discover (if you haven't already) that the medication-related needs of the patients in your practice are far more than you or even a small team of ambulatory care pharmacists can handle. Once the value of your services has been firmly established, you'll likely become overwhelmed by the patient volume, and you'll find new medication-related problems that need attention. And just when you think you've got it all figured out, things will change. No one can predict the future, but you can be certain that the world around you won't remain stagnant. New medications and technologies will bring new challenges. And the need for your services will grow and shift over time. Changes in health care financing may lead to a major transformation in the health care system as monetary incentives encourage health systems to adopt new methods, engage in new activities, and set new priorities. And there will be a continual need for new knowledge and understanding as we uncover new problems and attempt to find new solutions.

In this chapter we explore how to maximize your practice by

- growing and expanding your services,
- contributing to our knowledge,
- training the next generation of ambulatory care specialists,
- anticipating the future, and
- planning strategically for long-term success (**Figure 9-1**).

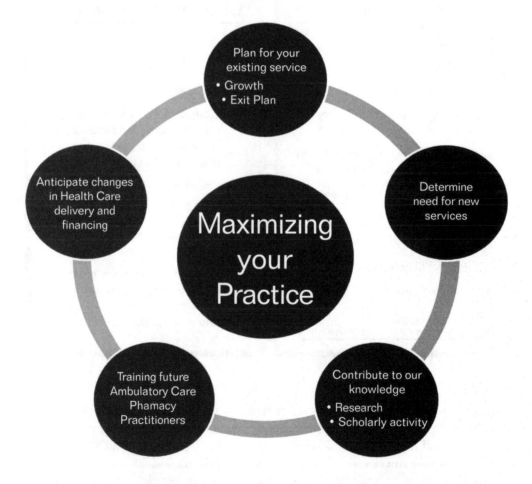

Figure 9-1. Maximizing Your Practice

Planning for Growth

CASE

You are now a board-certified ambulatory care pharmacist and have been working for Dr. Busybee for 3 years. The pharmacotherapy consult service you created initially to manage diabetes and anticoagulation patients is growing rapidly. You are now working at the clinic 5 days a week. Initially, referrals to the pharmacotherapy consult service came from Dr. Busybee, but soon word spread among the other providers regarding the availability and success of your service. In fact the referrals are now expanding to hypertension and dyslipidemia, as your work with diabetic patients has demonstrated your ability to assist with medication management of these conditions. Your growth has been fast, and you are struggling to meet the demands of the new, more complex patient health concerns. The following table illustrates the growth of the service and the change in its case mix.

36 Months Ago	24 Months Ago	12 Months Ago	Now
Total number of patient encounters (per month):			
200	325	400	550
New referrals (per month):			
37	71	80	99

INDICATIONS FOR REFERRAL

Anticoagulation

VTE prophylaxis (Ortho):			
20	59	72	70
Atrial fibrillation:			
15	50	82	90
VTE treatment:			
30	42	49	73
Prosthetic heart valve:			
3	6	14	32

Medication Management

Diabetes:			
2	8	15	20
Hypertension:			
0	0	5	10
Dyslipidemia:			
0	0	3	8

VTE = venous thromboembolism

With the growth and expansion of your service, you have updated your collaborative practice agreement to include hypertension and dyslipidemia. Additionally, the physicians are requesting your assistance in medication reconciliation for all patients seen in the office who were recently discharged from a hospital or extended care facility. Despite the growth, the majority of your practice still remains anticoagulation management. However, an increasing number of patients are being initiated or converted to the new oral anticoagulants for atrial fibrillation and postoperative orthopedic procedures. You have a sense that anticoagulation referrals seem to be declining, and there is more and more interest in your assistance with patients with other disease states. You have the following issues and concerns:

•   New oral anticoagulation therapies will change patient management and monitoring requirements. Dr. Busybee and his partners are interested in converting appropriate patients to the new oral anticoagulation medications. Initially, the use of the new oral anticoagulants may be limited by cost and the need to gain experience with the new medications in your population, but you anticipate that they will be prescribed more often over the next year. How should you approach and plan for this anticipated change? Should you ignore, reject, or accept these new drugs?

•   Continued growth of the service is unsustainable. With the increased referrals of more complex non-anticoagulation patients, you are finding you are becoming increasingly busy. You believe that you have reached the clinic's capacity with a single practitioner. You currently have a very limited amount of time for other responsibilities (e.g., administrative tasks). Indeed, you often work late to catch up on paperwork and make phone calls to patients. Moreover, finding coverage during periods of your absence (e.g., vacations, illness, and professional meetings) has become problematic. Although the number of new referrals continues to increase overall, the number of patients with long-term indications for warfarin therapy has decreased slightly. How should you approach and plan for this issue? Should you figure the decrease in patients on warfarin will offset the increase in other patient referrals? In the meantime how do you handle how busy you are? Are you expanding too quickly?

When you establish a new practice, it is certainly rewarding to finally "open" the clinic and begin to provide care for patients. Since provision of patient care was your ultimate goal and may be what most interests you in your job, it may be tempting to consider your task of building a successful practice complete. However, clinicians who fail to maintain their focus on managing the practice may find their practice faltering or exceeding their capacity.

When building your infrastructure, you thought carefully about determining not only the appropriate services to provide but also the resource needs (see Chapter 2). In determining the number of full-time equivalent (FTE) pharmacists needed to establish the service, you considered several factors, including the number of hours per day and days per week the service would be available, the predicted patient volume, the distribution of face-to-face patient visits and telephone encounters, and the availability of support staff. As your practice grows, it is important to monitor for changes in your original plan. Has your distribution of face-to-face visits increased over the projected plan? What about the volume of new referrals? For example, you may follow 100 patients, but there is 20% turnover every quarter as patients meeting their treatment goals are discharged and new referrals are accepted. Compared to a stable practice of 100 patients with few new referrals, this means substantially more new patient visits, which are more time consuming. (Updated Resources and Reimbursement Worksheet)

Key Point

Reevaluate your service and resource needs, including patient volume and staffing levels, at regular time intervals.

It is important to set aside some time at regular intervals, quarterly or semiannually, to critically examine the trends and shifts in your practice. This will prevent any gradual creeps in service volume from causing a staffing crisis. The most difficult time to deal with these issues is when you are busy caring for your patients, leaving little time to devote to administrative tasks. Alternatively, early identification of a fall in demand for your services should prompt you to perform a needs assessment and develop new services in areas of need rather than face scrutiny from administration regarding overstaffing. Since you should be reviewing your services on a quarterly or semiannual basis for quality assessment (Chapter 7, Quality Assurance for Ambulatory Patient Care), this is an ideal time to look at the overall needs of the service. Your quality report should contain information on service activity, such as the number of patients and the number of referrals as well as the number and type of patient encounters. Use this as an opportunity to think about what the numbers mean. Has your total patient load increased? What about the nature and type of patient encounters? (Example Measures to Examine Trends in Practice)

In addition to developing a set timeline for evaluating increases and decreases in service demand, it is important to consider your business plan. You should establish benchmark metrics that prompt staffing adjustments. For example, build into your business plan that when you reach 90% of capacity, the criteria and process to hire additional staff will already be established. Allow time for necessary administrative approvals for new positions, recruitment, hiring, and training new members of the team. Depending on the administrative structure at your institution, this may take 6 months or more. If your service is part-time, for example an anticoagulation clinic offered 2 days per week, establish a benchmark for when a third day will be added. Responsibilities of the pharmacist on service will need to be shifted to accommodate the added workload, and ideally this growth should be anticipated. If additional staff are not an option due to resource constraints, consider capping or closing the service at a prespecified number of patients.

You may even be able to anticipate swings in patient-care volume. Take a step back from your practice and think about your health system and changes in the local environment. If a large cardiology group is added to a health system, an antithrombosis clinic may experience a rapid increase in patient volume. If a nurse practitioner is hired by a key endocrinology group to assist in patient management, your diabetes service may experience a decline in referrals. Furthermore, if your health system decides to no longer accept a certain insurance plan and a large number of your patient population happens to have this plan, how will this impact your patient volume?

Not only does the volume of patient care encounters need to be considered in workload planning and resource needs, but non-patient care activities of the ambulatory care specialist must be considered in a growing service. Some of these elements are directly related to the patient care provided. In your original estimation of resource needs, did you adequately account for these elements, or do you find they are taking more time? You may have underestimated the amount of time administrative tasks related to patient care takes, and clinicians cannot be expected to provide direct patient care 40 hours per week. Time needs to be set aside for administrative tasks related to patient care, such as phone calls from patients with clinical concerns, rescheduling patients and contacting patients who do not show for appointments, coordinating care, and documentation. If you find this was not accounted for properly in your original plan, it may be worthwhile to track the time you devote to these ancillary tasks as your practice grows. A 1- to 2-week self-study tracking the number of hours devoted to non-patient care or the number of phone calls may help you get a better estimate of resource needs related to these tasks. This objective information will help you to rework your resource allocation and perhaps help you to justify adjusting clinic hours downward or hiring support staff for administrative tasks. (Tracking Tool for Non-patient Activities)

Key Point Non-patient care related activities must be considered in a growing service.

Since you first estimated your resource needs, the scope of non-patient care services may have shifted in your practice. Successful ambulatory care practices often become training sites for pharmacy students and residents. Leaders in the health care organization may look to a successful ambulatory care practitioner to fulfill key roles on committees within the organization or to serve as an advisor in a specific therapeutic area. For example, a clinician in a diabetes clinic may be asked to provide an assessment of a new drug being considered for inclusion on a formulary or to provide staff in-services. You may be extensively involved in developing quality metrics and reporting for your practice, as outlined in Chapter 7. If you are an ambulatory care pharmacy specialist, consider how your role has changed since the clinical service was developed and the initial needs assessment was outlined. Are you more or less involved in committee work? Do you chair any committees? Have you become involved in student precepting or resident training? Do you serve as a residency program director or teach in the classroom? How much of your time do you devote to quality reporting or scholarly activity? If you are the manager for a group of clinical pharmacy specialists, have your specialists become more engaged in these elements of pharmacy practice?

CASE

You face a common problem: anticipating a change and the growth of a successful but busy practice. You are concerned about the effect the new agents on the market will have on your workload coupled with the new referrals for non-anticoagulation patients and your staffing capacity. At this point you feel frustrated, overworked, overwhelmed, and underappreciated. Like most practitioners you have had little time to plan for future changes because you have been busy developing your practice and providing patient care. However, it is essential and wise that you develop both short-term and long-term plans to address the changes and problems that you face.

Just as you planned for the initiation of the new pharmacy service, any expansion in clinical services needs similar attention to careful planning. The good news is that now you have learned a great deal about the functions of your health care institution, the common barriers, and the factors that contribute to success. You first need to redefine your mission and vision statements to encompass a broader overall goal and guide your actions (Chapter 2, Planning and Steps to Building the Ambulatory Practice Model). Then, revisit your needs assessment. Were there other needs identified but not initially selected when you started your service? If so, gather the benchmark data again and perform a new SWOT analysis. In your daily practice, you may routinely be approached by other health care professionals to assist with drug therapy management in a particular area or with perceived pharmacotherapy needs. Lastly, during the quality improvement activities in which you have been involved, you may have identified gaps between institutional performance and goals. These are great areas in which to gather data to plan for growth. Essentially, you will need to revisit each of the steps in defining the service and building the practice and business model. This time, in developing of the model, consider how to sustain your current practice as you redefine resource needs and structure. This may also be a perfect opportunity to modify your existing services. For example, you can build in resource requests for ancillary staff or pharmacists for cross-coverage as discussed for a growing service. At this point, what are your short- and long-term solutions?

Short-Term Solutions

Ancillary Staff

In the short term, you can consider ways to maximize the use of current personnel to meet current needs. As you consider shifting your practice away from anticoagulation management, it may be possible to have the nursing staff provide point-of-care testing or vital signs for each visit as they take the vitals for each patient. This would allow you more time in another exam room where you may be conducting patient visits for hypertension or hyperlipidemia. Also, this is a good time to brainstorm to see if there are other administrative tasks with which nursing or office staff can assist. You are already using them to perform scheduling and medication refill tasks; review your daily workload; and be creative about what you can delegate.

Closing to New Referrals or Referring Back Patients

While closing to new referrals is always a difficult decision, you have to also consider that the quality of care that you provide may be impacted by a hurried clinician. As always, you need to consider what is best for the patient and your organization. A well-controlled anticoagulation patient could be managed by the physician or the nurse. Your value to patients and the organization may be in care of the more complex patient, that is, multiple medications or comorbidities. The physician and nurse may be able to handle stable patients without much added stress to their service, which would then allow you to provide the quality of care you need to give to the remainder of your patients. In essence, you could "close referrals" to a sub-set of patients and "refer back" a sub-set of patients. Trying to do it all may not be in the best interest of the patients you see or your organization. Even a 10% decrease in patient load may give you enough time to regroup. You can remain the provider's backup for those patients who develop new problems or who become more complex.

Redistribution of Responsibilities

In the short term, you may want to brainstorm what other types of non-patient care activities occupy your time. Do you serve on any committees within the organization or provide educational in-services to staff? If so, can these responsibilities be delegated as you work to improve your practice model? When you first initiated your practice 3 years ago, you probably did not have the level of commitments that you do today. You may have to reallocate your time even though you receive professional fulfillment and growth by being involved in committees and professional organizations. By taking a step back, you will be in a better position once your practice finds its new equilibrium.

Long-Term Plan

Cross-Training Pharmacists

This is a good time to address your problem of providing coverage for vacation and professional meetings so that your patients have uninterrupted care.

CASE

You approach Dr. Busybee about cross-training another pharmacist to manage patients in your absence and help you on certain, particularly busy days. You explain under your state's CDTM that you can assign an alternative pharmacist to work with the collaborating physician. As you look to change the scope and type of patients you care for, this may be the perfect time to integrate and cross-train a new pharmacist. Dr. Busybee agrees to this, but only if the pharmacist has the appropriate training and background (Chapter 7).

Adding Pharmacists

Another option to consider is the addition of a pharmacist as a new hire. You will need to reevaluate your resource and expense needs as it relates to your workload changes resulting from the new anticoagulation medications, medication reconciliation activities, and the increased patient referrals for medication management beyond diabetes (Chapters 2 and 3). An assessment of anticipated patient numbers for each service group and a reworked analysis (Chapter 3) will prepare you for the work-flow change that you are experiencing. The result of the reanalysis may indeed demonstrate a need for increased staffing levels. As an alternative, you can also consider a proposal to hire a temporary ambulatory care specialist until the future of the service is better defined.

Develop a Monitoring Plan

From here you should develop a plan to evaluate the service at regular intervals. This may coincide with quarterly or semiannual quality reports to streamline data collection. This will prevent any future surprises of dramatic shifts in workload and inform you so that you can *anticipate* needs instead of respond to changes. Establish milestones at which additional staff resources will be considered to expand services. Similarly, you will need to establish an exit plan should changes in pharmacotherapy or changes in the needs and priority of the practice occur. Use these regular time intervals to think about changes in your health system that may impact your ambulatory care practice.

Whether trying to sustain a service, grow a service, or expand into new therapeutic areas, you will find that all require careful planning and continual monitoring. The needs of your patients and the institution, changes in the environment, staffing, and finances all need to be constantly considered as you continue to build and revise your practice and business model.

Contributing to Our Knowledge

Undoubtedly, as you approached building an ambulatory care practice, you came across questions for which little information was available to guide you. Perhaps you wished that there was a published report of a successful diabetes care clinic in an institution similar to yours. You may have wished there was a better description of

how to overcome barriers that you encountered. Or, administrators may have requested more robust information documenting the value of pharmacist involvement
in patient care. The future of ambulatory care practice in part will be shaped by
descriptions of practice models and outcomes associated with these services. All
ambulatory care specialists have the capacity to contribute to this body of knowledge.

There are many elements of practice that you already do that can contribute to
our knowledge of ambulatory care practice. For example, the quality initiatives that
you developed and track likely yield a wealth of information that document the
value of pharmacy services (Chapter 7, Quality Assurance for Ambulatory Patient
Care). Documentation of the economic value of services may help to provide further evidence of the value of clinical pharmacy services in multiple health care
environments.[1,2] Unique cases encountered in practice can become case reports to
assist other clinicians provide optimal patient care, spark new research, or identify
new adverse reactions or drug interactions.[3] You should conduct a thorough review
of published literature to ensure it has not already been reported before investing a
significant investment of time and effort.[4]

For projects that you will be sharing with an outside audience, an institutional
review board (IRB) must review all of your research to minimize the risks to human
subjects posed by the research.[5] These risks are not limited to the use of investigational drugs. Survey research and case reports must be reviewed to ensure that the
identity and health information of subjects are protected. While data you collected
for your internal quality purposes does not require IRB oversight, if you decide you
want to share these data with an outside audience through a poster presentation or
publication, it will require IRB review. If your own institution does not have its own
IRB, you can find an IRB who will review your proposal for a fee. Ask physicians
involved in research at your institution if they have any experience with an IRB. Or,
you can ask local universities with health care programs if they allow external applications to their IRB. You can learn more about human subject protection and complete free online training in protecting human research participants through the
National Institute of Health Office of Extramural Research (http://
phrp.nihtraining.com). A primer on the role, function, and operation of the IRB,
informed consent, and criteria for review and approval will also be helpful.[5]

CASE

You are 6 months into the expansion of your practice, and it is going well.
The physicians understood your concerns and approved the hiring of an
additional pharmacist. You worked with them and the office team to
incorporate a number of creative work-flow changes during the interim.
You realize that by establishing a short-term and long-term plan and by
thinking through the process as a team you have created a successful
transition. Others may benefit from your story.

After you have worked on a project, there are a number of venues in which to share your work. Your local pharmacy organizations likely have poster sessions in conjunction with their meetings, and perhaps they have a local or statewide journal. National organizations have similar opportunities and often have "clinical pharmacy forum" or similarly titled poster session that will allow you to share the development, justification, or documentation of your unique clinical pharmacy service. Pharmacy journals have opportunities to present short pieces, including letters or notes, to highlight your service or unique observations. Lastly, do not forget about medical meetings and journals. It may be better to share your findings with primary care physicians or other health care professionals in your specialty. This could be through publication or presentation at local or national meetings. For example, sharing the success of a clinical pharmacy service with local physicians at a local meeting of a chapter of the American College of Physicians or American Academy of Family Physicians might be a great way to network with area physicians.

Another way to get involved is to contribute to a practice-based research network (PBRN).[6] A PBRN is a group of clinicians or clinical practice sites that provide patient care and network together to investigate real-world questions to understand and enhance the quality of care. Since PBRNs comprise clinicians from the community and not from a single academic medical center, PBRNs are uniquely suited to provide information that is externally relevant and applicable to day-to-day practice. PBRNs focus on investigating issues related to primary care, making them particularly suited for ambulatory care specialists.[7,8] PBRNs can be used to test interventions intended to improve the quality of medication therapy management and patient management processes. For example, one PBRN investigated the effect of physician and pharmacist collaboration on blood pressure control in hypertension.[9] (ACCP Web Site)

One of the challenges that ambulatory care pharmacists face is a lack of large, multicentered studies documenting the clinical and economic value of ambulatory care clinical pharmacy services.[6] You can contribute by becoming involved in a PBRN. A common misconception is that you must have an extensive research background to become involved. Since a PBRN is a network of both researchers and clinicians, each individual has a different role to play. The study design and data evaluation is typically performed by clinician-researchers, but a PBRN needs lots of clinicians who provide direct day-to-day patient care to be involved with these research projects. Pharmacy organizations are beginning PBRNs that may be of interest to you. For example, the American College of Clinical Pharmacy now has a national PBRN with participants from all practice settings (http://www.accpri.org/pbrn/).

Training Future Ambulatory Care Pharmacy Practitioners

To ensure the future of ambulatory care pharmacy, we need highly skilled clinicians to provide patient care and to expand the frontiers of clinical pharmacy.

And we will need a lot more of them—particularly in ambulatory care. One analysis conducted by the Pharmacy Manpower Project estimated that 165,000 primary (ambulatory) care pharmacists will be needed by 2020.[10] These pharmacists will be involved in direct patient-care activities, including medication management and patient assessment, not just prescription order fulfillment.[11] The vision of the profession as illustrated by the PPMI is that by 2020 residency training will be a prerequisite to enter these direct patient care roles in which pharmacists assume responsibility for managing drug therapy.[12-14] To achieve this vision, a 17% annual growth rate in residency training is needed.[15] To make the vision a reality, we all need to contribute to training future practitioners. The profession needs more residency-trained pharmacists, particularly pharmacists with training in ambulatory care, to be ready for the enhanced patient care responsibilities in an aging patient population with many chronic comorbidities.

CASE

Two years ago a nearby pharmacy school asked if you would precept pharmacy students. At the time, you were petrified; however, to date, you have acted as a preceptor for more than 10 students, and the experience has been gratifying. Dr. Busybee has noted the value of the students and would like you to increase the number rotating at the site. You agree because you see the possibility of recruiting new pharmacists needed for growth from this pool. Because you helped educate the students, they have worked at the practice and know the electronic medical record and work flow. Precepting enables you to identify candidates to join your pharmacotherapy practice model, which allows you to encourage those students to seek out a Postgraduate Year One residency for further training.

A first step toward the goal of becoming involved in residency training often starts by precepting pharmacy students in your practice. If you are not yet involved as a preceptor, contact your local college or school of pharmacy to indicate your interest. Get involved in the school's preceptor training programs and start by developing your rotation goals, objectives, and activities. A new preceptor should supervise only one student at a time, but consider precepting four to six students over the course of the year to build your experience. After you've been precepting students for 3 to 5 years, the next logical step is to become involved as a Postgraduate Year One (PGY1) pharmacy residency preceptor. If your practice site is part of health system, you may be asked to be a PGY1 pharmacy preceptor fairly early on. However, if your practice is not part of a large health system, you can become involved in PGY1 residency training through an affiliation agreement with a hospital, health system, or college/school of pharmacy in your area. Eventually, you may wish to become a PGY1 residency program director (RPD). As your practice develops into providing care for ambulatory care patients with complex diseases in multiple specialty areas, consider developing a Postgraduate Year Two (PGY2) pharmacy residency program. The value of providing residency training includes the personal satisfaction of giving back to the profession, plus a well-structured residency program can help you to expand services and enhance revenue generation.[4,16] Just as you developed a business plan for your pharmacy service, a well-designed residency program and budget will include expenses as well as direct and indirect revenues. Extensive resources are available from the American Society of Health-System Pharmacists to assist you in designing the program and formulating a business plan. As you become involved in training students and residents, remember to set aside time for teaching and residency program administration when planning workload. While serving as a preceptor, mentor, or RPD is professionally rewarding and serves the needs of the profession, providing high-quality training takes time.

Anticipating Changes in Health Care Delivery and Financing

Change is inevitable. For most of us, change is frightening because we feel as though we have little control over what's happening and we can't predict the outcome. In the book *Who Moved My Cheese*, Dr. Spencer Johnson uses a parable to examine how people and organizations deal with change.[17] In the story, four characters live in a maze and look for cheese to nourish them and make them happy. "Cheese" represents all the things that humans need and want in life: food, shelter, relationships, health, money, recognition, and possessions. And the maze is the environment around us: the organizations where we work, the communities where we live, and our families. As the story unfolds, the characters face an unanticipated change, and one character deals with this change more successfully than the others. The message is a simple one. Choosing to adapt when change occurs, and it will occur, leads to a richer and more fulfilling life.

Key Point
Learning to anticipate and adapt to change is a critical skill you'll need to develop to maximize your practice.

So what changes should you be anticipating in the years to come? We believe that changes are likely to occur in three broad areas: technical advances, health care reform and financing, and practice models.

Technical advances will come in many forms. New medications, especially new products that are significantly more effective, safer, and convenient to use, are the fundamental tools of our trade. Our professional lives are built on the premise that we are best prepared to help people use these tools in the wisest and most cost-effective manner possible. Occasionally, new medications will come along that will profoundly change what we do.[18,19] What if a new medication became available that no longer required coagulation testing or dose adjustments as noted in our case example? As readers of this book well know, this is not a hypothetical proposition; oral anticoagulant medications are now available that do not require routine coagulation status monitoring, are prescribed in fixed doses, and have fewer drug interactions. The introduction of these new agents *will* result in changes in prescribing patterns. And the pace of this change might be slow and gradual, or it might be sudden and cataclysmic.

CASE

You and Dr. Busybee have three choices when you realize your practice model needs to evolve:

Option 1: Ignore it. You can continue to conduct business as usual and turn a blind eye to the inevitable reduction in warfarin use that will occur. Eventually, the need for warfarin-monitoring services will dwindle along with the need to employ knowledgeable people. By ignoring the new technology, its use—when, how, and how often—is determined by others, and the fate of the anticoagulation management services will be decided by external forces.

Option 2: Resist. Don't let others decide your fate. Fight back. You can engage in a well-orchestrated campaign to thwart the use of these alternative agents, thus preventing the demise of warfarin. Block its inclusion on the formulary. Point out the potential dangers of using these agents. Highlight the lack of data and experience with these new drugs. Use scare tactics with patients and prescribers. As knowledgeable and respected experts, you will undoubtedly find receptive ears, and these strategies will work, at least in the short run.

Option 3: Adapt. Embrace the new technology and plan to engage in new activities. The *fundamental mission* of the anticoagulation management service, helping people use anticoagulation therapies wisely and in the most cost-effective manner possible, won't change. However, what we do to accomplish our mission should, will, and must change over time. This is the opportunity to expand your scope of service. There are plenty of therapeutic areas for which you can help patients use their medications wisely and cost-effectively. The process of adaptation will require using the same tools discussed throughout this book. Conduct a needs assessment, perform a SWOT analysis, consult with peers, experiment with new models of care, collect data, and disseminate your findings.

 Adaptation requires planning. Conduct a needs assessment, perform a SWOT analysis, consult with peers, experiment with new models of care, collect data, and disseminate your findings.

Technological advances won't be limited to the introduction of new drug therapies. New technologies will undoubtedly include new monitoring devices, new communication mediums, new data storage and retrieval systems, new medication delivery systems, and new practice models.[19] The indiscriminant use and automatic adoption of new technologies and models of care is costly and, all too frequently, results in little benefit in terms of outcomes or efficiency. On the other hand, resisting the use of all new technologies or models of care simply because they require changes in practice habits will deny patients access to truly worthwhile advances.

In addition to considering adding another pharmacist to your clinic, the team convenes to discuss how to use technology to the advantage of the practice. The anticoagulation monitoring services you created initially could be completely reconfigured using new technologies and rethinking what functions the pharmacist performs. The fundamental elements of warfarin management— a structured system of patient follow-up, accurate and readily available coagulation testing equipment, and a person knowledgeable about warfarin management—can be accomplished through patient self-management. Web-based health records and communication systems can be used to provide a structured system for ongoing patient follow-up. INR monitors can be used at home to provide patients (and clinicians) with accurate and timely information about the patient's anticoagulation status. And while we may believe that pharmacists are the only people knowledgeable enough to effectively collect and assess patient-specific data, make appropriate dose adjustments, anticipate problems, and coordinate care, there is ample evidence that most patients can handle these tasks after they've had some training and guided practice.[20] Patient self-management would require a major restructuring of what the pharmacists do in this model of care. Whether such a model is "better" than seeing patients face-to-face or calling them on the phone to discuss their test results is certainly open to debate. Considering this type of change allows more time to for the expanded services you are now providing. The fundamental point is that new technologies require us to rethink what we do. Evaluating, adopting (when appropriate), and using new technologies wisely is among our primary responsibilities.

New technologies are scary enough, but what about health care reform?[21] The financing of health care has a very substantial impact on how we practice by providing (and in some cases, failing to provide) monetary incentives to engage in specific activities.[22] If the state of Montana started paying pharmacists $500 to collect a comprehensive medication history at the time of admission to a hospital, we could anticipate the following:

- The pharmacy department would reorganize its work flow so that pharmacists could spend *a lot* more time gathering comprehensive medication histories.

- Hospitals would hire more pharmacists so that a comprehensive medication history could be collected from *every* patient.

- Training sessions on how to code and bill for comprehensive medication histories would be conducted.

- Patients would be admitted to hospitals more often, transferred between sister hospitals more frequently, and discharged more rapidly to be readmitted again.

- More people in Montana would apply to pharmacy school, the college of pharmacy would be pressured to increase enrollment, and more pharmacists would move to Montana.

The example is a bit far-fetched, but the concepts are simple. The financing of health care provides strong incentives to behave in specific ways.

 Health care reform efforts will likely have an enormous impact on what pharmacists in ambulatory care practice do.

The health care delivery system in the United States is essentially a cottage industry characterized by dedicated craftsmen and craftswomen who value autonomy, who disdain standardization, and whose efforts are poorly coordinated.[23] Such behavior is encouraged and inadvertently rewarded in most settings by the incentives built into our health care financing structures. According to the Kaiser Family Foundation's Annual Employer Health Benefits Survey, the average private health insurance premium was $4,825 for an individual and $13,375 for a family in 2009.[24] If these numbers aren't alarming enough, the Centers for Medicare and Medicaid Services (CMS) report that the U.S. national health expenditures were $2.3 trillion in 2008, or $7,681 per person, and accounted for 16.2% of gross domestic product (GDP). This amount is expected to grow to nearly 20% of GDP in 2019. This amount far exceeds the health care expenditures of all other developed nations. According to LECG, LLC, a global consulting firm that provides advisory services to large multinational corporations and local, state, and national governments, there are five megatrends in health care financing:[25]

- There will be continual shift from employer-based to federally provided coverage.

- Per unit reimbursement for health care products and services will decline.

- Health information technology will mature rapidly.

- Standardization of the health care industry will be led by the federal government.

- Providers will focus on efficiency improvements before they address quality-of-care improvements.

The implications, according to LCG, are that

[a]s health plans experience pressure to increase provider payments there will be increasing interest in more effectively managing medical care costs with specific emphasis on managing chronic care costs. As higher prevalence of diseases needing chronic care increase the volume of services, health insurers will need to manage volume as they address higher prices. Chronic care management may be the best way to affect volume

although current approaches need to be reviewed and evaluated for their efficacy. At the same time, government efforts at effectiveness measurement will identify new opportunities to standardize chronic care protocols.[25]

CASE

Dr. Busybee has just returned from an American Academy of Family Physicians meeting where he attended a session that discussed the patient-centered medical home model and Accountable Care Organizations. He had heard of this previously, but now it seems there could be financial gain from implementing this type of model within his practice. Based on the success you have had managing his patients, he would like you to be a part of this initiative but is unsure exactly how to differentiate your role and that of the nurse or nurse practitioner in the model. You assure Dr. Busybee there is a role on the team that only a pharmacist can fill. Now you have to use your skills acquired over the past 3 years to outline and show the pharmacy impact within this proposed model.

Health care delivery in the ambulatory care setting will undoubtedly be influenced by the movement to adopt the patient-centered medical home (PCMH) model in most primary care settings as well as the Patient Protection and Affordable Care Act (PPACA) passed by the U.S. Congress and signed by President Obama in April 2010.[26-28] A PCMH is a model of care that focuses on wellness and prevention as well as the management of chronic illness. This model of care is not yet available to most people in the United States but has been positively received by patients and physicians, has achieved better health outcomes, and resulted in lower costs.[29,30] The PPACA provides funding to evaluate elements of the PCMH model and independence at home (IAH) demonstration projects as well as creating accountable care organizations (ACOs).[27] Prior to the passage of the PPACA, several managed organizations and the Veterans Health Administration in the United States had already begun pilot programs examining the feasibility and impact of these models of care.[30] The seven core features of a PCMH include (1) a personal physician, (2) physician-directed medical practice, (3) whole person orientation, (4) care coordination and integration, (5) quality and safety, (6) enhanced access, and (7) payment reform.[28] In a PCMH, the care is directed by the patient's personal physician working collaboratively with a team of individuals who collectively are responsible for the quality, safety, and outcomes of the care provided. While such structures exist in an informal sense now, PCMH makes the relationships between the patient and the health care team members explicit, not implicit. Furthermore, the role of each team member is clearly articulated, not only to enhance the patient's understanding of "who's responsible for what" but also to organize the team's collective effort. Under a PCMH model, the roles and responsibilities of the team members are not confined to traditional professional functions. The care provided in a PCMH is driven by quality and safety; thus, health information systems will be a critical ingredient, providing meaningful data upon which to make informed decisions regarding the performance of the practice in relation to quality benchmarks. Enhanced access to care is another element of the PCMH model. The PCMH is community based and provides high-quality care in rural and underserved urban areas. Lastly, payment reform is a critical ingredient for the success of the PCMH model. The current payment system rewards consumption and use rather than quality and safety. Clinicians and hospitals are in competition to offer new technologies and procedures that garner more revenue, rather than practices that maximize the health of the population they serve. Moreover, the current payment system retrospectively reimburses specific practitioners (e.g., physicians, nurse practitioners) rather than prospectively paying a team of practitioners.

The experiences with Family Health Teams (FHT) in Ontario, Canada, and the medical home model in Group Health Cooperative of Seattle, Washington, demonstrate the potential benefits of the PCMH practice model.[29,30] Not only has patient satisfaction improved substantially, but also physician satisfaction has increased and clinician burnout has decreased.[29,30] Compared to other clinics within their system, the Group Health Cooperative has demonstrated that patients experience fewer hospitalizations and fewer emergency visits. Moreover, implementation of the model appears to save money.[30] A clinical pharmacist is an integral member of most FHTs in Ontario, and they play a key leadership role with regard to managing patients on complex, high-risk medications as well as monitoring medication use patterns, educating prescribers, and analyzing quality data. Similarly, in the Group Health Cooperative there is one pharmacist for every 10,000 patients to provide expanded care and manage medication therapy as part of the team. Clearly, ambulatory care pharmacy specialists can and should play key roles in the PCMH, but whether such a model will become the norm in the United States remains to be seen.

Keeping Up with Changes

Keeping up with new technologies, changes in health care delivery, and health reform is a major challenge.[31] Membership in professional organizations has been a time-honored method of keeping abreast of what's happening. In addition to face-to-face programming at local, regional, and national meetings, many professional organizations connect members to one another through list-servs, bulletin boards, and other interactive web-based communication tools. This is a great way to get alerts about what people are seeing and talking about in the field. However, belonging to professional organizations and attending meetings is no longer enough. You'll need to set aside time (e.g., weekly) and use information management resources to help you keep abreast of what's happening in ambulatory care pharmacy practice and chronic disease statement management.[31] Subscriptions to online resources that review and summarize the latest findings in the professional literature can be extremely helpful. Examples of resources the ambulatory care pharmacist might find most useful include the following: The Pharmacist's Letter (http://pharmacistsletter.therapeuticresearch.com/); JournalWatch (http://www.jwatch.org/);

Evidence-Based Medicine (EBM) for Primary Care and Internal Medicine (http://ebm.bmj.com/); and Medscape (http://www.medscape.com/). Really Simple Syndication (RSS) feed readers, such as Google Reader, FeedDemon, and NewzCrawler, are free services that can help you organize information and alleviate the amount of work involved in its management. Electronic tables of contents (eTOC) are available from most peer-reviewed journals, and most of these can be sent automatically to your RSS feed reader or e-mail. (Examples of eTOCs)

Staying current is crucial for your professional future as well as your responsibility. Recently, ASHP initiated a discussion on where health-system pharmacy practice should be by 2020. From their efforts, a new pharmacy practice model initiative was created with the goal of creating a framework to unify the profession with regard to how pharmacists provide patient care, how technicians are involved to support the pharmacists' role, and the use of automation and technology in the medication use system. A summit of pharmacy leaders drawn from across the country yielded 147 points of consensus about optimal pharmacy practice models in hospitals and health systems. These items were categorized according to major sections of the summit proceedings (Table 9-1). The recommendations constitute consensus advice and vision regarding how to create sustainable pharmacy practice models.

Table 9-1. Pharmacy Practice Model Initiative

Overarching Principles
- There is an opportunity to advance the health and well-being of patients by changing the practice model.
- Financial pressures will force changes in how resources are used.
- Every pharmacy department should identify drug therapy management services provided consistently by pharmacists.
- Investments in technology will be required to fully achieve optimal deployment of pharmacy resources.

Services
- Pharmacy practices play a critical role in medication-related national quality indicators and evidence-based practice guidelines.
- Pharmacy practices track and trend adverse drug events and treatment failures.
- Pharmacy practices manage prospective and retrospective medication use evaluation programs.
- Pharmacy practices track and trend pharmacist interventions.
- Essential elements of a pharmacy practice model can be developed for use in all hospital and health-system departments of pharmacy.
- All patients deserve the care of a pharmacist. It is recognized that resources will need to be allocated according to the complexity of patients and organizational needs.

Technology
- Technology is a tool that will enable pharmacists to better interact with patients and caregivers if implemented into the work flow correctly.
- Technology will allow for rapid access to patient information and variables, which will facilitate pharmacist development of a drug therapy management plan for individual patients.
- The priority of technology is in the following order of importance:
  - Electronic medical record systems
  - Use of barcode technology during medication administration
  - Real-time monitoring systems that provide a work queue of patients needing review and possible intervention

Table 9-1. Pharmacy Practice Model Initiative (cont'd)

Technicians
- Pharmacy technicians who have appropriate education, training, and credentials should be used to free pharmacists from drug distribution activities.
- Assigning medication distribution tasks to technicians would make it possible to deploy pharmacists to drug therapy management services.
- Uniform national standards should apply to the education and training of pharmacy technicians.
- To support optimal pharmacy practice models, technicians must be licensed by state boards of pharmacy.

Implementing Change and Responding to Challenges
- Critical components of change implementation are as follows:
    - Support from medical staff leadership
    - Department of pharmacy administrative leadership
    - Pharmacist electronic access to complete patient-specific data
    - Support from health care executives
    - Clinical pharmacy leadership

Source: Redefining the Practice Model: Shaping the Future for Pharmacy Practice: 2010 ASHP State Affiliate Presidential Officer Retreat.

The PPMI describes how you can allocate your resources to best provide optimal patient care; however, we all know one size does not fit all. As an ambulatory care pharmacist, your job will be to determine what aspects of the initiative work for your practice model. As a resource, the executive committee of the ASHP Section of Ambulatory Care Practitioners has updated and revised the guidelines for ambulatory care practice to reflect the recommendations within the PPMI that pertain to ambulatory care practice.

CASE

Conclusion: It has been 5 years since you approached Dr. Busybee with your business plan. In that time, you developed a plan, implemented the model, and adapted your practice to meet the needs of your patients. The tools that facilitated the plan helped you to manage the practice, and they continue to help you reevaluate practice needs and the potential for growth. News of your success has reached various professional organizations that contact you for help to educate their members about your successes and failures as you've worked through this process. But, this is not the end of your story; it is just the beginning!

There are areas of growth you still want to tackle, and after some thought, you present your ideas to Dr. Busybee on how to advance the practice in your setting. Because of all of your groundwork, preparation, and collaboration with Dr. Busybee over the past 5 years, he agrees. You can feel confident that the ambulatory care practice has a bright future.

Chapter Summary

Maximizing your practice requires strategic vision and careful planning while remaining flexible enough to adapt to changes in technology and practice models. The ambulatory care pharmacy specialist should be engaged in expanding the frontiers of practice by training the next generation of ambulatory care pharmacy practitioners through residencies and by generating the new knowledge that will improve the care of patients through practice-based research. The tools you'll need to maximize your practice include conducting periodic needs assessments and SWOT analyses, effectively using information-management resources, networking with peers through pharmacy organizations, and advocating for meaningful change in health care financing. (Sample Plan for Re-evaluating the Service) 🔎

References

1.   Perez A, Doloresco F, Hoffman JM, et al. ACCP: Economic evaluations of clinical pharmacy services: 2001-2005. *Pharmacotherapy.* 2009;29(1):128.

2.   Schumock GT, Butler MG, Meek PD, et al. Evidence of the economic benefit of clinical pharmacy services: 1996-2000. *Pharmacotherapy.* 2003;23(1):113-132.

3.   Cohen H. How to write a patient case report. *Am J Health-Syst Pharm.* 2006;63(19):1888-1892.

4.   Smith KM. Building upon existing evidence to shape future research endeavors. *Am J Health- Syst Pharm.* 2008;65(18):1767-1774.

5.   Byerly WG. Working with the institutional review board. *Am J Health-Syst Pharm.* 2009;66(2):176-184.

6.   Lipowski EE. Pharmacy practice-based research networks: Why, what, who, and how. *J Am Pharm Assoc.* 2008;48(2):142-152.

7.   Lindbloom EJ, Ewigman BG, Hickner JM. Practice-based research networks: The laboratories of primary care research. *Med Care.* 2004;42(4):III45-49.

8.   Nutting PA, Beasley JW, Werner JJ. Practice-based research networks answer primary care questions. *JAMA.* 1999;281(8):686-688.

9.   Carter BL, Ardery G, Dawson JD, et al. Physician and pharmacist collaboration to improve blood pressure control. *Arch Intern Med.* 2009;169(21):1996-2002.

10. Knapp DA. Professionally determined need for pharmacy services in 2020. *Am J Pharm Educ.* 2002;66(4):421-429.

11. Teeters JL, Brueckl M, Burns A, et al. Pharmacy residency training in the future: A stakeholder's roundtable discussion. *Am J Health-Syst Pharm.* 2005;62(17):1817-1820.

12. Murphy JE, Nappi JM, Bosso JA, et al. American college of clinical pharmacy's vision of the future: Postgraduate pharmacy residency training as a prerequisite for direct patient care practice. *Pharmacotherapy.* 2006;26(5):722-733.

13. Haines ST. Making residency training an expectation for pharmacists in direct patient care roles. *Am J Pharm Educ.* 2007;71(4):71.

14. American Society of Health-System Pharmacists. Requirement for Residency. Policy Position 0701, 2007. Available at: http://www.ashp.org/DocLibrary/BestPractices/policypositions2009.aspx. Accessed March 10, 2010.

15. Knapp KK, Shah BM, Kim HB, et al. Visions for required postgraduate year 1 residency training by 2020: A comparison of actual versus projected expansion. *Pharmacotherapy.* 2009;29(9):1030-1038.

16. Smith KM, Sorensen T, Connor KA, et al. ACCP white paper. Value of conducting pharmacy residency training—the organizational perspective. *Pharmacotherapy.* 2010;30:490e-510e.

17. Johnson S. *Who Moved My Cheese?* New York, NY: Putnam Press; 1998.

18. Nutescu EA, Spinler SA, Dager WE, et al. Transitioning from traditional to novel anticoagulants: The impact of oral direct thrombin inhibitors on anticoagulation management. *Pharmacotherapy.* 2004;24(10, Pt 2):199S-202S.

19. Bussey HI. The financial viability of an anticoagulation clinic: A discussion from the anticoagulation forum meeting, May 2009. *J Thromb Thrombolysis.* 2010;29(2):227-232.

20. Ansell J, Jacobson A, Levy J, et al. International Self-Monitoring Association for Oral Anticoagulation. Guidelines for implementation of patient self-testing and patient self-management of oral anticoagulation. international consensus guidelines prepared by international self-monitoring association for oral anticoagulation. *Int J Cardiol.* 2005;99(1):37-45.

21. Rittenhouse DR, Shortell SM, Fisher ES. Primary care and accountable care—Two essential elements of delivery-system reform. *N Engl J Med.* 2009;361(24):2301-2303.

22. American College of Physicians. Controlling Health Care Costs While Promoting the Best Possible Health Outcomes. Philadelphia, PA: American College of Physicians, 2009. Available at: http://www.acponline.org/advocacy/where_we_stand/policy/controlling_healthcare_costs.pdf. Accessed March 10, 2010.

23. Swensen SJ, Meyer GS, Nelson EC, et al. Cottage industry to postindustrial care—The revolution in health care delivery. *N Engl J Med.* 2010;362(5):e12.

24. Claxton G, DiJulio B, Finder B, et al., eds. *The Kaiser Family Foundation and Health Research & Education Trust. Employer Health Benefits 2009 Annual Summary.* Menlo Park, CA: Henry J. Kaiser Family Foundation; 2009.

25. Miller H, Vandervelde A, Russo G. Healthcare Megatrends: The future of healthcare financing and delivery. LECG, LLC., 2009. Available at: http://www.lecg.com/files/Publication/a703979e-c776-4608-a790-0ea356f5bc75/Presentation/PublicationAttachment/a558fc51-d976-4042-86ee-101c31fc08b5/HCMegatrends0423.pdf. Accessed March 10, 2010.

26. Lipton HL. Home is where the health is: Advancing team-based care in chronic disease management. *Arch Intern Med.* 2009;169(21):1945-1948.

27. Lipton HL. Pharmacists and health reform. Go for it! *Pharmacotherapy.* 2010;30:697-672.

28. The Patient Centered Medical Home. History, Seven Core Features, Evidence and Transformational Change. Washington, DC: Robert Graham Center; November 2007.

29. Rosser WW, Colwill JM, Kasperski J, et al. Patient-centered medical homes in Ontario. *N Engl J Med.* 2010;362:e7.

30. Reid RJ, Coleman K, Johnson EA, et al. The Group Health Medical Home at year two: Cost savings, higher patient satisfaction and less burnout for providers. *Health Affairs.* 2010;29:835-843.

31. Slawson DC, Shaughnessy AF. Teaching information mastery: Creating informed consumers of medical information. *J Am Board Fam Pract.* 1999;12(6):444-449.

Additional Selected Resources

American College of Physicians. Controlling Health Care Costs While Promoting the Best Possible Health Outcomes. Philadelphia, PA: American College of Physicians; 2009. http://www.acponline.org/advocacy/where_we_stand/policy/controlling_healthcare_costs.pdf.

Bates DW. Role of pharmacists in the medical home. *Am J Health-Syst Pharm.* 2009;66:1116-1118.

Patient-Centered Primary Care Collaborative. *Integrating Comprehensive Medication Management to Optimize Patient Outcomes. A Resource Guide.* Washington, DC: PCPCC; 2010. Available at: http://www.pcpcc.net/files/medmanagepub.pdf.

Robert Graham Center. *The Patient Centered Medical Home. History, Seven Core Features, Evidence and Transformational Change.* Washington, DC: Robert Graham Center; November 2007. http://www.graham-center.org/online/etc/medialib/graham/documents/publications/mongraphs-books/2007/rgcmo-medical-home.Par.0001.File.tmp/rgcmo-medical-home.pdf.

Sidorov JE. The patient-centered medical home for chronic illness: Is it ready for prime time? *Health Aff.* 2008;27:1231-1234.

Smith KM, Sorensen T, Connor KA, et al. American College of Clinical Pharmacy White Paper. Value of conducting pharmacy residency training—The organizational perspective. *Pharmacotherapy.* 2010;30:490e-510e.

Thomas P, Griffiths F, Kai J, et al. Networks for research in primary health care. *BMJ.* 2001;322:588-590.

Young PL, Olsen L, McGinnis JM, Roundtable on Evidence-Based Medicine. *Value in Health Care: Accounting for Cost, Quality, Safety, Outcomes, and Innovation.* Washington, DC: National Academies Press; 2009. http://www.nap.edu.proxy-hs.researchport.umd.edu/catalog.php?record_id=12566.

Research

Agency for Health-care Research and Quality. AHRQ Support for Primary Care Practice-Based Research Networks (PBRNs): http://www.ahrq.gov/research/pbrn/pbrnfact.htm

American College of Clinical Pharmacy Research Institute: Practice Based Research Institute Initiative: http://www.accpri.org/pbrn/

American Journal of Health-System Pharmacy Series: Research Fundamentals: http://www.ashp foundation.org/MainMenuCategories/ResearchResourceCenter/FosteringYoungInvestigators/AJHPResearchFundamentalsSeries.aspx.

A collection of articles originally published in the *American Journal of Health-System Pharmacy* designed to aid the reader in learning about research design, data collection and analysis, dissemination of research results, and applying research findings into your practice.

National Institute of Health Office of Extramural Research: http://phrp.nihtraining.com

A free series of online training modules. After you have successfully completed the corresponding quizzes, you can print a certificate of completion that may be required by your local IRB to show that you have completed training in protecting the rights of human subjects.

Residency Training

American Society of Health-System Pharmacists. Residency learning system: http://www.ashp.org/accreditation-residency

This site will provide you the tools to design and deliver a pharmacy residency training program, including the accreditation standards, goals and objectives for PGY1 and PGY2 pharmacy residency training programs, guidance for starting a residency program, and information on the Residency Learning System (RLS).

Health Care Reform and the Patient-Centered Medical Home

The Henry J. Kaiser Family Foundation. Health Reform Source: http://healthreform.kff.org/

The Kaiser Family Foundation (KFF) is a nonprofit, private foundation focusing on major health care issues in the United States. KFF develops and runs its own research and communications programs and serves as a nonpartisan source of facts, information, and analysis. KFF products are provided free of charge—from the most sophisticated policy research to basic facts and numbers. This website is a comprehensive information source regarding the Patient Protection and Affordable Care Act. You can sign up for an RSS feed that will alert you when new information is posted to the site.

The National Academies of Science, Institute of Medicine. http://www.iom.edu/

The Institute of Medicine (IOM) serves as adviser to the government agencies and the private sector to improve health. The IOM publishes books, monographs, and reports regarding a wide range of contemporary issues related to health and health care delivery. The IOM is an independent, nonprofit organization that works outside of government to provide unbiased and authoritative advice to decision makers and the public.

Information Mastery

ACP Journal Club. http://www.acpjc.org/

ACP Journal Club selects biomedical literature articles that report original studies and systematic reviews that warrant immediate attention by health care practitioners attempting to keep pace with advances in internal medicine. These articles are summarized in abstracts and commented on by clinical experts.

Cochrane Collaboration and Cochrane Library: http://www.cochrane.org/

The Cochrane Collaborative is a global network of volunteers who conduct authoritative and unbiased systematic reviews of the effects of health care interventions. These reviews are published in the Cochrane Library.

Evidence-Based Medicine for Primary Care and Internal Medicine: http://ebm.bmj.com/

> *Evidence-Based Medicine* is published bi-monthly and provides comprehensive coverage of primary care medicine by surveying a wide range of international medical journals. The editorial staff apply strict criteria for the quality and validity of research. The key details of these essential studies are presented in a succinct, informative abstract.

EvidenceUpdates: http://plus.mcmaster.ca/EvidenceUpdates/

> A great resource developed and maintained by The BMJ Group and McMaster University's Health Information Research Unit. This site provides access to the best evidence, tailored to your interests, to support evidence-based clinical decisions. All citations, from over 120 premier clinical journals, are rated for quality, clinical relevance, and interest by a worldwide panel of expert practitioners.

Journal Watch. Evidence that Matters: http://www.jwatch.org/

> Journal Watch is available in print and online. It is intended to help heath professionals save time and stay informed by providing brief, clearly written, clinically focused perspectives on the medical developments that affect practice.

TRIP (Turning Research into Practice) database– clinical search engine: http://www.tripdatabase.com/

> The TRIP Database is a clinical search tool designed to allow health professionals to rapidly identify the highest quality clinical evidence for clinical practice.

University of Virginia School of Medicine, Center for Information Mastery: http://www.healthsystem.virginia.edu/internet/familymed/information_mastery/info_mastery.cfm

> The Center for Information Mastery offers courses and other resources.

Web Resources

Updated Resources and Reimbursement Form to Show Growth (Form originally introduced in Chapter 2.)

Example Measures to Examine Trends in the Practice

A Tracking Tool for Non-patient Activities

Examples of eTOCs

A Sample Plan for Re-evaluating the Service

http://www.ashp.org/ppmi

http://www.ashp.org/menu/MemberCenter/SectionsForums/SACP.aspx

http://www.accpri.org/pbrn/index.aspx

 Web Toolkit available at
www.ashp.org/ambulatorypractice

Glossary

Accountable Care Organization (ACO): A health care organization and a related set of providers that can be held accountable for the cost and quality of care. They consist of providers that meet specific criteria and work together to coordinate care.

Capitated Payments: A payment method for health care services. The physician, hospital, or other health care provider is paid a contracted rate for each member assigned, referred to as "per-member-per-month" rate, regardless of the number or nature of services provided. The contractual rates are usually adjusted for age, gender, illness, and regional differences.[1]

Certified Diabetes Educator: A health care professional [clinical psychologist, registered nurse, occupational therapist, optometrist, pharmacist, physical therapist, physician (MD or DO), podiatrist, dietician, physician assistant, exercise physiologist or master's in social work] with a minimum of 2 years' clinical practice in his or her profession, 1,000 hours of diabetes self-management education, and 15 continuing education hours of diabetes education during the preceding 2 years who has successfully completed a certification exam.[2]

Collaborative Drug Therapy Management (CDTM): A collaborative practice agreement between one or more physicians and pharmacists wherein qualified pharmacists work within the context of professional responsibility to do the following: perform patient assessments; order drug therapy-related laboratory tests; administer drugs; and select, initiate, monitor, continue, and adjust medication regimens.

Compliance Officer: The person responsible within an organization for the process of helping our health care professionals understand and meet the expectations of those who grant us money, pay for our services, regulate our industry, etc. Health care compliance includes numerous issues such as reimbursement, grant accounting, managed care, OSHA and Joint Commission on Accreditation of Healthcare Organizations regulations, licensure, and due diligence to prevent and detect violations of the law. (Definition from the Association of Health Care Compliance Association)[3]

Consumer Behavior: Psychological processes individuals go through in recognizing needs and finding products or services that will meet their specific needs.

Current Procedural Terminology: Description of medical, diagnostic, and procedural health care services; codes are maintained by the American Medical Association CPT Editorial panel, and utilized as a uniform method of communicating health care information between health care providers and entities.

Current Procedural Terminology (CPT) Codes: Numbers assigned to every task and service a medical practitioner may provide to a patient, including medical, surgical, and diagnostic services. They are then used by insurers to determine the amount of reimbursement that a practitioner will receive by an insurer.

Employer-Sponsored Wellness Program: Specific type of employer-based reimbursement where pharmacists contract with an employer to provide chronic disease management to improve the health outcomes of employees.

Evaluation and Management (E&M) Codes: Codes used by medical providers to indicate the level of visit billed based on history, physical exam, and medical decision of the visit.

Facility Fee Billing: A method of billing technical fees for services rendered by ancillary personnel in a hospital-based/owned facility.

Fee-for-Service: Service referring to the traditional form of reimbursement for health care, where a fee is paid to a provider, according to the service performed, by a patient or a conventional indemnity insurer, after a service is rendered.[4]

Fiscal Intermediary: A private company that has a contract with Medicare to pay Part A and some Part B bills (for example, bills from hospitals and other providers). These companies are responsible for set regions of the country and are responsible as agents of the federal government to administer the Medicare program, including reimbursement and medical coverage review, and payment of claims.

Hospital-Based Outpatient Clinic: Clinic providing "outpatient service" as listed on the hospital's general acute-care license issued by the State Department of Public Health. The clinic may be located on or off the main grounds of its hospital, but must be owned and operated by a hospital or system. The clinic must be formally organized as a Federally Qualified Health Center (FQHC) [county owned and operated], Federally Qualified Health Center Look-Alike (FQHC-LA) [county owned and operated], Rural Health Clinic (RHC), Outpatient Primary Clinic, or Specialty Care Clinic. It must be primarily engaged in providing outpatient health services that furnish diagnostic and therapeutic care. This includes medical history, physical examinations, and assessment of health status and treatment monitoring for a variety of medical, dental, or behavioral health conditions.

"Incident-to" Physician's Professional Services: The services or supplies that are furnished as an integral, although incidental, part of the physician's personal professional services in the course of diagnosis or treatment of an injury or illness. (Medicare Carriers Manual Part 3-Claims Process. Transmittal 1764, August 28, 2002.)

Institutional Review Board (IRB): Board that provides oversight for research to protect the rights and welfare of human subjects.

Marketing: Processes for creating, communicating, delivering, and exchanging offerings that have value for customers, clients, partners, and society at large.[1]

Marketing Mix: Executable plan and strategy based on marketing research and planning that has taken place. For a service, it consists of the 7 Ps (product, price, place, promotion, people, physical evidence, and process).

Marketing Research: Process of gathering and analyzing information for use in the market planning process. It can be qualitative or quantitative.

Medically Necessary: Services or supplies that are considered medically necessary if they:

- Are proper and needed for diagnosis or treatment of your medical condition.
- Are provided for the diagnosis, direct care, and treatment of your medical condition.
- Meet the standards of good medical practice in the medical community of your local area.
- Are not mainly for the convenience of you or your doctor.

Medicare Administrative Contractors (MAC): People independently contracted by Medicare to answer questions and process enrollment applications for Medicare. As of April 2010, they are divided into 14 areas across the United States.

Medicare Current Year Conversion Factor: A scaling factor that converts a geographically adjusted relative value unit for services listed in the Medicare physician payment schedule to a dollar payment amount.

Medication Reconciliation: The comprehensive evaluation of a patient's medication regimen any time there is a change in therapy in an effort to avoid medication errors such as omissions, duplications, dosing errors, or drug interactions, as well as to observe compliance and adherence patterns. This process should include a comparison of the existing and previous medication regimens and should occur at every transition of care in which new medications are ordered, existing orders are rewritten or adjusted, or if the patient has added non-prescription medications to his or her self-care.

Patient-Centered Medical Home (PCMH): A model of care that focuses on wellness and prevention and the management of chronic illness with care directed by the patient's personal physician working collaboratively with a team of individuals who collectively are responsible for the quality, safety, and outcomes of the care provided.

Pay-4-Performance: Aligning payment amounts for health care services provided based on certain goals achieved by patient receiving those services, or aligning financial incentives with the best interest of the patient.[5,6]

Payer Mix: The number of and the proportion of patients covered by different payers represented in a health care setting or practice.

Pharmacy Practice Model Initiative (PPMI): ASHP's effort to move pharmacists more completely into patient care roles that foster the best use of medications.

Physician-Based Outpatient Clinic: Office or clinic owned and operated by a physician or a group of physicians. Traditionally the setting is not affiliated with a health system; however, it can be associated with a network of other outpatient settings, such as a consortium.

Point Tool: A tool used in hospital-based clinics to tabulate points assigned to various tasks, assessments, and education provided by ancillary hospital employees in order to determine the level of service billed to a patient.

Postgraduate Year One (PGY1) Pharmacy Residency: An organized, directed residency program for graduates from professional pharmacy degree programs designed to enhance general competencies in managing medication therapy outcomes for patients within a wide range of therapeutic areas and medication-use system management.

Postgraduate Year Two (PGY2) Pharmacy Residency: A residency designed to be completed after a PGY1 residency. This second-year residency program is focused in a specific area of practice historically called a "specialty" residency program.

Practice-Based Research Network (PBRN): A group of clinicians or clinical practice sites that primarily serve to provide patient care, but network together to investigate real-world questions to understand and enhance the quality of care.

Quality Gap: The difference in performance between the top 10% of and industry and the national average for that industry.

Quality Measure: A quantitative reflection of the characteristics or attributes of an entity, a service, process, product, etc. In its most simplistic form, data is presented as a percentage based on a numerator that describes the number of entities that have an attribute or characteristic being looked at and a denominator that is the number of that particular entity being studied.

Reproducible: The ability to exactly replicate the function and process of the program in a new setting.

Return on Investment: A financial measure of a project or program that compares the financial gain to the financial costs by creating a ratio between revenue and costs. The goal is to achieve the best positive ROI or a number greater than 0.00. The formula used is:

$$ROI = \text{financial gain} - \text{program costs}$$

Scalable: The ability for a resource to increase in capacity in order to meet increasing workloads over a period of time. In a scalable model, regardless of the setting, the base concept is consistent.

Scope of Practice: Term that defines the procedures, actions, and processes permitted for a licensed individual or practitioner.

Self-Insured Employer: A business that administers its own health care plan.

Sliding Fee Scale: A tool to be used with self-pay patients to discount patient fees in a uniform manner, typically based on the federal poverty income guidelines.

Stakeholders: Individuals involved in or affected by a course of action; the people who have a vested interest in the service.

Superbill: A form completed and submitted to an insurance company for reimbursement of medical provider services.

Value: A fair return or equivalent in goods, services, or money for something exchanged; the relationship of quality to cost.

Value Based Insurance Design: A policy design provided by health care insurers that rewards high-quality providers who manage patients using those procedures and treatments that are more clinically beneficial and cost effective based on evidence, i.e. a higher value; with higher payments or bonuses. It also incentivizes patients to adopt and adhere to these procedures and treatments with a reduction or elimination of co-payments.

References

1. Mosby's Medical Dictionary, 8th edition. Elsevier; 2009.
2. http://www.ncbde.org/eligibility.cfm
3. Accessed from http://www.hccainfo.org/AM/Template.cfm?Section=About_HCCA&Template=/TaggedPage/TaggedPageDisplay.cfm&TPLID=23&ContentID=10393 4/23/2011.
4. McGraw-Hill Concise Dictionary of Modern Medicine. The McGraw-Hill Companies, Inc.; 2002.
5. American Medical Association. Quality of care. *J Am Med Assoc.* 1986;256:1032–1034.
6. Wharam JF, Sulmasy D. Improving the quality of health care: who is responsible for what? *J Am Med Assoc.* 2009;301:215–217.

Index